Problem Behaviors in Long-Term Care

Recognition, Diagnosis, and Treatment

Peggy A. Szwabo, R.N., A.C.S.W., C-CS, is the Director of the Geriatric Psychiatry Education Center and the Outpatient Services of Geriatric Psychiatry, Department of Psychiatry and Human Behavior, Saint Louis University School of Medicine. Ms. Szwabo is a therapist with the elderly and their families, provides consultation in-services to agencies and nursing homes in care and treatment of the older adult. Her area of interest is staff caregiver burnout.

George T. Grossberg, MD, is Director of the Division of Geriatric Psychiatry and Professor, Department of Psychiatry and Human Behavior, Saint Louis University School of Medicine. Dr. Grossberg is past president of the American Association of Geriatric Psychiatry. He has been a leader in developing mental health programs, treatment, and research in geriatrics.

Problem Behaviors in Long-Term Care

Recognition, Diagnosis, and Treatment

Peggy A. Szwabo
George T. Grossberg
Editors

Springer Publishing Company
New York

Springer Publishing Company, Inc.
536 Broadway
New York, NY 10012

93 94 95 96 97 / 5 4 3 2 1

Library of Congress Cataloging-in-Publication Data

Problem behaviors in long-term care : recognition, diagnosis, and
   treatment / Peggy A. Szwabo, George T. Grossberg, editors.
      p.   cm.
   Includes bibliographical references and index.
   ISBN 0-8261-7820-0
   1. Nursing home patients—Mental health. 2. Geriatric psychiatry.
I. Szwabo, Peggy A. II. Grossberg, George T.
   [DNLM: 1. Chrone Diseases—psychology. 2. Long-Term Care—
psychology. 3. Mental Disorders—in old age. WT 1560 P962]
RC451 . 4 . N87P76   1993
618 . 97'689—dc20
DNLM/DLC
for Library of Congress   92-2322
                                                       CIP

Printed in the United States of America

Contents

PART II   Medical Disorders

PART III   Ethical and Legal Issues

Foreword

Rosalie A. Kane

This is an ambitious book. Assembled here is a comprehensive examination of mental health topics for those who work in, plan for, or simply care about nursing homes. As the title suggests, the focus is on problem behavior of residents, which the various contributors examine from multiple perspectives.

Problem behaviors are seen as secondary to psychiatric or medical problems, and even to common treatments. The section on Psychiatric Disorders contains chapters organized by diagnostic categories—dementia, depression, personality disorders, and sleep disorders, but it also has a chapter on psychotropic drugs, which reminds us that the treatment of psychiatric disorders also can cause behavior problems. Another cluster of chapters remind us that medical conditions and common related symptom syndromes (delirium, eating disorders, and pain) can result in behavior problems. Wandering, that quintessential problem in long-term care, has its own chapter, which emphasizes strategies to manage the problem. Chapters on interventions describe physical restraints and their alternatives, drug treatment for aggression, special care units, design features, family programs, and programs to alleviate distress of the staff. Taken together, these chapters provide clear and basic information that might be helpful to a neophyte, but they also review research in a way helpful to a person experienced in long-term care.

The contributors avoid the too common problem of putting all behavior of all nursing home residents under the microscope. Indeed, it is too easy to medicalize the lives of nursing-home residents. Too readily, talking can become verbalizations (capable of being counted), friendships can become socialization (as though they can be prescribed), and decisions to pass up activities can be labeled withdrawal. Too often, it is forgotten that the marvelously varied human responses that we call behavior occur in reaction to social environments; that behavior is a private choice; and that any of us might react with anger, frustration, or depression to being transported into nursing-home life. It would add insult to injury to have understanding professionals chronicling our behavior to help us toward "adjustment." But, in this book, the focus is on behavior that undisputably causes difficulty in group-living situations, and that tends to have its etiology in neurological or psychiatric problems. The behavior of cognitively intact residents is not up for dissection, except perhaps in the helpful chapter on sleep disorders, in which the focus is still on the relationship between anxiety and sleep disturbance. Even so the chapter properly prompts one to ask whether all "nocturnal awakenings" are problems, and, if so, for whom?

Perhaps in a foreword, especially to a book on mental health problems, I am permitted free associations. I think of two. The first concerns the definition of a problem. There are dozens of variations on the joke about the physician who is unconcerned about the patient's gall-bladder or knee, to take examples, and reassuringly indicates that he sees no problem, whereupon the patient's rejoinder is: "I know it's not a problem for you, doc; if it were *your* knee, I wouldn't have a problem either." In the area of behavior problems among nursing-home residents, the reverse of that joke may be pertinent. The problem can be perceived by caregivers—family and staff—and, perhaps, by other residents, yet not be experienced as a problem by the person manifesting the behavior. The long-term care field has yet to sort out when behavior modification efforts are justified in the name of efficient and cost-effective nursing home routines? In the name of safety and protection? In the name of pleasant group living? The field must consider when environmental modifications and separation of persons with antisocial behavior secondary to dementia should be used rather than trying to eliminate behaviors, such as noisemaking, pacing, or wandering. This, in turn, requires us to understand when a behavior may have a negative long-range effect—for example, physical exhaustion from pacing—and when it exposes the resident to unreasonable risks of injury, as opposed to being a harmless, and perhaps enjoyable, behavior that staff should learn to accept.

It would help, of course, if we could understand when certain behavior among persons with Alzheimer's disease and other dementias causes distress to the resident. At present, we rely on intuition. It seems quite clear that the tearful, anguished quest "to go home" is the behavor of someone who is suffering, even if the reality base for the suffering is distorted. It is also clear that many behaviors that are bothersome to staff because they make messes or noise are not problems for the persons behaving in that way, and may even be pleasurable. Conversely, it is not always clear which behaviors disturb others. For example, repeated crying out on the part of a resident, behavior that drives cognitively intact residents to distraction, may not be disturbing to a group of moderately demented persons on a Special-Care Unit. These issues can be illuminated by painstaking research, the kind that requires detailed observation to record both the behaviors and the reactions. Some such work is going on now, and it would be enhanced by common language to refer to the behavior in question, common measures, and accepted measures of emotion in residents who are cognitively impaired.

My other free association takes the form of a fantasy. In this vision, nursing-home residents are having a conference on problem behaviors of nursing home staff. I wonder what their list might be. To turn the tables, the list might include short attention span, depression, aggressiveness, and unexpected ambulation and wandering into residents rooms. It could include gossiping and secret-telling; rudeness and roughness; prying and inquisitiveness; and insensitivity. There might even be a behavior called "over-labelling," or "vocalization in jargon," for the propensity of professionals to categorize the residents' behavior. It is certain that we, as the subjects of this effort, would not enjoy having our behavior classified. It would belittle our reactions and make them less ours. This image, of course, is most relevant to the many cognitively intact residents who have both brief and long stays in nursing homes. It is less pertinent to the many other residents who suffer from dementia, and whose behavior is something of an enigma to those who help them. I like the analogy, nonetheless, because it promotes humility in the quest to understand behavior problems. At least some of the problems—even in relation to persons with dementia—may be our own.

In summary, the editors have performed a useful service by assembling between two covers so much information about problem behaviors and their possible causation and alleviation. The challenge now for readers and the long-term care field in general is to take the next steps in considering the proper goals, as well as the proper techniques, for modifying behavior.

ROSALIE A. KANE

Preface

This book is intended to be a vehicle for disseminating state-of-the-art practical information and practice approaches to health care professionals committed to the care of older adults in nursing homes. Health care professionals providing care for older adults face an important challenge to provide quality care in a dynamic atmosphere of change, new knowledge, and regulatory mandates.

The text takes a comprehensive approach in addressing the many issues facing long-term-care providers today and is divided into psychiatric and medical conditions and treatments. Special populations such as the younger resident and behavior problems are also addressed. A particularly valuable chapter involves the role of the family in the nursing-home setting. In response to concerns about restraints, several authors present issues and suggestions for chemical and nonchemical options. The book rounds out with discussions of ethical and legal issues facing the elderly, their families, and their caregivers.

Unique and important chapters are those on pain management and eating disorders. Two very difficult management problems challenging caregiving staff. The chapter on personality offers insight into the issues in working with personality styles and disorders and provides concrete suggestions for intervention. The in-depth chapter on psychotherapy in long-term care assists the caregivers in providing a comprehensive review of approaches toward meeting residents' psychological needs.

As the body of knowledge about care of older adults in long-term care grows, so does the need for information to be disseminated in practical, usable form for those who are involved in providing that care. It was with that goal in mind that Dr. George T. Grossberg and I set out to plan this book. In looking at the final product, I am confident that we have achieved our goal of providing state-of-the-art approaches and treatments in a format that will be readily utilized in the nursing-home setting.

PAS

Acknowledgment

Many people are responsible for the completion of this book. Jane Colt deserves special thanks for the hours, the details, and the help she gave in its production. She did it all with dedication, humor, and grace.

Contributors

Donna L. Algase, PhD, RN, is an Assistant Professor of Gerontological Nursing and an Associate Research Scientist at the University of Michigan School of Nursing.

Susan Bass, MA, CTRS, is a Recreational Therapist for the Saint Louis University Hospital and works exclusively on the geriatric psychiatry inpatient unit, specializing in functional and leisure skill assessments for geriatric patients.

Karen R. Boesch, MD, is currently a fellow in the Geriatric Psychiatry Department of Psychiatry and Human Behavior at Saint Louis University School of Medicine. In August 1992 she will join the department as Clinical Instructor.

Carl W. Bretscher, MSW, ACSW, is a Social Worker with the Geriatric Psychiatry Inpatient Unit, Saint Louis University Hospital.

Christopher T. Cahenzli, MD, is currently an Instructor in Psychiatry at Cornell University Medical College and a Staff Psychiatrist at New York Hospital-Cornell Medical Center-Westchester Division.

Gloria A. Crumpton, RN-C, is Charge Nurse, Surrey Place, St. Louis, Missouri. She is a member of the Alzheimer's Association Speaker's Bureau and is a Captain and Training Officer in the United States Army Reserves Nurse Corps.

Jean de Blois, CSJ, RN, PhD, is presently the Associate Director of the Center for Health Care Ethics; Assistant Professor of Medical Ethics, Department of Internal Medicine; and Assistant Professor of Hospital and Health Care Administration at Saint Louis University Medical Center.

Sanford I. Finkel, MD, is the President of the International Psychogeriatric Association. His current positions are: Director, Gero-Psychiatry Services at Northwestern Memorial Hospital; Associate Director of the Buehler Center on Aging of Northwestern University; and Associate Professor of Northwestern University Medical School.

Leah F. Friedman, PhD, is currently on the research staff of the Department of Psychiatry and Aging Clinical Research Center at Stanford University working in the general area of the psychology of aging with special interest in treatments for insomnia and memory training interventions.

Barbara J. Gilchrist, JD, is Associate Director and Adjunct Assistant Professor of Law, Saint Louis University School of Law, and is the Director of the Health Law Clinic which provides legal services to elderly homebound persons with Alzheimer's disease.

Linda K. Griffin, RN-C, is Charge Nurse, Geriatric Psychiatry Inpatient Unit, Saint Louis University Hospital; serves on the faculty of the Geriatric Psychiatry Education and Consultation Center; is a member of the Alzheimer's Association and Alzheimer's Speakers Bureau; and serves on the Retention and Recruitment Committee at Saint Louis University Hospital.

Mary S. Harper, PhD, RN, FAAN, is Coordinator for Long-Term-Care Programs, Center for the Studies of the Mental Health of the Aging, National Institute of Mental Health, Rockville, Maryland.

Rakhshanda Hassan, MD, is an Instructor in the Division of Geriatric Psychiatry, Department of Psychiatry and Human Behavior at Saint Louis University School of Medicine.

Rev. Herbert E. Hohenstein, ThD, MA, STM, is Pastor of Unity Lutheran Church, St. Louis, Missouri. He is also a member of the Geriatric Psychiatry Advisory Board of the Saint Louis University Medical Center.

Rosalie A. Kane, DSW, is a Professor of social work and public health at the University of Minnesota. She directs the University of Minnesota's Long-Term Care DECISIONS Resource Center, one of six National Resource Centers on Long-Term Care funded by the Administration on Aging.

David V. Kromm, AIA, is an architect whose professional experience includes programming special needs for special care units, nursing homes, assisted living facilities, congregate care apartments, and independent living cottages.

Young-Hie Nahm Kromm, AIA, is an architect whose professional experience includes design of facilities for special care units, nursing homes, assisted living facilities, congregate care apartments, and independent living cottages.

Helen W. Lach, RN, MSN, CS, is a Clinical Nurse Specialist, Program on Aging, Jewish Hospital at Washington University. She is also a Clinical Instructor in Nursing, Department of Gerontological and Psychiatric/Mental Health Nursing at Saint Louis University Medical Center.

Jothika Manepalli, MD, is an Instructor and Director of the Refractory Depression Unit, Division of Geriatric Psychiatry, Department of Psychiatry and Human Behavior at Saint Louis University School of Medicine.

Barnett S. Meyers, MD, is Associate Professor of Clinical Psychiatry at Cornell University Medical College and Chief of the Geriatric Specialty Clinic, New York Hospital-Cornell Medical Center, Westchester Division, White Plains, New York.

Douglas K. Miller, MD, is currently an Associate Professor of Medicine at Saint Louis University and the St. Louis Department of Veterans affairs and is board certified in internal medicine and geriatric medicine.

John E. Morley, MB, BCh, is Dammert Professor of Gerontology and Director of the Division of Geriatric Medicine at Saint Louis University Medical Center and Director of Geriatric Research, Education and Clinical Center, St. Louis Department of Veterans Affairs, St. Louis. He is board certified in internal medicine, endocrinology and geriatrics.

James C. Romeis, PhD, is Associate Professor and Director, Doctoral Program in Health Services Research, Saint Louis University School of Public Health and Coordinator, Health Services Research & Development [Great Lakes Field Program], St. Louis VA Medical Center.

Raymond F. Rustige, CFACHCA, is Assistant Director and Assistant Professor of the Center for Health Services Education and Research, Saint Louis University Medical Center. He is a Certified Fellow on the American College of Health Care Administration and serves on many boards for long-term care and health planning.

Javaid I. Sheikh, MD, is an Assistant Professor, Medical Director, General Psychiatry and Geriatric Psychiatry Inpatient Programs at the Stanford University Medical Center. He is also a member of the task force on nomenclature of the American Association for Geriatric Psychiatry and chair of the Geriatrics Committee of the Northern California Psychiatric Society. He currently received a grant from the Teaching Nursing Home Project at Stanford.

Andrew Jay Silver, MD, is currently an Assistant Professor of Medicine, Saint Louis University School of Medicine, and an Associate Investigator, St. Louis Department of Veterans Affairs.

Adam J. Sky, MD, is a fellow in the Division of Geriatric Psychiatry, Department of Psychiatry and Human Behavior, Saint Louis University School of Medicine. He is currently involved in both inpatient and out-patient care as well as participating in several research studies.

Kenneth Solomon, MD, is currently Associate Professor, Division of Geriatric Psychiatry, Department of Psychiatry and Human Behavior, Saint Louis University School of Medicine and Chief, Geriatric Psychiatry Unit, St. Louis Department of Veterans Affairs Medical Center-Jefferson Barracks Division.

Amy L. Stein, MSW, is a mental health specialist with the Division of Geriatric Psychiatry, Department of Psychiatry and Human Behavior, Saint Louis University Medical Center.

Pamela J. Swales, PhD, is presently completing a postdoctoral research training fellowship, sponsored by a National Institute of Mental Health Grant (MH16744), at Stanford University School of Medicine, Department of Psychiatry and Behavioral Medicine. Her present research focuses on cognitive-behavioral aspects and treatment of anxiety disorders with special interest in geriatric panic disorder.

Raymond C. Tait, PhD, is Director of the Pain Management Program and Associate Professor of Psychiatry and Human Behavior at the Saint Louis University School of Medicine.

Laura Wehrenberg, M. Arch, holds a master's degree in architecture from Washington University in St. Louis. Her professional experience includes rehabilitation and adaptive re-use of historic housing, health-care work, and public relations from Kromm, Rikimaru & Johansen, Inc., an architectural firm specializing in the design of elderly care facilities.

George H. Zimny, PhD, is a Professor (Psychology) in the Department of Psychiatry and Human Behavior of the Saint Louis University School of Medicine.

Special Populations in Extended Care Facilities: Psychosocial and Cultural Perspectives

Mary S. Harper

Special populations in this chapter include racial and ethnic minority elderly, elderly persons who are mentally retarded, the elderly who are poor and underserved, and the rural elderly. The author will focus on cultural, psychosocial, behavioral observations, and problems associated with these special groups in extended care facilities.

Minority elderly are the fastest growing population in the nation. The U.S. Bureau of the Census (1990) figures on race and ethnic statistics show dramatic growth in the numbers and percentage of black and Hispanic elders over the next 60 years. According to their projections, the number of black elders will grow from the current 8.3% of the 65 and over population to 14.0% of that population. The elderly Hispanic population is projected to more than triple from the current 3.6% of the 65 and over population to 11.5% (U.S. Bureau of the Census, 1988).

Referring to minorities can be confusing because of the different names used, that is, nonwhite, culturally deprived, disadvantaged. Actually, these terms convey more about societal attitudes than provide a description of the special population. The terms may cause misrepresentation and poor allocation of resources. The term nonwhite "lumps" all Asian/Pacific Islanders together. Asian Americans really encompass 40 or more ethnic groups (Liu & Yu, 1985). There are several black groups (African-Americans; Haitians, Jamaicans, and other groups from the Caribbean and Nigeria). The Hispanic label is used as a substitute for the more specific ethnic identifiers (Mexican, Puerto Rican, Cuban, Salvadoran, and so on). Although Cubans comprise about 4% of the total U.S. Hispanic population, they represent 14% of the Hispanic elderly. Central and South Americans, Spaniards and others account for 24% of the Hispanic elderly (Cuellar, 1990).

MINORITY, ETHNICITY, AND CULTURAL RELATIVISM

Minority has been defined as a group of people who, because of their physical or cultural characteristics, are singled out from others in the society in which they live for differential and unequal treatment, and who therefore regard themselves as objects of collective discrimination. Minority status carries with it the exclusion from full participation in the life of the society (see Table 1.1). Statistical under-representation does not, in itself, account for groups being considered a minority in the sociological sense. It is not even a necessary condition for those groups who have uneven access to power.

Ethnicity has been defined as social differentiation based on such cultural criteria as a sense of peoplehood, shared history, a common place of origin, language, dress, food preferences, and participation in particular clubs and associations which engender a sense of exclusiveness and self-awareness that one is a member of a distinct and bounded social group. Ethnic ideologies tend to pursue cultural norms not shared by others in society. What ethnic membership thus implies for the elderly is the opportunity to sustain continuity in their repertoires of familiar lifestyle and culturally stylized patterns of social involvement (Holzberg, 1982).

TABLE 1.1 Minority Characteristics

Each minority group has a special history.
The special history has been influenced by discrimination.
A subculture has developed.
Coping structures have developed.
Rapid change is occurring with aging members.

TABLE 1.2 Profile of the Health Behaviors of Minority Elderly

Onset of chronic illnesses is usually earlier.

Frequent delay in seeking treatment and help.

Underutilize mental health services (Lopez, 1981).

Primary care physicians (nonpsychiatrists) are the primary providers of mental health services.

High rate of treatment dropout.

Increased tolerance to illness/discomfort that has been ignored, normalized, or left to develop.

Attribute symptoms to old age.

Under-reporting and incomplete reporting are common until trust established.

Over-representation in mental institutions.

Increased rate of commitment to mental hospitals. Blacks three times more likely than whites to be committed.

Linton (1945) has defined culture as a shared, learned behavior which is transmitted from one generation to another for purposes of human adjustment, adaptation, and growth. Culture shapes virtually all aspects of human behavior. It impacts the way one defines reality and interprets experiences; it also shapes one's coping style. It includes sense of time, space, causality, morality, personhood, and interpersonal processes. These dimensions of human behavior are not inborn but are shaped by socialization. This understanding of culture should assist in providing and evaluating treatment, care plans and planning health policies. As practitioners, planning care or treatment should never occur without consideration of an individual's culture (see Table 1.2). Knowledge of the individual's culture can greatly influence treatment outcome.

In summary, most of the conditions of the elderly are equally influenced by lifestyle, sociocultural, and psychosocial factors as well as by genetics and biology. Lifestyles are modifiable. Treatment outcomes are frequently more favorable from a change in lifestyle and behavior than they are from treatment medication alone. Patient and family education and monitoring are equally as important as the prescription.

AMERICAN INDIANS AND ALASKAN NATIVES

In the United States, there are 1.4 million American Indians and Alaskan Natives (AIAN); 5.3% (109,000) are age 65 and over; 7.7% (6,100) are 85 years of age and over. Twenty-five percent of the AIAN elderly live on reservations. In the United States, there are 500 Indian tribes, organizations, villages and rancherias. Each tribe represents a unique culture. AIAN speak 250 distinct languages, some of which are written; however, most are not (Manson & Galloway, 1990).

Little is known about the epidemiology of major mental disorders among the AIAN elderly. Depression among American Indians appears to be a prevalent problem (Neligh, 1988) and often is difficult to diagnose because of the cultural factors influencing its presentation and the lack of appropriate diagnostic tools for American Indians. One such tool, the American Indian Depression Schedule (AIDS) developed by Mason, Shore and Bloom (1985), addresses cultural validity and ethnicity. AIAN elderly are stoic, and they may be more willing to communicate a physical symptom than a psychological or behavioral symptom. Psychological symptoms are viewed as a sign of weakness, and a strong person can control them (Neligh, 1988). Depression sometimes presents as pseudodementia in Indian elderly like their non-Indian counterparts. Behavioral changes which produce a picture of agitation, anger and irritability are frequently seen in major depressive illness in the elderly Indian population.

Anxiety associated with major depression is often seen in elderly Indians. Neligh (1988) observed that the onset of anxiety is later than it is for non-Indians, and that patients frequently present as if they had cardiovascular symptoms even though evaluation reveals little. Increased prevalence of suicide and alcoholism has been addressed in the American Indian population but is less common in the over 55 age group. Not addressed is the large number of elderly Indians who are addicted to prescribed narcotic analgesics and sedative hypnotics (Manson & Galloway, 1990).

Although tribes differ from one another, Table 1.3 describes some common characteristics of AIAN elderly.

TABLE 1.3 American Indian/Alaskan Native Elderly: Common Characteristics

Disproportionately high rate of poverty.

Poor access to quality health care.

Changing family structure and family functioning.

High prevalence of diabetes mellitus, obesity, stroke, cardiovascular disease, alcohol abuse, delirium & arthritis (Manson & Galloway, 1990; Mink, 1983).

Multiple morbidity; several medical conditions which are more related to lifestyle than biological impairment.

High rate of unemployment.

Social isolation, loneliness, delirium/confusion and depression.

Frequent use of a dual system of care, namely, Indian and Western medicine.

Underutilization of mental health services.

Low participation in Medicare and Social Security.

ASIAN AMERICANS AND PACIFIC ISLANDER ELDERLY

Asian Americans

There are 40 Asian groups (Liu & Yu, 1985). The percentage of elderly in each group varies. It is lowest in the Indochinese (2% are 65 years and over) where predominantly refugee status has limited elderly immigration and the highest is from the Phillipines, comprising 20.3% of Asian/Pacific Americans (Liu, 1985). The characteristics of Asian/Pacific Americans are unique for each group.

At the present time there are no accurate breakdowns of prevalence rates of psychopathology in Asians (Sakauye, 1990). Folk beliefs, culture, ethnicity, and folk medicine must be considered in the care, diagnosis, and treatment of Asian/Pacific Island Americans. Emotional illness may present in culturally unique ways. Recognized, culturally bound syndromes include Latah, an exaggerated startle response to minimal stimuli in Japanese and Southeast Asian women; Amok, Southeast Asian males showing sudden assaultive behavior; and Byung, a Korean response to prolonged, suppressed anger causing epigastric distress and fears of death. Suicide rates differ among Chinese Americans. Liu and Yu (1985) found suicide rates three to ten times higher for Chinese women compared to their white counterparts. Chinese American women's suicides are often a response to a culturally insolvable problem, such as frequent, long-term family quarrels. Liu and Yu (1985) found that 80% of the women who committed suicide could not speak English and they frequently lived in meager circumstances. Japanese women 75 years and older and Issei men 85 years and older have a much higher rate of suicide relative to white Americans (Liu & Yu, 1985). For the Southeast Asian, depression has been reported as a major problem in addition to the problems of malnutrition and infection (Mueke, 1983). Mueke postulates the depression is related to a residual effect of post-traumatic stress disorders among refugees.

Korean immigrants have the highest incidence of depression among their counterpart Asians (Kuo, 1984). Korean elderly appear to be independent and too proud to seek help outside their immediate family. They acknowledge loneliness, and are concerned with preserving traditional values and tend to internalize their problems. They are highly competitive among their family members, and thus their mutual support systems are much weaker than those of other Asians.

One preliminary report suggests that like the Chinese American, the prevalence of multi-infarct dementia among the Japanese and Japanese-American populations may be higher than that found in the general population (Hasegawa, 1989). The relative prevalence of multi-infarct dementia and Alzheimer's disease was examined in a Chinese-American nursing home and compared to American nursing home populations. There was a four to six times greater prevalence of multi-infarct dementia than Alzheimer's dementia in the Chinese-American sample. (Serby, Chon, & Franssen, 1987).

Pharmacology

Important differences exist between Asian/Pacific and white Americans relative to the pharmacokinetics and pharmacodynamics of drugs. Tien (1984) studied the antihypertensive and cardiac medication, propranolol, in a small sample of white and Chinese men ages 20–40. The investigator found that the Chinese subjects had at least a twofold greater sensitivity to the beta-blocking effects of the drug in reducing heart rate, a greater sensitivity to its effect in lowering blood pressure in both supine and upright positions, a higher free fraction of propranolol in plasma, and more rapid metabolism of the drug. In Tien's review (1984) of psychotropic drug responses of Asian Americans and non-Asians, she also found that Asian patients require a lower dosage and manifest side effects readily with what is perceived as a typically low dosage in the United States. Similarly, Lin Fu (1988) quotes a recent study that found that the effective weight-standardized neuroleptic drug dose for Asian-American elderly was significantly lower than for white elderly.

Asian Americans are reported to experience extrapyramidal effects at lower neuroleptic doses than do blacks or whites (Binder & Levy, 1981). In another study, plasma antidepressant levels for a given dose of desipramine were higher for the Chinese than for white volunteers (Rudorfer, Lane, & Chang, 1984). However, Asians require lower plasma antidepressant levels. Asians also reportedly require lower oral dosages and blood levels of lithium (Takahashi, 1979), and tend to show higher plasma levels of diazepam at a given oral dose in comparison with white elderly (Ghoneim, Korrtila, & Chiang, 1981), and tend to better tolerate the sedative effects of diphenhydramine, presumably because of lower plasma levels for a given oral dose (Spector, Choudhury, & Chiang, 1980).

HISPANIC AMERICAN ELDERLY

Hispanics are the fastest growing segment of the U.S. population. While the total U.S. population grew by almost 12% between 1970 and 1980, the total Hispanic population grew by approximately 61% (U.S. Bureau of the Census, 1987). At the same time, the population of Hispanic elderly age 65 and over increased 75%, triple the 25% growth rate among the white elderly and more than double the 34% increase among older blacks. It is projected that the elderly will account for 25% of the total Hispanic population growth in the next 20 years. It is also projected that the older U.S. Hispanic population would total 11.5 million in 1992 and be as high as 13 million by the year 2000.

From a demographic perspective, Hispanics within the United States can be considered as being composed of five (5) major groups: Hispanics of Mexican American descent who are the largest sub-group (62.3%), of which 55% were born in the U.S.A. and only 4% migrated after age 50; Puerto Ricans (12.7%); Cubans (5.3%); Hispanics from Central America and South America (11.5%); and other Hispanic origin (8.1%). Hispanic elderly live predominantly in urban areas. Only 11% live in rural areas.

There is a great deal of heterogeneity among the Hispanic elderly. The profile of Hispanic elderly is impacted by the normative expectations, beliefs, customs, lifestyles and values of the host society, and the acculturation process. This profile is also influenced by socioeconomic status, intermarriage, inter-generational factors, status of health, family status, relationships, status of citizenship, migration, and chronic unemployment.

Health and Mental Health

In a study of mortality rates of the three major first-generation U.S. Hispanic populations between 1979 and 1981, it was found that Puerto Ricans had the highest age-adjusted death rates, and Cubans had the lowest. Puerto Ricans had the highest mortality rate from chronic liver disease and cirrhosis, a leading cause of death among heavy users of alcohol. This rate was twice the rate among Mexicans and nearly three times the rate among Cubans.

Currently, there is controversy regarding health status and gender. Although older Hispanic women tend to outlive and outnumber older Hispanic men, older Puerto Rican and Mexican women have higher mortality rates due to diabetes. Older Hispanic women age sooner and die younger than whites and other minorities. One study in East Los Angeles reported a high degree of disability among retired Hispanic males when compared to females, while a large-scale survey in Texas found the health of Mexican-American women to be significantly worse than that of men (Thompson, 1991). The most common disorders and conditions of the Hispanic elderly include: obesity, late-onset diabetes mellitus among women, hypertension, arthritis, and dysphoria or depression.

Early researchers reported Mexican Americans, in general, had lower levels of stress than whites (Antunes, Gordon, Gaitz, & Scott, 1974). More recent researchers report that depression and dysphoria associated with physical disability were more prevalent in an elderly Hispanic population than in an elderly non-Hispanic white population. In another study of 700 older Hispanics living in Los Angeles County, the same researchers found 26% of elderly Hispanics had major depression or dysphoria and that these affective disorders were strongly correlated with medical disability, including dementia. Without physical health complications, the rate was 5.5%, equivalent to other non-Hispanic populations. The biggest difference was in dysphoria, not major depression, suggesting more of a demoralizing effect upon the older Hispanic due to physical and probably socioeconomic factors. The many correlates associated with affective disturbances in elderly Hispanics include being female, being unable to speak English, being a widow, having low income, having family with serious health problems, and feeling lonely even when living with an adult child (Thompson, 1991).

Language

In the National Needs Assessment Study (1987), 94% of older Cubans, 91% of Puerto Ricans, 86% of Mexicans and 76% of other older Hispanics reported Spanish is spoken primarily. Only 10% of all older Hispanics reported speaking English at home. Although 57% of all older Hispanics could speak English well or very well, estimates are that more than half of older Hispanics are actually functionally illiterate in both Spanish and English due to their low educational attainment. The fields of mental health, diagnosis and assessment are heavily dependent on language and ability to communicate. Many of the psychometric test outcomes are dependent on language proficiency.

AFRO-AMERICAN (BLACK) ELDERLY

About 2,381,313 (2 million metropolitan and 397,573 nonmetropolitan) of the black population in the U.S. were 65 years of age and over as of 1990 (U.S. Bureau of the Census, 1990). Of that group, about 230,188 (7.7%) were age 85 or over (U.S. Bureau of the Census, 1990). The number of blacks aged 85 plus grew by an astonishing 33.9% between 1980 and 1986, a gain of 10 percentage points more than that for similar-aged whites and very similar to the 35.9% gain observed between 1970 and 1980. Regional differences in black population growth have changed very little since 1970. Today, 54.2% of all blacks live in the South, with 17.7% in the Northeast, 19.7% in the Midwest and 8.5% in the West (O'Hare, 1989).

Most blacks who achieve old age in the urban United States do so after passing through a life beset with economic and social health hazards. Consequently, it is not surprising that elderly blacks are more likely to be sick and disabled (Huntley et al., 1986), more likely to show cognitive impairment on standardized testing but not more depression (Kramer et al., 1985), and generally have less access to health services (U.S. Department of Health and Human Services, 1985).

On the other hand, there is some evidence to suggest that after the age of 75, blacks may experience certain health-related advantages. A so-called "crossover" of white and black mortality rates has been reported, such that black mortality rates, which are consistently higher than white rates from birth to age 75, become lower, with the difference widening progressively in advanced old age (Jackson, 1985; Manton, 1982). As a result of these changes in mortality, the proportion of black elderly in the population is increasing more rapidly than is the case for the white population. Also, since favorable mortality rates are occurring particularly among the oldest black males, sex ratios are becoming higher (i.e., relatively more males) among the oldest blacks. In addition, elderly blacks are less likely to be institutionalized (Hing, 1987).

It must be remembered that current elderly blacks have had 45 years of separate but not equal "segregated" health services. The black elderly's expectation of the health care system is based on a segregated health care system. Health care services were generally received in public clinics and emergency rooms. It was hard to find a physician who would treat a "colored" patient. The few "colored" physicians seldom had "visiting" privileges in white hospitals. Seldom was consent for surgery sought from black patients in white hospitals when they were admitted in the 1950s and 1960s. With an annual income of about $4,500, few blacks could afford health care services; therefore, they frequently used folk healers (Baker, 1990). The present black elderly frequently distrust the health care system in terms of safety and quality of care.

Biological differences appear to explain very little of the difference in health status between blacks and whites. There were 58,942 excess deaths for blacks in 1980. Only 379 of these deaths, less than 1%, were attributable to hereditary conditions such as sickle-cell anemia, for which genetic patterns among blacks have been established (U.S. Department of Health and Human Services, 1985). Instead, the major risk factors appear to be socioeconomic and physical environment, personal health habits and lifestyle. Five of the problems which contribute to the black and white differentials are: homicide, AIDS, substance abuse, hypertension, and cancer. Socioeconomic factors have been shown to be strongly related to the incidence, survival and mortality from cancer (Page & Kuntz, 1980).

Mental Health, Mental Illness, and Behavioral Disorders

The concept of mental health is difficult to define for black elderly. Most concepts and definitions of mental disorders in the literature focus on the individual and psychopathology. Definitions of mental health for black elders must consider the impact of slavery, racism, poverty, segregated and disorganized communities, an inadequate health care system, and an elaborate system of denial and avoidance, the latter having survival and adaptational value.

Recently, social scientists and psychiatrists have begun to focus on the mechanisms underlying "positive" mental health and adaptive coping styles of blacks. Black elderly live with great stress, but they have the personal, religious and social resources to maintain a perspective which keeps the stress external and does not permit it to become internalized or to disrupt personal integration (Veroff, Donovan, & Kulka, 1981). The subpanel on the Mental Health of Black Americans of the President's Commission on Mental Health (1978) states: "It is largely the environment created by institutional racism, rather than intrapsychic deficiencies in black Americans as a group, that is responsible for the over-representation of blacks among the mentally disabled." The racist attitude of many Americans causing and perpetuating tension, stress and hostility is patently a most compelling mental health hazard for black elderly. Mental health among blacks has generally been measured against white middle-class norms. This has continued to be a problem in clinical diagnosis and the use of psychological and intellectual assessment instruments (Bass, Wyatt, & Powell, 1982). Evaluated against such norms, blacks have frequently been pictured as deviant or deficient. Misdiagnosis is frequent. Black inpatients are diagnosed with schizophrenia at almost twice the rate of white inpatients (56.3%–31.5%). Yet only 7.7% of blacks are diagnosed with affective disorders, compared to 15.6% of white inpatients (National Institute of Mental Health, 1986). Misdiagnosis may lead to mistreatment and erroneous use of psychotropics. A study of 272 black manic-depressive outpatients in Chicago found these patients had been previously misdiagnosed as schizophrenic at a rate of 71.7% in a public hospital and at a rate of 52.2% in a private hospital (Bell & Mehta, 1980, 1982).

Overall, reports show increasing instances of depression, dementia (Alzheimer's and multiple infarct), and schizophrenia among black elderly. The exact incidence and prevalence of mental disorders among the black elderly is difficult to state because of: (1) vague definitions and conceptualization of mental disorders for the black elderly; (2) biases of white psychiatrists in clinical assessment; (3) lack of assessment instruments normed on blacks according to social class; (4) misdiagnosis; (5) lack of a culturally sensitive health care system, racially and ethnically sensitive health care professionals, physicians, social workers, et al.; and (6) the black elderly's underutilization of mental health services—the primary providers of mental health services to the black elderly are nonpsychiatrists (primary care, emergency room, and outpatient physicians).

Pharmacokinetics and clinical response are not the only factors that determine dosage of psychotropic drugs. Psychosocial factors should not be ignored; i.e., blacks receive more pro re nata (PRN) medication (Flaherty & Meagher, 1980) and may spend more time in seclusion than whites (Soloff & Turner, 1982). Actual doses of medication may be determined by the hospital or clinic staff's perceptions of blacks at least as much as by biological factors such as blood levels or by clinical improvement (Lawson, Yesavage, & Werner, 1984). Even though overt racism is not as prevalent in today's psychiatry, the consequences of ignoring racial and ethnic factors can be important (Lawson, 1986).

Assessment and Diagnostic Issues

Several researchers have questioned the usefulness of the Mini Mental State Examination (Folstein, 1975) in older African-American populations with limited formal education (Robinson, Stewart, & Baker, 1990). Similarly, Robinson et al. (1990) found limited use for the 15-item Geriatric Depression Scale (GDS) with community-dwelling African-American elderly, particularly if the original cut scores are used. When a revised score of 4 or more was used as the threshold suggestive of depression, the sensitivity improved. Several recent studies have demonstrated not only that patients' extrapsychic characteristics affect diagnosis and treatment but also that the social characteristics of psychiatrists, race and gender may influence diagnostic and treatment decisions (Loring & Powell, 1988; Rosenfield, 1984).

MENTALLY RETARDED AND DEVELOPMENTALLY DISABLED ELDERLY

In 1982 it was reported that there were 196,000 persons age 55 and older and 150,000 persons age 60 and older who were mentally retarded (Jacobson, Sutton, & Janicki, 1985). Colkins and Kultgen (1990) estimate the number of elderly persons who are mentally retarded/developmentally disabled (MR/DD) fall between 200,000 and 500,000 with an expectation of nearly double that amount in the year 2020. Before 1979 the mentally retarded elderly were rarely mentioned in the gerontology or mental retardation literature. There are 200,000 elderly persons with MR/DD in institutions, nursing homes (intermediate-care facility/mentally retarded), board and care homes, and institutions for MR/DD. Older persons with MR/DD constitute a growing population.

Mental Illness, and Behavioral Problems

It is difficult to define emotional disturbance in mental retardation. The co-existence of mental retardation and mental illness in the same person presents unique challenges to the professionals in mental health and mental retardation. Diagnosis and assessment are challenges, because the development of a diagnosis is very dependent on the individual's ability to verbally describe his or her stress and dysfunction. The verbal ability of MR/DD elderly is frequently impaired; therefore, the clinician must rely on observational skills especially in those persons with severe degrees of mental retardation.

It is estimated that the prevalence of psychosis and neurosis in the MR/DD elderly ranges from 40–60% (Rowitz, 1990; Menolascino, 1977). Campbell and Malone (1991) report the prevalence of co-morbidity of psychiatric disorders and mental retardation in the community and institutions ranges from 14.3% to 67.3%. In a six-year study (1979–1985), Menolascino (1990) noted 543 cases with a dual diagnosis. The highest frequency of diagnoses were: 25% schizophrenia, 19% organic brain disorders, 19% adjustment disorders, 13% affective disorders, 6% psychosexual disorders, 4% anxiety disorders, and 6% other mental disorders. The elderly with MR/DD represent a challenge in diagnosis because "masked" depressive features are so often noted. Frequently noted delayed language development in the retarded produces a major diagnostic roadblock in eliciting vegetative and somatic symptoms. Thirty-four percent were found to have one or more major medical disorders, such as diabetes mellitus, epilepsy, hypothyroidism, and cerebral palsy.

Sovner and Hurley (1983) identified four factors in identifying psychiatric symptoms in persons with mental retardation: psychological masking, cognitive disintegration, intellectual distortion, and exaggerated baseline behavior demonstrated by diminished capacities for abstract thinking and communicating feelings or experiences. Psychological masking is evident secondary to segregation from the general public. With limited life experience, the content of their conversation may resemble delusions or fantasies. Cognitive disintegration occurs when coping mechanisms fail. When intellectual functioning deteriorates, behavioral regression may result and may be accompanied by hallucinations. The hallmark of this syndrome is remission of these symptoms when the depression is treated. Stress alone can also produce cognitive disintegration in persons with mental retardation. Some individuals with mental retardation exhibit exaggeration of their baseline behaviors such as distractibility, poor judgment, stereotopic or aggressive behaviors (Gualtieri, 1987).

Pharmacology

Overall, psychopharmacological agents can be used as an adjunct to alleviate some symptoms of mental illness. Research and knowledge of the pharmacokinetics of these drugs on the MR/DD elderly are inadequate. Despite a lack of research, there are some facts to be gleaned from some of the previous research, such as:

1. Neuroleptic agents appear to be effective in ameliorating hostile and aggressive behaviors, self-mutilation behaviors, and hyperactivity.
2. If the neuroleptic agents are prescribed in high dosages and for prolonged periods of time, there is a noted serious interface with learning and performance abilities.
3. The anxiolytics have not been adequately evaluated in MR/DD population.

To assist in diagnosis, standardized instruments for assessing depression in individuals with MR/DD have been developed. The Self Report Depression Questionnaire (Reynolds, 1990) and the Psychopathology Instrument for Mentally Retarded Adults (Kazdin, Matson, & Senatore, 1990) are examples. Both tools demonstrate validity measures comparable to the Hamilton Depression Scale.

RURAL ELDERLY

According to the 1990 census, there are 31,241,834 persons 65 years of age and over. Approximately seven (7) million elderly (31%) live in rural/nonmetropolitan areas. Of the aged 65+ elderly in the rural/nonmetropolitan approximately 3,831,159 are minorities (U.S. Bureau of the Census, 1990). The rural elderly are generally underserved. Rural elderly are among those hardest hit by inadequate housing, poor transportation, poverty, and lack of indoor plumbing and refrigeration (American Association for Retired Persons (AARP), 1990). Fifty percent of rural elderly are poor. Rural elderly receive less than 25% of all Medicaid, and receive only 29% of Medicaid funds for hospital and posthospital care (Hill, 1988). Black and Hispanic rural elderly living alone have an income range from $4,600 to $6,000 per year (Kasper, 1988).

Mental Health

Difficulties in the last decade have created increasing stress for the elderly and other Americans living in rural areas. Financial hardships have increased due to struggling farms and businesses. The quality of family and community life has declined. Evidence shows that elderly in rural areas have significantly higher rates of various mental disorders than elderly in urban areas (Schlesinger, 1989). Other studies have noted moderate to large increases in numbers of dysfunctional adults, exceptionally large increases in child, spouse, and substance abuse, and increases in cognitive impairments, depressions and anxiety disorders (McCoy & Brown, 1978; National Institute of Mental Health Announcement, 1990). A study of the quality of life for seriously mentally ill persons by Schlesinger (1989) observed that 73% lived in rural areas and 78% of these individuals were black. The blacks were extremely poor, receiving $340 per month from Social Security. Eighty-five percent received Social Security benefits. Only 25% had completed high school. In 50% of the households, no family member had been employed in the past year.

At the same time, rural areas have unusual difficulties in providing mental health services, because of high rates of poverty, lack of available mental health services, and lack of transportation. Additionally, rural hospitals are reimbursed at lower rates (Schlesinger, 1989). Attitudes of rural residents toward mental health services and lack of incentives for providers to live in rural areas are often additional barriers to obtaining needed services.

RESEARCH

Research on minority aging has been of poor quality with flawed research methodology. Most studies have not utilized adequate control or comparison groups. Further studies are needed with a particular focus on the impact of socioeconomics in the development of psychopathology.

SUMMARY

There are over two and one-half million racial and ethnic minority elderly in the United States, comprising 10% of all persons 65 years or older. Racial and ethnic minority elderly have been increasing at faster rates than white elderly in recent years and we can expect this trend to continue into the next century. By the year 2025, 15% of this population is projected to be nonwhite and by 2050, one in five older persons is likely to be nonwhite, a total of almost 13 million. Kramer (1986) observes that the greatest increase in nursing home populations will be among blacks and other minorities. The rate for white persons increased from 26.6 per 1,000 persons age 65 and over in 1963 to 49.7 in 1977, an increase of 87%, while the corresponding rate for blacks and other races increased from 10.3 to 30.4 per 1,000, an increase of 195%.

For minority elderly and other special groups in extended care facilities, special attention must be given to a group of diseases and conditions which are not fatal, but which may increase with age, and cause excessive disability, such as diabetes mellitus, obesity, hypertension, depression, poverty, certain cancers, cardiovascular disease, and various dementing diseases (multi-infarct dementia and Alzheimer's disease).

Health care providers must learn the pathophysiology of the processes as well as the lifestyle which leads to the array of age-dependent conditions to postpone their onset and allow the increased years to be increasingly free of these nonfatal and often preventable and modifiable conditions. Although multiple factors contribute to the persistent health disadvantages of minority groups, poverty and lifestyle may be the most profound and pervasive determinants. Another determinant of the risk for poor health among minority elderly is the interacting and complex relationships between lifestyle, personal behavior, knowledge, poverty, and social policy. The deleterious effect of poverty, ignorance, environment, hazardous working conditions, and lifestyle upon the aging processes and the experience of aging are as influential in the health and quality of life for minority elderly as biological, social and genetic risk factors. Researchers have viewed the excessive disabling and aging processes of minority elderly as genetically hard-wired and biologically determined. Therefore, they seldom conduct research pertaining to the impact of lifestyle, poverty, or lack of access on the health profile of the minority elderly.

Mental illness and behavioral problems are frequently manifested in minority elderly. The conditions are late onset as well as early onset. Research is critically needed for special populations of older people. Of the older population, those who are institutionalized are the least understood but have the highest prevalence of mental disorders (National Institute of Mental Health, 1990). Mental illness in minority elderly is often untreated, unrecognized, misdiagnosed, and neglected. Understanding the effects of gender, class, ethnicity, and race is salient to every priority area listed. Ethical issues must be thoughtfully analyzed and researched in each priority.

It is important for all health care providers to recognize that people arrive at the end of life by different routes, and societies influence these routes in varied but consequential ways. The goal is to prevent and postpone morbidity and to add years of healthy life. The extended care facility can create a culturally competent system of care by having an understanding of individual culture and by developing skills in differentiating between symptoms of intrapsychic stress and stress from social and cultural backgrounds.

REFERENCES

American Association of Retired People (AARP). (1990). *A profile of older Americans*. Washington, DC. Author.

Antunes, G., Gordon, D., Gaitz, C. M., & Scott, I. (1974). Ethnicity, socioeconomic status and the etiology of psychological distress. *Sociological Research, 58*, 360–368.

Baker, F. M. (1990). Ethnic minority elders: Differential diagnosis, medication, treatment and outcomes. In M. S. Harper (Ed.), *Minority aging: Essential curricula content for selected health and allied health professionals* (pp. 549–577). Washington, DC: U.S. Government Printing Office.

Bass, B. A., Wyatt, G. E., & Powell, E. (1982). *The Afro-American family: Assessment, research and treatment issues*. New York: Grune and Stratton.

Bell, C. C., & Mehta, H. (1982). Misdiagnosis of black patients with manic-depressive illness. *Journal of The National Medical Association, 72*(2), 141–145.

Bell, C. C., & Mehta, H. (1980). Misdiagnosis of black patients with manic-depressive illness: second in a series. *Journal of The National Medical Association, 73*(2), 101–107.

Binder, R. L., & Levy, R. (1981). Extrapyramidal reactions in asians. *American Journal of Psychiatry, 138*(6), 1243–1244.

Campbell, M., & Malone, R. P. (1991). Mental retardation and psychiatric disorders. *Hospital and Community Psychiatry, 42*(4), 374–379.

Colkins, C. F., & Kultgen, P. (1990). Enhancing the life changes and social support networks for older persons with developmental disabilities. In S. F. Gilsons, T. L. Goldsbury, & E. H. Faulkner (Eds.), *Three populations of primary focus: Persons with mental retardation and mental illness, persons with mental retardation who are elderly and persons with mental retardation and complex medical needs* (pp. 131–135). Omaha, NB: University of Nebraska.

Cuellar, J. B. (1990). Hispanic Americans aging: Geriatric education curriculum development for selected health professionals. In M. S. Harper (Ed.), *Minority aging: Essential curricula content for selected health and allied health professions* (DHHS/PHS/HRHSA Publication No. HRS-P-D.V. 90-4, pp. 365–413). Washington, DC: U.S. Government Printing Office.

Flaherty, J. A., & Meagher, R. (1980). Measuring racial bias in inpatient treatment. *American Journal of Psychiatry, 137*(2), 679–682.

Folstein, M. F., Folstein, S., & McHugh, P. R. (1975). Mini mental state: A practical method of grading the cognitive state of patients for the clinician. *Journal of Psychiatric Research, 12*, 189–198.

Ghoneim, M. M., Korrtila, K., & Chiang, C. K. (1981). Diazepam effects and kinetics in caucasians and orientals. *Clinical Pharmacology and Therapeutics, 29*(2), 749–756.

Gualtieri, C. T. (1987). *American Psychiatric Association task force on treatment of psychiatric disorders of the mentally retarded.* Washington, DC: American Psychiatric Association.

Hasegawa, K. (1989, March). Research update of cross-cultural aspects of Alzheimer's disease in Japan. Paper presented at the Asia-Pacific Alzheimer's disease Conference, Honolulu, Hawaii.

Hill, C. E. (1988). *Community health system in the rural American south.* Boulder, CO: Westview Press.

Hing, E. (1987). *Use of nursing homes by the elderly: Preliminary data from the 1985 National Nursing Home Survey* Hyattsville, MD: U.S. Government Printing Office. NCHS Advance Date, No. 135, (DHHS Publication No. PHS 87-1250).

Holzberg, C. S. (1982). Ethnicity and aging: Anthropological perspectives on more than just minority elderly. *The Gerontologist, 22*(3), 249–257.

Huntley, J. C., Dwight, B. B., Ostfeld, A. M., Taylor, J. O., & Wallace, R. B. (1986). *Established populations for epidemiologic studies of the elderly: Resource data book* (NIH Publication No. 86-2443). Bethesda, MD: U.S. Department of Health and Human Services, Public Health Service.

Jackson, J. J. (1985). Race, national origin, ethnicity and aging. In R. H. Binstock & E. Shanas (Eds.), *Handbook of aging and the social sciences* (2nd ed.). New York: Van Nostrand Reinhold.

Jacobson, J., Sutton, M., & Janicki, M. (1985). Demography and characteristics of aging and aged mentally retarded persons. In M. Janicki & H. Wisniewski (Eds.), *Aging and developmental disabilities—Issues and approaches.* Baltimore, MD: Paul H. Brookes Publishing.

Jones, B. E., & Gray, B. A. (1986). Problems in diagnosing schizophrenia and affective disorders in blacks, *Hospital and Community Psychiatry, 37,* 61–65.

Kasper, J. D. (1988). *Aging alone.* New York: The Commonwealth Fund Commission.

Kazdin, J., Matson, J., & Senatore, K. (1990). Psychopathology instrument for mentally retarded adults. *Dialogue on drugs, behavior and developmental disabilities, 2*(3), 10, Kansas City, MO: University of Missouri.

Kramer, M. (1986). Trends of institutionalization and prevalence of mental disorders in nursing homes. In M. S. Harper & D. B. Lebowitz (Eds.), *Mental illness in nursing homes: Agenda for research* (pp. 7–26). Washington, DC: U.S. Government Printing Office.

Kuo, W. H. (1984). The prevalence of depression among Asian Americans. *Journal of Nervous and Mental Disease, 172*(6), 449–457.

Lawson, W. B. (1986). Racial and ethnic factors in psychiatric research. *Hospital and Community Psychiatry, 37*(1), 50–54.

Lawson, W. G., Yesavage, J. A., & Werner, P. A. (1984). Race, violence and psychopathology. *Journal of Clinical Psychiatry, 45*(3), 294–297.

Lin Fu, J. S. (1988). Population characteristics and health care needs of Asian/Pacific Americans. *Public Health Reports, 103*(6), 18–27.

Linton, R. (1945). *The cultural background of personality.* New York: Appleton-Century-Crafts.

Liu, W. T. (1985). Asian/Pacific American elderly: Mortality differentials, health status, and use of health service. *Journal of Applied Gerontology, 4*(1), 35–64.

Liu, W. T., & Yu, E. (1985). Asian-American elderly: Mortality differentials, health status and use of health services. *Journal of Applied Gerontology, 4*(6), 34–64.

Loring, M., & Powell, B.(1988). Gender, race and DSM III: A study of the objectivity of psychiatric diagnostic behavior. *Journal of Health and Social Behavior, 29*(3), 1–22.

Manson, S. M., & Galloway, D. G. (1990). Health and aging among American Indians: Issues and challenges for the geriatric sciences. In M. S. Harper (Ed.), *Minority aging: Essential curricula content for selected health and allied health professions* (pp. 63–119). Washington, DC: U.S. Government Printing Office.

Manton, K. G. (1982). Differential life expectancy, possible explanation during the later ages. In R. C. Manuel (Ed.), *Minority aging: Sociological and social psychological issues.* Westport, CT: Greenwood Press.

Mason, M., Shore, J. H., & Bloom, J. D. (1985). The depressive experience in American Indian communities; A challenge for psychiatric theory and diagnosis. In A. Klunmon & G. B. Berkley (Eds.), *Culture and depression: Studies in the anthropology and cross-cultural psychiatry of affective disorders,* Berkeley, CA: University of California Press.

McCoy, J., & Brown, D. (1978). Health status among low income elderly persons: Rural-urban differences. *Social Security Bulletin, 41*(6), 14–26.

Menolascino, F. J. (1977). *Challenges in mental retardation: Progressive ideology and services.* New York: Human Sciences Press.

Menolascino, F. J. (1990). Mental illness in the mentally retarded: Diagnostic and treatment issues. In S. F. Gilson, T. L. Goldsbury, & E. H. Faulkner (Eds.), *Three populations of primary focus: Persons with mental retardation and mental illness, persons with mental retardation who are elderly and persons with mental retardation and complex medical needs* (pp. 165–175). Omaha, NB: University of Nebraska.

Mueke, M. A. (1983). Caring for Southeast Asian refugee patients in U.S.A. *American Journal of Public Health, 73*(4), 431–438.

National Institute of Mental Health (NIMH) (1990). Program announcement—*Research on mental disorders in rural populations.* Washington, DC: Author.

National Institute of Mental Health. (1986). *Characteristics of admissions to the inpatient services of state and county mental hospital, 2988.* (Mental Health Statistical Note, No. 117, DHHS Publication No. ADM 86-1476). Rockville, MD: Author.

Neligh, G. (1988). Major mental disorders and behavior among American Indians and Alaskan Natives. In S. Manson & N. Dinges (Eds.), *Behavior health issues among American Indians and Alaskan Natives: Explorations on the frontiers of biobehavioral Sciences, 1*(Whole No. 1), 116–159.

O'Hare, W. P. (1989). Black demographic trends in the 1980s. In D. P. Willis (Ed.), *Health policies and black Americans* (pp. 35–55). New Brunswick, NJ: Transaction Publishers.

Page, W. F., & Kuntz, A. J. (1980). Racial and socioeconomic factors in cancer survival: A comparison of Veterans Administration results with selected studies. *Cancer*, *45*(3), 1029–1040.

Reynolds, R. (1990). Self report depression questionnaire (SRDQ). *Dialogue on Drugs, Behavior and Developmental Disabilities*, *2*(3), 9–10.

Robinson, B., Stewart, B., & Baker, F. M. (1990). *Screening for cognitive impairment and depressive illness in African American elders.* Unpublished manuscript, University of Texas, Departments of Psychiatry and Nursing, San Antonio.

Rosenfield, S. (1984). Race differences in involuntary hospitalization: Psychiatric vs. labeling perspectives. *Journal of Health and Social Behavior*, *25*(1), 14–23.

Rowitz, L. (1990). Survey of services used by the elderly retarded. In S. F. Gilson, T. L. Goldsbury, & E. H. Faulkner (Eds.), *Three populations of primary focus: Persons with mental retardation and mental illness, persons with mental retardation who are elderly and persons with mental retardation and complex medical needs* (pp. 105–127). Omaha, NB: University of Nebraska.

Rudorfer, M. V., Lane, E. A., & Chang, W. H. (1984). Desipramine pharmacokinetics in Chinese and Caucasian volunteers. *British Journal of Clinical Pharmacology*, *17*(2), 433–440.

Sakauye, K. (1990). Differential diagnosis, medication, treatment and outcomes: Asian American elderly. In M. S. Harper (Ed.), *Minority aging: Essential curricula content for selected health and allied health professions* (DHHS/PHS/-HRHSA Publication No. HRS-P-D.V. 90-4). Washington, DC: U.S. Government Printing Office.

Schlesinger, M. (1989). Paying the price: Medical care, minorities and the newly competitive health care system. In D. P. Willis (Ed.), *Health policies and Black Americans* (pp. 270–296). New Brunswick, NJ: Transaction Publishers.

Serby, M., Chon, J. C. Y., & Franssen, E. (1987). Dementia in an American Chinese nursing home population. *American Journal of Psychiatry*, *144*(3), 811–812.

Soloff, P. H., & Turner, S. M. (1982). Patterns of seclusion: A prospective study. *Journal of Nervous and Mental Disease*, *169*(3), 37–44.

Sovner, R., & Hurley, A. H, (1983). Do the mentally retarded suffer from affective illness? *Archives of General Psychiatry*, *140*(3), 1539–1540.

Spector, R., Choudhury, A. K., & Chiang, C. K. (1980). Diphenhydramine in Orientals and Caucasians. *Clinical Pharmacology and Therapeutics*, *28*(3), 220–234.

Sue, S. (1982). *The Mental Health of Asian Americans* (pp. 22–38). San Francisco, CA: Jossey-Bass Publishers.

Takahashi, R. (1979). Lithium treatment in affective disorders: Therapeutic plasma level. *Psychopharmacology Bulletin*, *15*(3), 32–35.

Thompson, L. (1991). Examining the health status of Hispanics. *Washington Post*, January 15, 1991, 7.

Tien, J. L. (1984). Do Asians need less medication? *Journal of Psychosocial Nursing*, *22*(6), 10–22.

U. S. Bureau of the Census. (1987). *Hispanic population in the United States, The national needs assessment, March 1986 and 1987: advanced report.* Washington, DC: Author.

U. S. Bureau of the Census. (1989, 1990). Population of the United States for metropolitan/nonmetropolitan areas by age, race and sex. Washington, DC: Author.

U. S. Department of Health and Human Services. (1985). Report of the Secretary's Task Force on Black and Minority Health (Vol. I, Summary). Washington, DC: Author.

U.S. Department of Health Education and Welfare: The Federal Council on Aging (1978). Report of the President's Commission on Mental Health: Task Panel on the Elderly (Subpanel on the Mental Health of Black Americans). Washington, D.C., U.S. Government Printing Office, p. 823.

Veroff, J., Donovan, E., & Kulka, R. A. (1981). *The inner American: A self-portrait from 1957 to 1976.* New York: Basic Books.

2

Problem Behaviors among Younger Adult Nursing Home Residents

James C. Romeis

In this chapter the author describes problem behaviors among nursing home residents aged 35–55. Data were derived from a series of secondary analyses using the 1987 National Medical Expenditure Survey—Institutional Population Component public use data to examine health services use among the long-term-care population in the U.S. (Romeis, 1991), to acquire some perspective on the younger adult population as compared to nursing home residents aged 65 to 75 and to nursing home residents over age 75. The rationale for the comparison relates to two sets of overlapping policies. One concerns the 1987 Omnibus Budget Reconciliation Act (OBRA) provisions regarding nursing homes as inappropriate places for younger adults. The other is that after three decades of deinstitutionalization, state mental health facilities have decreased in capacity by a third and nursing homes have trebled in number, yet nursing homes still offer inappropriate services for residents with mental heath problems, independent of age (Talbott, 1988). It may be that contrary to OBRA intentions, younger adults in nursing homes should be seen as special populations, rather than inappropriate admissions, where the place for care and costs could be appropriate. This line of inquiry is similar to the development of innovative long-term-care facility programs for Alzheimer's patients (Ohta & Ohta, 1988).

BACKGROUND

It is often useful to categorize nursing home residents into "short stayers" and "long stayers." Short stayers generally reside in nursing homes between 1 and 6 months and may be divided into two sub-groups; the terminally ill and those who need short-term rehabilitation or have subacute illnesses. Long stayers reside between 6 months and 2 years or longer and are further divided into three general groups: those with only cognitive impairments, those with only physical impairments, and those with significant impairments in both cognitive and physical functioning (Ouslander & Martin, 1987). These generalizations are not necessarily age dependent and do not usually include behavioral problems unless they are linked to the physical or mental impairment. From both cost and appropriateness perspectives, younger nursing home residents who are long stayers are a concern for policy officials.

Admissions to nursing homes occur for predictable reasons that usually have to do with an individual's decline in health or functional abilities (Greene & Ondrich, 1990; Liu, Korbin & Kenneth, 1984; Kane & Matthias, 1984). Unless there is some major shift in the industry, the reasons for admitting people to nursing homes may not vary significantly over time. Once admitted, health and functional status generally are expected to decline with tenure in the nursing home. Nursing homes may try to minimize the rate of decline but length of time in nursing homes and health status should be inversely related; as tenure increases, health status should decrease, but the rate of decrease is highly variable among nursing home residents. It could be expected that for a given distribution of long stayers, residents with the most recent admission dates would have fewer health, functional, cognitive and other types of deficits than residents who had lived in nursing homes for several years. These generalizations are more apt to apply to elderly nursing home populations and may not apply to younger adults.

METHODOLOGY

The data for this analysis are a subset of the 1987 National Medical Expenditure Survey—Institutional Population Component (NMES-IPC) conducted by the Agency for Health Care Policy and Research, formerly the

National Center for Health Services Research and Technology Assessment. The primary objective of the IPC is to estimate "the use of and expenses for health services and health insurance coverage for all of 1987 for all persons who reside in a nursing home or personal care home or facility for the mentally retarded at any time during the survey year" (Edwards & Edwards, 1989). The data are derived from nursing and personal care homes with more than three beds ($n = 3,347$), intermediate care facilities for the mentally retarded and all other facilities for the mentally retarded with more than 15 beds ($n = 3,618$). Additional data obtained included census region, certification status, ownership type, number of beds, and number of admissions. The selection of sampled individuals was twofold—those who were current residents of facilities and those who were admitted during the calendar year of 1987. The key admission date refers to the "most recent admission date in the person's record that did not follow discharge solely for an acute hospital stay" (Edwards & Edwards, 1989). This operational definition is intended to minimize differences in practices by administrators and residents who move between hospitals and nursing homes for very short stays. The baseline data refer to admission dates that range between 1932 and 1986 and do not include individuals admitted in 1987.

The data for this paper were extracted from the baseline Phase 1 of the nursing home sub-sample and refer to younger adults aged 35–55 ($n = 150$), older adults aged 65–75 ($n = 542$), and the oldest adults aged 76 and older ($n = 2,391$). The age of the younger adults cohort is partly arbitrary but was intended to focus on adults who were beginning their middle years. The younger adults represent approximately 54,000 individuals residing in nursing homes at the end of calendar year 1986. These residents represent approximately 3.36% of the total nursing home population in 1986, while the latter two age groups represent 90.5% of the total nursing home population. For the baseline questionnaire, the response rate was 98.67% because nursing home personnel (usually nursing) provided data from residents' records. The data are pre-OBRA and therefore we can ask, if younger people in nursing homes may be inappropriately placed, then what would be alternatives for OBRA era residents?

The first set of comparisons helps to describe younger adults in nursing homes and is compared to the two older reference groups. These demographic comparisons also include selected characteristics of facilities. The second set of comparisons consists of their health status characteristics including medical and psychiatric diagnoses. The diagnoses are broadly categorized and were obtained from residents' medical records and nursing home personnel most familiar with the residents.

Another set of health status characteristics refers to the residents' functional status, cognitive, communication, continence, and memory deficits. The measure of functional status is an eight-item summated scale of six

Activities of Daily Living (ADLs), e.g., bathing, dressing, toileting, walking, feeding, and bed; and two Independent Activities of Daily Living (IADLs), e.g., shopping and transportation items; plus an item referring to the ability to walk across a room. This measure of functional status parallels measures of active life expectancy (ALE) reported by Katz et al. (1983, 1985) and Spector, Katz, Murphy, & Fulson (1987). The scale is conceptualized as a generalized functional status measure and varies between 0, or no functional status deficiencies, and 8, or deficiencies in all of the ADL and IADL areas.

Cognitive deficits refer to the resident's ability to identify and recognize the number of friends, family, and staff. Communication deficits refer to the resident's cumulative ability to see and hear even with appliances, be understood, and talk with others. The level of incontinence refers to no problems, urinary or bowel incontinence, and incontinent in both. Memory function refers to no memory problems, forgetting things that just happened or forgetting important past events.

Problem behaviors refer to a set of dichotomous variables associated with: getting upset, yelling, crying, hurting others or self, hoarding, wandering, stealing, exposing self, or dressing inappropriately. All of these data were recorded from interviews with nursing home staff most familiar with the resident and the resident's records and refer to deficits and behaviors at the time of the survey.

RESULTS

Demographic and Nursing Home Characteristics

Table 2.1 has two parts: demographic and facility characteristics. Unlike their older nursing home resident counterparts, the data indicate that younger residents are slightly more likely to be males. Younger residents are slightly more likely to be racial and minority group members than their older counterparts. The gender differences probably reflect differences in life expectancy and institutionalization patterns, e.g., women live longer and older women are more likely to be admitted to nursing homes. The racial and minority group member data await further study.

The marital and family status characteristics of the residents indicate that more than half of the younger residents only have siblings, although almost one-fourth have siblings and children, but less than 5% have a spouse. While these differences are important, they probably reflect stage-of-life-cycle difference and health problems at birth or early onset.

Relative to facility characteristics, an interesting comparison is the admission date. Approximately 21% of the younger population was admit-

TABLE 2.1 Demographic and Long-Term-Care-Facility Characteristics: Percent Comparisons Between Younger Adults and Older Adults

Demographic characteristics	Age group		
	35–55	65–75	76 plus
Race (% white)	79.3	87.1	92.1
Gender (% female)	56.0	63.1	76.9
Marital & Family Status			
Alone	12.3	13.5	20.2
Siblings only	55.7	36.0	15.9
Kids and siblings	23.0	21.5	18.3
Kids only	4.9	14.8	34.6
Spouse and kids	0	4.9	5.0
Spouse only	0	1.3	1.8
Spouse and siblings	1.6	1.6	1.6
Spouse, kids & siblings	2.5	6.5	2.6
Facility Characteristics			
Admission Year			
< 1980	20.7	13.7	9.8
1980–1983	23.3	21.6	25.2
1984–1985	21.3	29.2	32.8
1986	34.7	35.6	32.2
Certification			
ICF only	44.4	63.0	65.1
ICF-MR only	2.1	0.6	0.0
ICF & ICF-MR	0.0	0.0	1.5
Neither	53.5	36.4	33.3
Ownership			
For profit	70.0	75.4	67.2
Nonprofit	20.7	15.2	25.0
Government	9.3	9.4	7.9
Part of Chain (% yes)	44.7	55.7	50.6
Total Beds			
50 or less	28.7	15.1	12.6
51–100	23.3	25.3	28.1
101–150	18.0	27.3	29.7
151–200	14.7	12.4	12.9
201 or more	15.3	19.9	16.6

ted prior to 1980 and compares to approximately 14% for the 65–75 age group and 10% for the over 75 age group. For convenience of reporting, the 1980–1983 and 1984–1985 admission years were grouped and indicate that approximately 20% of the younger age group were admitted in each of these periods. Approximately one-third of each age group was admitted in 1986. The younger age group was more likely to have been admitted from hospitals and other health-related facilities (60%), including group homes, compared to the other age groups which were more likely to have been admitted from independent living settings (44%) and hospitals and other health-related facilities, excluding group homes (36%).

When the remaining facility characteristics are compared, younger residents appear slightly more likely to live in nursing homes that have neither a licensed intermediate care facility (ICF) nor beds for the mentally retarded (MR) and slightly less likely to live in facilities that have only ICF beds. No demonstrable differences appear relative to nursing home ownership type, but younger adults are less likely to be living in facilities that are organizationally linked to nursing home chains. This latter finding may be related to the finding that 52% of the younger residents appear to be more likely to live in smaller nursing homes (less than 100 beds) compared to 40% of the 65–75 age group and 41% of the over 75 age group.

HEALTH STATUS CHARACTERISTICS

Table 2.2 compares each age group by the list of active medical diagnoses in the residents' records. Residents may have more than one reported diagnosis. In general, and as might be expected from a cross section of the population in nursing homes, older residents are more likely to have medical diagnoses and younger residents are more likely to have psychiatric diagnoses. However, there are younger long stayers who have medical problems, in particular, cardiovascular system problems. Almost 25% are mentally retarded and an additional 11% have seizure disorders.

As suspected, younger residents are more likely to have classic psychiatric diagnoses compared to their older counterparts. Specifically, 34% of the younger age group had a current diagnosis of schizophrenia compared to 13% of the 65–75-old age group and 3% of the 76-plus age group. The percentage difference is not as great with personality disorders and anxiety disorders, but younger nursing home residents appear to be more likely to have these diagnoses than the two older cohorts. The age group differences are negligible for depressive disorders, other psychoses, and mental disorder categories.

The younger residents have some functional ability deficits but as expected fewer deficits than the older groups. Similarly, they are less likely to be incontinent than the older groups. Almost two-thirds of the younger nursing home residents do not have any communication deficits or cognitive deficits. Finally, over two-thirds of the younger group do not have short-term or long-term memory problems, compared to 55% of the 65–75 age group and only one-third of the 76-plus age group.

Problem Behaviors

Table 2.3 compares the list of problem behaviors for each age group. Those printed in bold type are statistically significant differences. Other than the drowsy/dull/sluggish behavior, the increased percentages associated with behaviors for the younger nursing home residents suggest that younger patients may be more difficult to provide services to than their older counterparts. Although not shown in Table 2.3, it is important to report that 24% of the younger age group did not have any problem behaviors listed in their records compared to 28% of the 65–75 age group and 26% for the over 75 age group. In general, the listed problem behaviors for the younger age group may be direct correlates of their mental or psychiatric problems including medication compliance, e.g., getting upset/yelling, a history of hurting themselves, stealing, dressing inappropriately, or exposing themselves. Alternatively, they may also be indirect correlates of being young nursing home residents, living in an environment where there are no age mates, thus making social interaction and quality of life difficult. For the remainder of the list there do not appear to be any striking differences by age group. Moreover, when all the behaviors are summed, the younger age group has slightly more problem behaviors than the older residents but this difference is not statistically significant ($p < .05$). Therefore, these specific behaviors appear related to the younger age group.

SUMMARY AND CONCLUSIONS

This secondary analysis was designed to describe and compare the younger adult nursing home resident population and their problem behaviors to older nursing home patients and their problem behaviors. The data were drawn from Phase I of the 1987 National Medical Expenditure Survey—Institutional Population Component. While the resulting survey data base is not technically suitable for estimating true population variance, it is suitable for crude estimates, descriptive comparisons as well as developing a heuristic perspective regarding the admission provision of OBRA for long-term-stayer nursing home resident less than age 65.

In general, what was found was expected. Younger nursing home residents are not short-stayers. Rather, they are part of the long-stayer population, but make up less than 5% of the total nursing home resident population. They have some medical problems, but compared to older nursing home residents, they are more likely to have either neurologic or psychiatric problems. Also unlike older nursing home residents, younger residents on the average have fewer functional, cognitive, communication,

TABLE 2.2 Health Status Characteristics: Percent Comparison Between Younger Adults and Older Adults in Long-Term Care Facilities

	Age group		
	35–55	65–75	76 plus
Medical diagnoses			
Hypertension	17.0	34.3	29.2
Arteriosclerosis	5.4	23.5	43.0
Rheumatism	0.7	5.8	7.7
Emphysema	2.0	9.0	4.6
Arthritis	6.2	23.8	37.6
Diabetes	8.8	21.2	14.8
Cancer	1.4	6.3	9.5
Heart Disease	8.8	33.0	50.4
Stroke	8.1	23.5	21.6
Heart Attack	1.4	7.1	9.1
Neurologic Diagnoses			
Retarded	26.0	8.3	1.2
Epilepsy	10.9	7.1	2.4
Cerebral Palsy	8.7	1.8	0.2
Autism	0.7	0.2	0.1
Spina Bifida	0.7	0.0	0.0
Psychiatric Diagnoses			
Schizophrenia	34.0	13.3	2.7
Personality Disorder	20.8	14.7	6.9
Anxiety Disorder	19.4	12.4	9.7
Depressive Disorder	18.2	18.7	13.6
Other Psychoses	7.6	6.4	3.3
Senile Dementia	6.2	33.8	46.3
Other Mental Disorder	8.4	7.3	3.8
Functional Status			
ALE[a]+WALK[b] mean	3.56	5.07	5.96
(SD)	(2.97)	(2.67)	(2.22)
Incontinence			
No Problem	75.2	56.5	39.6
Urinary or Bowel	7.8	11.5	16.6
Both	17.1	32.0	43.7
Communication Deficits			
No deficits	58.6	56.4	42.8
One deficit	23.3	27.0	32.4
Two deficits	16.5	13.3	17.4
3–4 deficits	1.5	3.2	7.5
Cognitive Deficits			
No deficits	74.6	60.7	37.8
One deficit	13.8	12.3	14.1
Two deficits	6.5	8.7	14.8

[a]ALE = Active life expectancy.
[b]WALK = Ability to walk across a small room.

	Age group		
	35–55	65–75	76 plus
Cognitive Deficits			
Three deficits	2.9	7.9	12.1
Four deficits	2.2	10.4	21.3
Memory Deficits			
No deficits	69.0	54.8	33.4
One deficit	13.5	13.2	17.5
Two deficits	17.5	32.0	49.0

memory, and continence problems. On the average, younger residents do not have significantly more behavioral problems than their older counterparts. However, when individual behaviors are compared across age groups, there are some important age cohort differences. Younger residents have behavior problems that are socially inappropriate if it is assumed that the behaviors preceded the institutionalization and that they were related to their neurologic or psychiatric problems. It could be that some of the problem behaviors surfaced or became exacerbated after they were institutionalized and these were related to the nursing home environment, e.g., living in a setting where the younger resident is unlike the rest of

TABLE 2.3 Problem Behaviors: Percent Comparison Between Younger Adults and Older Adults in Long-Term-Care Facilities

	Age group		
Problem behaviors	35–55	65–75	76 plus
Gets upset/yells*	39.3	32.0	29.3
Hurts other people	14.7	12.5	10.3
Hurts self*	8.0	3.2	2.6
Dresses inappropriately*	16.7	9.9	8.0
Cries without reason	8.0	10.6	8.4
Hides things/hoards*	13.3	11.9	7.2
Gets lost/wanders	8.7	10.6	11.9
Unable to avoid danger	12.1	9.7	11.5
Steals*	10.7	3.7	2.7
Exposes self*	10.7	6.3	5.4
Worried/apprehensive	32.9	34.0	33.9
Drowsy/dull/sluggish*	15.1	17.1	21.6
Unresponsive/withdrawn	17.0	18.3	17.6
Easily annoyed	37.7	38.4	34.4
Suspicious/not trusting	23.8	20.2	18.7
Total Behaviors mean	2.65	2.34	2.20
(SD)	(2.58)	(2.37)	(2.23)

*= $p < .05$.

the population. It is in this context where the rationale for special treatment programs may have some merit.

When the demands of caregiving exceed the resources of the family, institutionalization is a rational response (Romeis, 1989; Perlin, Mullan, Semple, & Skaff, 1990). Younger residents' families may be less equipped to cope with the individual's mental health and behavior problems than the facility. The facility is at least able to meet some of the younger adults' needs, but as mental health providers argue, nursing homes too often do not meet the mental health needs of the younger adult.

It would seem that rather than set up rigid Federal and state policy prohibitions to divert younger patients from nursing homes to community settings, it may be prudent to establish incentives for nursing homes to provide age-appropriate, special treatment programs focusing on the problem or inappropriate behaviors of younger residents. If these behaviors could be modified, and other health and mental health problems could be managed outside the nursing home, then the magnitude of the current younger long-stayer nursing home resident population might be reduced. Moreover, younger residents in the future might be short-stayers rather than long stayers.

REFERENCES

Edwards, W. S., & Edwards, B. (1989). *Questionnaires and data collection methods for the institutional population component, Methods 1 National Medical Expenditure Survey* (NCHSR, DHHS Publication No. (PHS 89-3440). Washington, D.C.: U.S. Government Printing Office.

Greene, V. L., & Ondrich, J. I. (1990). Risk factors for nursing home admission and exits: A discrete-time hazard function approach. *The Gerontologist, 45*, S250–258.

Kane, R. L., & Matthias, R. (1984). From hospital to nursing home: The long term care connection. *The Gerontologist, 24*, 604–609.

Katz, S., Branch, L. G., Branson, M. H., Papsidero, J. A., Beck, J. C., & Greer, D. S. (1983). Active life expectancy. *New England Journal of Medicine, 309*, 1218–1224.

Katz, S., Greer, D. S., Beck, J. C., Branch, L. G., & Spector, W. D. (1985). Active life expectancy: Societal implications (pp. 57–72). In *America's aging: Health in an older society*. Institute of Medicine/National Research Council. Washington, DC: National Academy Press.

Liu, K., & Manton, K. (1984). The characteristics and utilization pattern of an admission cohort of nursing home patients (II). *The Gerontologist, 24*(1), 70–76.

Ohta, R. J., & Ohta, B. M. (1988). Special units for Alzheimer's disease patients: A critical look. *The Gerontologist, 28*(6), 803–808.

Ouslander, J. G., & Martin, S. (1987). Assessment in the nursing home. *Clinics in Geriatric Medicine, 3*(1), 155–174.

Perlin, L.I., Mullan, J. T., Semple, S. J., & Skaff, M. M. (1990). Caregiving and the stress process: An overview of the concepts and their measures. *The Gerontologist, 30*(5), 583–594.

Romeis, J. C. (1989). Caregiver strain: Toward an enlarged perspective. *Journal of Aging and Health, 1*(2), 188–208.

Romeis, J. C. (1991). (in press.) Nursing home population composition in the PPS-era. *Health Services Administration Review.*

Spector, W. D., Katz, S., Murphy, J. B., & Fulton, J. P. (1987). The hierarchical relationship between activities of daily living and independent activities of daily living. *Journal of Chronic Diseases, 40*(6), 481–489.

Talbott, J. A. (1988). Nursing homes are not the answer. *Hospital and Community Psychiatry, 39*(2), 11.

PART I
Psychiatric Disorders

3

Psychiatric Disorders: Overview of Behavior Problems and the Dementing Illnesses

George T. Grossberg
Kenneth Solomon

Older Americans, or those over 65 years of age, constitute more than 13% of our population. Those over the age of 85 are the most rapidly growing segment. It is the latter group which is increasingly found in community nursing homes in our country. As nursing homes see older and older residents, the prevalence of diagnosable psychiatric syndromes in nursing homes is increasing, primarily due to the growing numbers of residents with dementing disorders. The dementias are the most commonly found psychiatric syndromes in the nursing home with a prevalence of 67–78% (Rovner et al., 1990; Chandler & Chandler, 1988; Rovner, Kafonek, Filipp, Lucas, & Folstein, 1986). The prevalence of major depression in the nursing home is almost 12.4% if those with dementia are also included (Parmelee, Katz, & Lawton, 1989). Rovner and associates (1990) found that of 454 consecutive new admissions to a group of community nursing homes, 10% had major depression. Others have found that undiagnosed depression occurs in almost 40% of nursing home residents (Grossberg et al., 1990).

TABLE 3.1 Prevalence of Psychiatric Diagnoses Among Nursing Home Residents (In Decreasing Order of Frequency)

Progressive dementias
   Probable Alzheimer's disease
   Probable multi-infarct dementia
Delirium
Mood disorders
   Major depression
   Dysthymia
Sleep disorders
   Insomnia
   Hypersomnia
Anxiety disorders
   Generalized anxiety disorder
Adjustment disorder
   with anxious mood
   with depressed mood
Schizophrenia

Much less is known relative to the prevalence of anxiety disorders and personality disorders. Chronic mental disorders such as schizophrenia in nursing home residents have also not been well studied. If all the diagnosable psychiatric syndromes are included, between 60% and 94% of nursing home residents carry psychiatric diagnoses (Rovner et al., 1990; Chandler & Chandler, 1988; Rovner et al., 1986). Table 3.1 lists the most common psychiatric diagnoses found among nursing home residents in decreasing order of frequency.

In this chapter, the authors will review the types of behavioral problems manifested by residents with dementia in the nursing home. As we shall see, there is little doubt that the typical nursing home in the United States is becoming a psychiatric nursing home. Consequently, it behooves all health care professionals working in nursing homes to become familiar with the major psychiatric syndromes seen in older adults and their treatment approaches.

DEMENTIA IN THE NURSING HOME

It has been noted as far back as 1962 by Goldfarb that the dementias or "chronic brain syndromes" are the most commonly found psychiatric diagnoses in nursing homes. In his study of 506 residents in nine nursing homes, Goldfarb found 87% to be so afflicted (1962). As our understanding of cognitive disorders in later life has increased, we are now able to more precisely diagnose patients with presumed dementias. According to most studies, Alzheimer's disease accounts for about 75% of all progressive dementias seen in the elderly, with multi-infarct dementia, also call "mini-strokes," seen in about 15%. Together, these two conditions account for nearly 90% of all dementias seen in older adults both in community as well as nursing home settings (Chandler & Chandler, 1988; Rovner et al., 1986; Barnes & Raskind, 1980).

Often, residents in the nursing home are admitted with or carry diagnoses of organic brain syndrome (OBS), chronic brain syndrome (CBS), dementia, senile dementia, senility, cerebrovascular disease, or other "wastebasket" diagnoses. It is important to review the resident's previous medical history to make sure that a workup for potentially remediable causes of cognitive decline in older adults was done. Table 3.2 lists the most common causes of potentially reversible dementia.

Diagnostic specificity is also important. Recently, Alzheimer's disease has become a catchall diagnosis, and it may not be uncommon for depression or delirium to be misdiagnosed as Alzheimer's disease (Grossberg & Nakra, 1990). A firm diagnosis of probable Alzheimer's disease versus a condition such as multi-infarct dementia is also vital in understanding the cause of behavior changes or problems in the demented nursing home resident and in instituting treatment.

Behavioral Problems in Dementia

The behaviorally disordered resident with dementia, usually of the Alzheimer's type, may be the most challenging of all residents in the nursing

---

TABLE 3.2 Common Causes of "Reversible Dementia" in the Elderly

Delirium
Depression
Drugs— prescribed, OTC, alcohol, e.g., anticholinergic,
         sedative/hypnotics, anxiolytics
Hypothyroidism
Nutritional deficiency, e.g., B_{12} or folate
Chronic infections
Metabolic change—Sodium/potassium imbalance
Hypo/hyperglycemia
Hematologic—Chronic anemia
Sleep deprivation—Chronic

**TABLE 3.3 Common Behavioral Problems
in Alzheimer's Disease**

Agitation/aggression
  Physical
  Verbal—e.g., screaming
Problem wandering
Socially unacceptable behaviors
Psychotic symptoms
  Delusions
  Hallucinations
Depression
Sleep disorder
Activity disturbance
  Cognitive abulia
  Hoarding/hiding things

home setting. No wonder special care, or dementia units have become so popular (see Chapter 16). Table 3.3 lists the most common behavioral problems seen in residents with Alzheimer's disease.

AGITATION AND AGGRESSION

These are among the most common and most distressing of the behavioral manifestations of the dementias. Winger et al., (1987) studied 43 residents in a VA nursing home and found that if both verbal and physical aggressive acts were included, 91% of the residents demonstrated one or another behavior. Even if disturbing behaviors were eliminated, 84% of the residents were found to have agitation/aggression problems of significant severity to pose a danger to themselves or to others. Other studies have found lower percentages. In Zimmer's study (1984) aggression occurred in 8.3% of nursing home residents while Burgio et al., found 20% of their residents showing physical aggression, and 22% with verbally abusive behavior (Burgio, Jones, Butler, & Engel, 1988). In Chandlers' (1988) study, 48% had significant agitation or aggression. Agitation and physical aggression may be more commonly seen in male nursing home residents and, in particular, those with more advanced cognitive impairment. High staff turnover may also be a contributing factor.

Only a handful of studies have addressed verbal agitation, noise-making, and screaming among demented residents in the nursing home. In a study by Ryan, Tainsh, Kolodny, Lendrum, and Fisher (1988) of 400 nursing home residents, 297 were found to be noise makers. However, this study also included nondemented residents as well as varying degrees of noise-making. Cariaga (1988) reported disruptive vocalizations in 11% of nursing home residents, with severe cognitive impairment being a risk factor. Cohen-Mansfield (1989) found screaming to be correlated with aggressive behavior as well as excessive verbal output. In a separate study, she found that 25% of nursing home residents screamed at least four times per week. Screaming was associated with cognitive impairment, depressed affect, poor-quality social networks, and severely impaired ability to carry out activities of daily living. A more detailed observation of five "screamers" showed that they screamed particularly if left alone in their rooms during evening hours (Cohen-Mansfield, Werner, & Marx, 1990). The disparity in prevalence rates of both physical and verbal aggression in nursing home studies relates primarily to problems in defining, quantifying and rating these behaviors. Without a doubt, the nursing home resident with progressive dementia who manifests a new onset of agitated, aggressive, or screaming behaviors needs a head-to-toe evaluation, initially to rule in or rule out delirium (see Chapter 9). Previously undiagnosed painful states, e.g. silent heart attack, arthritis, etc., also need to be considered. As well, depression, manifested by agitation or screaming, needs to be entertained.

PROBLEM WANDERING

This is a common problem among demented nursing home residents and is treated in detail elsewhere in this text (Chapter 13). Suffice it to say that 11.4% of nursing home residents are considered wanderers by staff (National Center for Health Statistics, 1979). Unfortunately, modern medicine has not invented an "anti-wandering pill," consequently, nursing homes need safe wandering areas (preferably indoor and outdoor) where these behaviors can be tolerated rather than medicated. Physical restraints are not an appropriate treatment for wandering behavior.

SOCIALLY UNACCEPTABLE BEHAVIORS

Residents with progressive dementia may have problems with sexual impulse control or other problems such as spitting, urinating in public, or fecal smearing. Burgio et al. (1988) in their study of 160 nursing home patients found spitting a problem in 3%, inappropriate sexual behavior in 7%, and fecal smearing in 11%. In the authors' experience, these problem behaviors respond best to nonchemical, behavioral interventions (see Chapter 12).

PSYCHOTIC SYMPTOMS

Psychotic symptoms are not uncommon among demented nursing home residents. The Chandlers (1988) found that 14/65 (22%) of nursing home residents studied had some evidence of psychosis. The most common psychotic symptoms seen are delusions. Morriss et al., (1990), studied 125 residents newly admitted to nursing homes and found 21% to have delusions. All were cognitively impaired. A delusion is a firm, false, persistent belief that an individual maintains that does not correlate with our sense of reality. By this definition, most delusions in demented individuals seem to be a consequence of or are driven by their forgetfulness. An example would be the demented nursing home resident who accuses her roommate or a staff member of having taken her sweater, who in reality has forgotten where she has put it. Another example would be the cognitively impaired, disoriented resident who maintains, even after being in the nursing home for years, that "I don't live here." One may also occasionally encounter delusions of infidelity as well as Capgras Syndrome, the notion that the demented resident's spouse, family member, or friend is really an imposter.

Hallucinations are less well studied in demented residents in nursing homes. Visual as well as auditory hallucinations may occur, with the former perhaps being more common. Generally, the more systematized and elaborate the delusion, the better it responds to antipsychotic medication. Nonsystematized delusions, usually related to cognitive errors, respond poorly to antipsychotics but are short-lived (Morriss, Rovner, Folstein, & German, 1990).

DEPRESSION

Depression in the nursing home is covered elsewhere (Chapter 4) in this book. However, it is important to keep in mind that individuals with probable Alzheimer's disease are particularly prone to becoming depressed. Depression in the face of dementia may be difficult to recognize and diagnose; consequently, one needs to have a high index of suspicion, particularly in an individual with dementia who takes a rapid turn for the worse. Depression may occur at any stage of the dementing process and seems to respond well to aggressive antidepressant treatment. There is some evidence that depression in Alzheimer's disease may respond preferentially to the Monoamine oxidase inhibitor (MAOI) type of antidepressants (Grossberg, Manepalli, & Solomon, 1992). In the authors' experience, serious suicide attempts can occur in the nursing home if severe depression in a demented resident is not diagnosed and treated. This seems to be a particular problem with depression complicating infarctive or multi-infarct dementia.

SLEEP DISORDERS

Residents with Alzheimer's disease have been documented to have severe alterations in sleep architecture with more fragmented sleep and disrupted diurnal rhythms. This may result in night-time awakenings and restlessness and at times daytime somnolence (Prinz, Peskind, Vitaliano et al., 1982). Initially, depression and delirium need to be considered as causes of the sleep disturbance. Residents may also awaken at night secondary to a need to urinate. Decreasing fluids after dinner and changing or eliminating diuretics may help improve quality of sleep. Sleep may also be affected by a painful medical condition such as arthritis. However, the demented patient may not be able to communicate pain effectively. Judicious use of an analgestic/anti-inflammatory drug may be beneficial. Often, night-time awakenings can be diminished by keeping the resident active during the day and minimizing daytime naps. Allowing the resident to have a later bedtime when he or she is more likely to be tired is also helpful.

ACTIVITY DISTURBANCE

Often, residents with progressive dementia manifest activity disturbances. Cognitive abulia or purposeless activity, usually of a repetitious nature, may involve things such as packing and unpacking, folding and unfolding a towel, etc. Hoarding and hiding of mostly worthless objects such as tissues, empty bottles, etc., is also encountered. Again, no medications have been proven to be successful in this type of behavior. The best approach is to be able to tolerate these behavior. If they become severe, distraction may be best, i.e., gently disrupting the patient's attention away from the repetitive behavior and refocusing it to another area. Often the original activity will be abandoned and forgotten.

As one can see, a whole array of psychiatric diagnoses are to be found in the typical community nursing home in the United States. The dementias with their behavioral symptoms are the ones most commonly encountered and account for an increasing proportion of staff concerns in community nursing homes.

REFERENCES

American Psychiatric Association. (1987). *Diagnostic and statistical manual of mental disorders* (3rd ed., rev.). Washington, DC: American Psychiatric Association.

Barnes, R. D., & Raskind, M. A. (1980). DSM III criteria and the clinical diagnosis of dementia: A nursing home study. *Journal of Gerontology, 36,* 20–27.

Burgio, L. D., Jones, L. T., Butler. F., & Engel, B. T. (1988). Behavior problems in an urban nursing home. *Journal of Gerontological Nursing, 14*(1), 31–34.

Cariaga, J., Burgio, L., Flynn, W., & Martin, D. (1988). Disruptive vocalization in institutionalized geriatric patients. *The Gerontologist, 28*, 264A.

Chandler, J. D., & Chandler, J. E. (1988). The prevalence of neuropsychiatric disorders in a nursing home population. *Journal of Geriatric Psychiatry and Neurology, 1*, 71–76.

Cohen-Mansfield, J., Werner, P., & Marx, M. S. (1990). Screaming in nursing home residents. *Journal of the American Geriatrics Society, 38*(7), 785–792.

Cohen-Mansfield, J., Marx, M. S., & Rosenthal, A. S. (1989). A description of agitation in a nursing home. *The Gerontologist, 44*, M77.

Goldfarb, A. (1962). Prevalence of psychiatric disorders in metropolitan old age and nursing homes. *Journal of the American Geriatrics Society, 10*, 77–84.

Grossberg, G. T., Hassan, R., Szwabo, P. A., Morley, J. E., Nakra, B. R. S., Bretscher, C. W., Zimny, G.H., & Solomon, K. (1990). Psychiatric problems in the nursing home: St. Louis University geriatric grand rounds. *Journal of the American Geriatrics Society, 38*, 907–917.

Grossberg, G. T., Manepalli, J., & Solomon, K. (1992) Diagnosis of depression in demented patients. In J. E. Morley, R. Strong, R. Coe, & G. T. Grossberg (Eds.), *Memory function and aging-related disorders.* New York: Springer. 237–247.

Grossberg, G.T., & Nakra, B. R. S. (1990). Psychiatry in the nursing home. In D. Bienenfeld (Ed.), *Verwoerdt's clinical geropsychiatry* (pp. 285–297). Baltimore: Williams & Wilkins.

Morriss, R. K., Barry, W., Folstein, M. F., & German, P. S. (1990). Delusions in newly admitted residents of nursing homes. *American Journal of Psychiatry, 147*(3), 299–302.

National Center for Health Statistics. (1979). *The national nursing home survey.* Summary for the United States. Washington, DC: U.S. Department of Health, Education and Welfare.

Parmelee, P. A., Katz, I. R., & Lawton, M. P. (1989). Depression among institutionalized aged: Assessment and prevalence estimation. *Journal of Gerontology: Medical Sciences*, pp. M22–M29.

Prinz, P., Peskind, E., Vitaliano, P., Raskind, M. A., Eisdorfer, C., Zemcuzinikov, N., & Gerber, C. J. (1982). Changes in sleep and waking EEG in non-demented and demented elderly. *Journal of the American Geriatrics Society, 30*, 86–93.

Rovner, B. W., German, P. S., Broadhead, J., Morriss, R. K., Brant, L. J., Blaustein, J., & Folstein, M. F. (1990). The prevalence and management of dementia and other psychiatric disorders in nursing homes. *International Psychogeriatrics, 2*(1), 13–24.

Rovner, B. W., Kafnek, S., Filipp, L., Lucas, M. J., & Folstein, M. F. (1986). Prevalence of mental illness in a community nursing home. *American Journal of Psychiatry, 143*, 1446–1449.

Ryan, D. P., Tainsh, S. M., Kolodny, V., Lendrum, B. L., & Fisher, R. H. (1988). Noise-making amongst the elderly in long term care. *The Gerontological Society of America, 28*(3), 369–371.

Teeter, R. B., Garetz, F. K., Miller, W. R., & Hailand, W. F. (1976). Psychiatric disturbances of aged patients in skilled nursing homes. *American Journal of Psychiatry, 133*, 1430–1434.

Winger, J., Schirm, V., & Stewart, D. (1987). Aggressive behavior in long-term care. *Journal of Psychosocial Nursing, 25*(4), 28–33.

Zimmer, J. G., Watson, N., & Treat, A. (1984). Behavioral problems among patients in skilled nursing facilities. *American Journal of Public Health, 74*(10), 1118–1124.

Recognition and Treatment of Depression

Jothika Manepalli
George T. Grossberg

INTRODUCTION

Nursing homes have become the major focus of care for the aged with chronic disabling physical conditions. Currently about 1.5 millon older adults reside in nursing homes, and this number is expected to increase synchronously with the increase in the elderly population. Many nursing home residents suffer from incurable disorders, for example, dementia, cancer, Parkinson's disease, arthritis, end-stage renal and cardiac disease, etc. Hence, it is important to identify potentially curable disorders, such as depression, and treat them aggressively in order to enhance the quality of life of older adults in the nursing home (Rovner, German, & Grant, 1991).

EPIDEMIOLOGY

Depression is among the most common psychiatric disorder in old age. In the older patient, chronic illness, functional disability and stressful life events are all associated with depression. The prevalence is thought to be between 2% and 14% in the elderly living in the community (Blazer &

William, 1990; Snowdon, 1990). Common precipitants are losing one's spouse, physical illness, lack of social interaction, and poor socioeconomic condition. The most common precipitant is felt to be a medical illness; depression is thought to affect between 6% and 14% of primary care patients and about 10% to 40% of medical inpatients (Kalyanam & Shamoian, 1990). Several reports estimate that the prevalence of depression is high in nursing home residents: 10.4% for affective disorders (Rovner, German, Broadhead, Morriss, Brant, Blaustein, & Folstein, 1990), 18%–20% for major depression, 27%–40% dysphoric states (Katz, Leshner, Kleban, Jethanandai, & Parmelee, 1989), 21% for major depression (Grossberg, et al., unpublished data 1991). About 14% of the nursing home residents are recognized by nursing home physicians, and 65% are recognized by nursing staff and family, to suffer from depression (Rovner et al., 1990).

CLINICAL FEATURES

The common symptoms encountered in a depressed older adult are listed in Table 4.1. Atypical depression, sometimes referred to as masked depression, is also common in the elderly. There may be an increase in somatic complaints, for example, vague feelings of being sick or other nonspecific complaints. Older adults may also deny feelings of sadness, depression or anxiety and attribute their symptoms to the worsening of a medical illness. They may complain of easy fatiguability even after mild activity, decreased interest in family, friends and pleasurable activities. They may complain of being forgetful, of misplacing things and start worrying that they are losing

TABLE 4.1 Sypmtoms of Late Life Depression

Change in mood, particularly if listless, apathetic, angry, hostile, irritable, depressed, sad or withdrawn.
Expression of fear and anxiety without apparent reason.
Change in sleep pattern (e.g., insomnia or hypersomnia).
Change in eating pattern, especially loss of appetite, with weight loss.
Extreme fatigue (e.g., frequent complaints of feeling tired and inability to participate in activities).
Concentration and memory problems.
Increased concern with bodily functions (e.g., frequent complaints of constipation, loose bowels, aches and pains, dizziness, increased heart rate).
Low self-esteem or self-concept, feelings of worthlessness, negativism.
Thoughts of death or suicide.

Note. From "Suicide in the Elderly: Clues and Prevention" by N. Osgood, 1988, *Carrier Letter* #133. Copyright *May 20, 1992* by *N. J. Osgood.* Adapted by permission.

their memory. They may worry excessively about finances, for example, doctors' bills or grocery bills, and become inappropriately frugal.

Nursing home residents may feel demoralized, helpless and perceive that they lack control or autonomy. This may lead to dysphoria or mild depression which, if not recognized or treated, may lead to major depression. In a study by Katz et al. (1989), about 43%–44% of the dysphoric residents in nursing homes had high scores on the Geriatric Depression Scale (Yesavage, 1983) perhaps indicating major depression.

Late-onset depression is often triggered by medical illness and is more frequently associated with sleep disturbance, hypochondriacal symptoms, agitation and delusions (Alexopoulos, Young, Meyer, Abrams & Shamoian, 1988). Eliciting delusional symptoms in the elderly is difficult, as they tend not to verbalize such symptoms. However, they may appear to be preoccupied with certain issues that may not be important to the examiner, may complain of guilt feelings or of being tormented without voicing a reason, or they may become hyper-religious. They may appear to be anxious or agitated without an explainable cause. It is important to recognize delusional depression as it may respond better to a combination of medications or to electroconvulsive therapy (ECT).

DIAGNOSIS

Depression is a heterogenous disorder. It can occur discretely or as a complication of other disorders. Identifying and diagnosing depression in a chronically ill and frail older adult is a difficult and challenging job. However, it is assumed that the principles of evaluation of depression in the elderly are in most respects similar to that in the younger population and that the DSM III-R criteria for mood disorders have equal validity in the elderly. The most common confounding factors in the diagnosis of depression in the elderly are: 1) medications/polypharmacy, 2) medical illness, 3) memory loss, 4) alcohol abuse (Sunderland, Molchan, Martinez, & Vitiello, 1990).

Medications/Polypharmacy

Older adults may be victims of polypharmacy by virtue of their multiple chronic medical problems. The average nursing home resident receives four to seven medications. Side effects of certain drugs and interactions between drugs can precipitate depression. Drugs that commonly contribute to depression are shown in Table 4.2 (Wood, Rizos, & Harris, 1988).

TABLE 4.2 Drugs That Can Cause Depression

Propranolol, reserpine, clonidine, guanethidine,
alpha methyldopa, levodopa, digitalis, cimetidine,
morphine, codeine, barbiturates,
chloral hydrate, diazepam,
steroids, estrogens,
cancer chemotherapeutic agents

Medical Illness

The various illnesses associated with depression are summarized in Table 4.3. Of particular interest in the elderly will be hypothyroidism as well as the association with certain malignancies such as pancreatic carcinoma. Cardiac disease and renal disease are also risk factors. There are several reports of a higher rate of depression in postmyocardial infarction. Suicide rates are higher in renal patients undergoing dialysis, and depression may remain undiagnosed in this patient population (Koenig, Meador, Cohen, Blazer, 1988). Higher rates of depression are also seen in patients after a stroke, particularly involving the left frontal hemisphere (Robinson & Szetela, 1981). Depression can commonly occur with Parkinson's disease as well as in Alzheimer's disease and may be the earliest or the only presenting symptom of the underlying disorder.

Memory Loss

Depression and dementia in the elderly can be secondary to the same underlying disorders, for example, thyroid disease, multiple sclerosis, Huntington's disease, Parkinson's disease, cerebrovascular disease, Acquired Immune Deficiency Syndrome (AIDS), etc. In Alzheimer's disease,

TABLE 4.3 Medical Causes of Depression

Hypothyroidism, Hyperthyroidism, adrenal disease
Anemia, hypokalemia, hyponatremia, vitamin B_{12} deficiency
Diabetes, hepatic disease, renal disease
Postmyocardial infarction, congestive heart failure
Cancer of pancreas, cerebral tumor
Stroke, Parkinson's disease
Huntington's disease, Alzheimer's disease
Multi-infarct dementia

depression may be associated with loss of noradrenergic neurons (Zweig, Ross, & Medrien, 1988). Depression and dementia, can coexist or present discretely. Older adults with depression frequently complain of memory loss and sometimes present with a dementia-like syndrome (referred to by several terms such as pseudodementia, dementia syndrome of depression, depressive pseudodementia, or depression with cognitive impairment). It is important to differentiate between depression and dementia and when this is difficult, aggressive treatment for depression is warranted. Aiding differential diagnosis is the fact that the depressed patient may have an abrupt onset and rapid progression of memory difficulty, rather than a slow deterioration as seen in dementia. Also with depression, some of the typical symptoms include impaired concentration, apathy, decreased interest in answering questions and frequent responses of " I don't know," "I don't remember" (Nakra & Grossberg, 1990). Mild confusion and forgetfulness is more common than actual memory loss in depression. Controversy exists regarding the prevalence of depression coexisting with dementia, with the reported prevalance ranges from 0%–50% (Rovner, Broadhead, Spencer, Carson, & Folstein, 1989). Currently there are no definitive methods for making the differential diagnosis. However, feelings of worthlessness, feelings of not being wanted, hopelessness, helplessness, demanding and becoming dependent, increased irritability, and suicidal ideation are common with depression and, when noted in a patient with dementia, should be considered as depressive symptoms and treated accordingly.

Alcohol Abuse and Depression

Alcohol abuse may not be an obvious problem in the nursing home but may be common in residential care facilities (RCF). This area is not often considered by clinicians when evaluating for depression in older adults. Patterns of use as an adult may continue, or the habit may start after retirement; other causes may be bereavement, depression, social isolation, physical illness, or poor education (Abrams & Alexopoulos, 1987). Depression and anxiety can be seen in early withdrawal of alcohol use and should be considered as a possible cause, especially in a new resident of the nursing home.

PAIN AND DEPRESSION IN NURSING HOMES

Pain due to rheumatoid arthritis and osteoarthritis as well as other chronic conditions is common in the elderly. Several studies indicate a relationship between pain and depression in the younger population. Chronic pain syndromes may represent a masked depression and respond to treatment with antidepressants. Dworkin, Von Korff and LeResche (1990) demonstrated that patients with pain complaints in two regions were six times more likely to be depressed, and patients with pain complaints in three regions are eight times more likely to be depressed. Some studies show that patients with depression report more intense pain and a greater number of localized pain complaints. A recent study of nursing home residents by Parmelee, Katz, and Lawton, (1991) demonstrated a significant association between depression and pain among the elderly residents, especially when there was a presence of physical disorder to which pain might be logically attributed (e.g., chest pain possibly related to cardiac, respiratory or upper gastrointestinal disorders). It is hypothesized that depressed residents are more sensitive to pain and this may explain the increased intensity and number of somatic complaints and somatic preoccupations in the elderly (Parmelee et al., 1991).

CONSEQUENCES OF NOT TREATING DEPRESSION

With the increase in prevalence of depression in the medically ill and frail elderly, there is a concomitant increase in the incidence of morbidity and mortality associated with unrecognized and untreated depression. A recent study of depression and mortality in the nursing home by Rovner, et al., (1991) reported that there is a 59% increase in the likelihood of death at one-year follow-up of patients with depression as compared to nondepressed elderly. In another study, at a four-year follow-up, elderly patients with depression, and in particular older males, had significantly higher mortality rates (Murphy, Smith, Lindesay & Slattery, 1988). This was not due to initial differences in physical health alone. In a 12-month follow-up, depressive disorder was the best predictor of major cardiac events like myocardial infarction, coronary bypass surgery, angioplasty, etc. (Carney, Rich, Freedland, teVelde, Saint, Clark, 1988). There is increased risk of mortality in previously healthy patients as well as in those with chronic medical disorders who suffer from depression. The usual causes of death are cardiovascular disease, pulmonary disease and cancer.

Morbidity is usually associated with depressed patients being noncompliant with the care of their physical illness, being forgetful in taking their medication, refusing treatment, or not being motivated in adhering to the care of their chronic illness, for example, uncontrolled diabetes. Depressed patients also perceive their general health to be poorer and limit their activities or give up easily due to feelings of fatigue, leading to physical and social inactivity. They are also sensitive to pain and other symptoms of their pre-existing illness and have multiple somatic complaints, make more phone calls to their family and or physician regarding their physical health, and also may request more doctor visits. These behaviors may lead the physician to suspect worsening of a physical illness which might result in medication changes and overtesting, leading to iatrogenic morbidity. Overall, there is increase in health care utilization and cost (Katon & Sullivan, 1990).

SUICIDE AND DEPRESSION

Suicide is a known complication of major depression. Older adults attempt suicide 50% more frequently than the young. Older persons tend not to communicate their intentions and are usually successful in their attempts. At-risk individuals are white males, widowed, and living alone. Those people over 75 years of age are at an increased risk (Conwell, Roenberg, & Caine, 1990; Osgood, 1988). Conwell et al., (1990) studied completed suicide in those age 50 and older and reported that physical illness and real or perceived loss of function are the most identifiable precipitants to suicide in the elderly. The trend toward violent methods, especially the use of guns, is on the increase in geriatric patients. The trend toward suicide is also increasing in the widowed and the physically ill. In Conwell's study 8.1% (6/62) of the 74-plus age group died of suicide in the institutional setting. Being in the nursing home does not protect a person from suicide; consequently, the clinicians and staff need to be aware of the risk factors. There are no reliable studies relative to the prevalence of suicide attempts and completed suicides in the nursing home. When attempts occur, the would-be suicides are usually those who hide pills. Occasionally residents will attempt to hang themselves (Grossberg & Nakra, 1990). Table 4.4 provides some guidelines to identify people at risk (Osgood, 1988).

EVALUATION OF DEPRESSION

As noted above, there are several clues to diagnosing depression in the elderly. A complete evaluation should include a history and physical, neurological, and psychiatric examination, as well as a review of the patient's current medication, a review of current physical problems (noting any change in the severity of the present illnesses), and also laboratory investigations to rule out metabolic or endocrine causes for depression. There are several examiner-rated or self-rated scales which can aid in the diagnosis of depression in the elderly. The most well-studied scale is the Geriatric Depression Scale (GDS); a score of 11 or more on this 30-item

TABLE 4.4 Clues and Warning Signs of Suicide in the Elderly

Verbal Clues
  I'm going to kill myself.
  I'm going to commit suicide.
  I'm going to end it all.
  I want to end it all.
  I just want out.
  You would be better off without me.

Behavioral Clues
  Donating body to a medical school.
  Purchasing a gun.
  Stockpiling pills.
  Putting personal and business affairs in order.
  Making or changing a will.
  Taking out insurance or changing beneficiaries.
  Making funeral plans.
  Giving away money and/or possessions.
  Changes in behavior, especially episodes of screaming or hitting, throwing
    things, or failure to get along with family, friends, or peers.
  Suspicious behavior, for example, going out at odd times of the day or night,
    waving or kissing goodbye (if not characteristic).
  Sudden interest or disinterest in church or religion.
  Scheduling of appointment with doctor for no apparent physical cause or very
    shortly after the last visit to the doctor.
  Loss of physical skills, general confusion, or loss of understanding, judgement, or
    memory.

Situational Clues
  Recent move.
  Death of spouse.
  Diagnosis of terminal illness.
  Flare-up with relative or close friend.

Note. From "Suicide in the Elderly: Clues and Prevention" by N. Osgood, 1988, *Carrier Letter* #133. Copyright *May 20, 1992* by *N. J. Osgood*. Adapted by permission.

scale may indicate depression. This scale is useful in screening for depression, even in the presence of dementia and physical illness (Yesavage & Brink, 1983). Other scales devised with the elderly in mind are the National Institute of Mental Health (NIMH) dementia mood assessment scale and the Cornell scale, but these have not found such wide usage as the Yesavage Depression Scale (Grossberg et al., 1991, in press).

TREATMENT OF DEPRESSION

Treatment of depression is essential. However, there are many myths which surround depression and aging. At times clinicians, nursing staff and families may assume that depression is part of aging, or "normal" in the person suffering with a major illness, or in anyone who has suffered a loss or is in the nursing home, and that nothing needs to be done. However, irrespective of the underlying or precipitating cause, when depression is noted it should be treated.

ANTIDEPRESSANT DRUG THERAPY

Antidepressants together with psychotherapy are usually the treatment of choice. However, physiological changes in the body occur due to the normal aging process, changes which affect the absorption, metabolism, and elimination of drugs, and the elderly become more susceptible to the adverse side effects of drugs. A reasonable practice is to choose a drug with a benign side effect profile and start at an initial dose which is one half to one third the normal younger-adult dose. As a general rule, the dose should be increased slowly, and patients should be carefully observed for side effects. Since geriatric patients may be taking other medications as well, possible drug interactions should be considered in selection of psychotropics, for example, cardiac conduction is decreased when a tricylic and quinidine are given together. Giving an antidepressant with clonidine inhibits activity of either agent. Fluoxetine may effect prothrombin time in someone on warfarin. There is an increased vulnerability to hypotension and an increase in Parkinsonian side effects when two or more psychotropics are given together. Drugs that have high anticholinergic side effects should be avoided as they cause dry mouth, constipation, urinary retention, and mental confusion. Another potential side effect is orthostatic hypotension, which may increase the risk for falls. Table 4.5 illustrates the commonly used antidepressants and their dose ranges in older adults. Antidepressants possess equal efficacy in younger as well as older individuals. Drugs such as imipramine, amitriptyline, and doxepin are best avoided because of their high anticholinergic side effects, except in cases where there is evidence of previous favorable response or family history of response to these drugs. Of the tricyclic antidepressants, desipramine and nortriptyline have the least anticholinergic side effects and are the best tolerated (Jenike, 1989; Nakra & Grossberg, 1990; Young & Meyers, 1991). The therapeutic blood level of nortriptyline is established to be between 50 and 150 mg; levels below 50 mg and beyond 150 mg are not effective. One study has shown that in elderly individuals, nortriptyline levels of 86.8+42.3 mg may produce a higher incidence of side effects. Adverse events include delirium, paranoid symptoms, and orthostatic hypotension (Katz et al., 1990). Trazodone lacks anticholinergic side effects and is less cardiotoxic and usually well tolerated. Newer drugs such as fluoxetine,

TABLE 4.5 Antidepressant Medications

	Side effect profile				mg per day suggested for elderly >65 years
	Sedation	Hypotension	Anticholinergic	Cardiotoxic	
Amitriptyline	++++	+++	++++	+++	25–150
Nortriptyline	++	++	+	++	10– 75
Imipramine	+	+++	+++	++	25–150
Desipramine	+	++	+	++	25–150
Doxepin	+++	+++	++++	++	25–150
Amoxapine	++	+++	++	+	15–150
Protriptyline	+	++	++++	++	5– 30
Maprotiline	+++	+++	+	+	25–150
Trazodone	++	+++	+/-	+	100–300
Fluoxetine	0	0	0	0	20– 40
Buproprion	0	0	0	0	150–300
Sertraline	0	0	0	0	50–150

sertraline, and buproprion have virtually no anticholinergic side effects and may be least cardiotoxic. Fluoxetine has a long half-life, so dosing may need to be modified in the elderly. It may be better to give this drug every two to three days rather than every day, with gradual increases in dosage, for example, once a month.

MONOAMINE OXIDASE INHIBITORS (MAOIs)

Many clinicians avoid the use of MAOIs in elderly patients because of a fear of adverse reactions. The common MAOIs are Phenelzine (15–90 mg daily), Tranylcypramine (10–60 mg daily), Isocarboxazid (10–50 mg daily). Phenelzine and Tranylcypromine are most often used. These agents can be safely used for the elderly and are effective in treating depression. Doses should, again, be less than what is used to treat younger adults. These agents have been found to be effective in depression associated with dementia, as demented patients have higher levels of monoamine oxidase than age-matched, nondemented controls. They are also effective in treating depression that does not respond to traditional and newer antidepressants. Dietary restrictions apply to the use of this group of drugs. Food products that contain high tyramine levels should be avoided, as a hypertensive reaction is a potential side effect (see Table 4.6) (Nakra & Grossberg, 1990; Young & Meyers, 1991). This should not be a problem as monitoring is not difficult in the nursing home. The most common side effect is hypotension, and consequently blood pressure monitoring is indicated.

TABLE 4.6 Food and Drug Restrictions for Patients Taking MAO Inhibitors

Foods that must be avoided
    All cheese, aged cheese
    Concentrated yeast extracts
    Fava or broad bean pods
    Sauerkraut, summer sausage, liver
    Over-ripened food—fermented or aged food
    Sour cream
    Red wine, sherry, all alcohol

Drugs that must be avoided
    Cold medications, ephedrine, pseudoephedrine
    Meperidine (Demerol)
    Amphetamines, Methylphenidate
    Tyramine, Fluoxetine (Prozac)
    L-Dopa, methyldopa
    Epinephrine, norepinephrine
    Local anesthetic agents containing vasoconstrictors

LITHIUM

Lithium can be used as an adjunct to antidepressants in certain antidepressant nonresponders. Doses of lithium should be low, and may begin with 150 mg p.o. B.I.D. rather than the usual 300 mg T.I.D. When lithium is used as augmentation, a reduction in depressive symptoms usually occurs in 48 hours to two weeks. Maintenance levels can be in the range of 0.4 to 1.0 mg/L. Response appears to be unrelated to lithium levels within this range (Craig, 1990). Lithium may also have some primary antidepressant effects.

PSYCHOSTIMULANTS

The medically ill, depressed elderly may not be able to tolerate antidepressant drugs. In such cases, psychostimulants such as dextroamphetamine or methylphenidate may be safer alternatives. Many studies show that depression improves with psychostimulants. Most show response after 48 hours. For dextroamphetamine, the dose range is 2.5 to 30 mg, with an average of 10 mg a day. For methylphenidate, the beginning dose is 5 to 10 mg, and the maximum daily dose is usually 30 to 50 mg (Frieson, Wey, & Tabler, 1991).

ELECTROCONVULSIVE THERAPY (ECT)

ECT can be safely used in the elderly and sometimes is a treatment of first choice, particularly in medically ill individuals and patients who cannot tolerate the antidepressants. ECT may also be life saving when there is an active risk of suicide, or with the development of electrolyte imbalance, dehydration, and inanition in a depressed older adult. It is also effective in treating psychotic depression. A review of the literature indicates its safety and efficacy in the elderly population, even in medically ill patients, and in patients with dementia (Hay, 1989). Nonetheless, ECT is generally underused in the treatment of geriatric depression (American Psychiatric Association Task Force, 1990).

COMBINED TREATMENT WITH ANTIPSYCHOTICS

Delusional depression carries a higher risk for suicide, and many elderly do not openly verbalize overt psychotic thoughts. They usually feel guilty for some perceived misdeed or just convey feelings of being "tormented," often without cause. Pharmacotherapy in these patients often requires combined antidepressant and antipsychotic medication. High-potency drugs such as haloperidol are preferred, as they have less potential for sedation and orthostatic hypotension. The dosage generally ranges from 0.5 to 2 mgs in divided doses.

PSYCHOTHERAPY

Many nursing home residents feel demoralized, helpless, and discontent, and feel that they lack control of their lives. Low levels of social participation may predispose to depression and also predict poor response to treatment of depression. Psychotherapy may be valuable in nursing home residents with depression to help them achieve some level of mastery and control of their lives. Treatments such as cognitive therapy, interpersonal expressive psychotherapy, and behavior therapy are helpful (Jenike, 1989; Lazarus, Sadavoy, & Langsley, 1991). Social contact is very important to the well-being of the nursing home residents. Recreational activity and intergenerational intermingling should be encouraged. Psychotherapy can maintain the alliance between the patient, the family, and the clinician.

DURATION OF TREATMENT

When a patient does well early in treatment, clinicians should continue maintenance treatment for a period of 6–18 months. Several recent reports state that whatever dose or blood level was required for acute treatment should be used for maintenance; otherwise, early relapse and recurrent episodes of major depression can occur. Maintenance on a lesser dose than needed for acute treatment, or the principle of least effective dose for maintenance therapy after acute treatment, appears not to be as effective in preventing relapses. Combined treatment with psychotherapy and medication is more effective than either treatment alone in preventing relapse of major depression (Frank et al., 1990).

In summary, depression in the elderly, especially the frail elderly living in nursing homes, should be recognized early and treated aggressively to prevent chronicity and associated morbidity and mortality.

REFERENCES

Abrams, R. C., & Alexopoulos, G. S. (1987). Substance abuse in the elderly: Alcohol and prescription drugs. *Hospital Community Psychiatry, 38,* 1285–1287.
Alexopoulos, G. S., Young, R. C., Meyer, B. S., Abrams, R. C., & Shamoian, C. A. (1988). Late-Onset Depression. *Psychiatric Clinics of North America, 11,* 101–115.

American Psychiatric Association. (1990). *Task force report on electroconvulsive therapy: The practice of ECT: Recommendations for treatment, training and privileges.* Washington, DC: Author.

Blazer, D., & William, C. D. (1980). Epidemiology of dysphoria and depression in an elderly population. *American Journal of Psychiatry, 137,* 439–444.

Carney, R., Rich, M. W., Freedland, K., teVelde, A., Saint, J., & Clark, K. (1988). Major depressive disorder predicts cardiac events in patients with coronary artery disease. *Psychosomatic Medicine, 50,* 627–633.

Conwell, Y., Roenberg, M., & Caine, E. D. (1990). Completed suicide at age 50 and over. *Journal of the American Geriatrics Society, 38,* 640–644.

Craig, N. (1990). Lithium augmentation in refractory depression. In S. P. Roose & A. H. Glassman (Eds.), *Treatment strategies for refractory depression* (pp. 35–49). Washington, DC: American Psychiatric Press.

Dworkin, S. F., VonKorff, M. R., & LeResche, L. (1990). Multiple pains and psychiatric disturbance: An epidemiologic investigation. *Archives of Geriatric Psychiatry, 47,* 239–245.

Frank, E., Kupfer, D. J., Perel, J. M., Cornes, C., Jarrett, D. B., Mallinger, A. G., Thase, M. E., McEachran, A. B., & Grochocinski, V. J. (1990). Three-year outcomes for maintenance therapies in recurrent depression. *Arch Ger Psych, 67,* 1093–1099.

Frieson, R. L., Wey, J. J., & Tabler, J. B. (1991). Psychostimulants for depression in the medically ill. *American Family Physician, 43,* 163–170.

Grossberg, G. T., & Nakra, B. R. S. (1990). Psychiatry in the nursing home. In D. Bienenfeld (Ed.), *Verwoerdt's clinical geropsychiatry* (3rd. ed. pp. 285–297). Baltimore, MD: Williams & Wilkins.

Grossberg, G. T., Manepalli, J., & Solomon, K. (1991). Diagnosis of depression in demented patients. In J. E. Morley, R. Strong, R. Coe, & G. T. Grossberg (Eds.), *Memory function and aging-related disorders.* New York: Springer.

Hay, D. (1989). Electroconvulsive therapy in the medically ill elderly. *Convulsive Therapy, 5*(1), 8–16.

Jenike, M. A. (1989). Affective disorders in the elderly. In *Geriatric psychiatry and psychopharmacology: A clinical approach* (pp. 33–126). Chicago, IL: Yearbook Medical Publishers, Inc.

Kalyanam, B., & Shamoian, C. A. (1990). Geriatric psychiatry: An update. *Journal of Clinical Psychiatry, 51,* 177–183.

Katon, W., & Sullivan, M. D. (1990). Depression and chronic medical illness. *Journal of Clinical Psychiatry, 51*(Suppl. 6), 3–11.

Katz,, I. R., Leshner, E., Kleban, M., Jethanandani, V., & Parmelee, P. (1989). Clinical features of depression in the nursing home. *International Journal of Geriatric Psychiatry, 1,* 5–15.

Koenig, H. G., Meador, K. G., Cohen, H. J., & Blazer, D. G. (1988). Depression in elderly hospitalized patients with medical illness. *Archives of Internal Medicine, 148,* 1929–1938.

Lazarus, W. L., Sadavoy, J., & Langsley, P. (1991). Individual psychotherapy. In J. Sadavoy, L. W. Lazarus, & L. Jarvik (Eds.), *Comprehensive review of geriatric psychiatry* (pp. 487–512). Washington, DC: American Psychiatric Association/ American Association of Geriatric Psychiatry.

Murphy, E., Smith, R., Lindesay, J., Slattery, J. (1988). Increased mortality rates in late life depression. *British Journal of Psychiatry, 152,* 347–353.

Nakra, B. R. S., & Grossberg, G. T. (1990). Mood disorders. In D. Bienenfeld (Ed.), *Verwoerdt's clinical geropsychiatry* (3rd. ed., pp. 107–124). Baltimore: Williams & Wilkins.

Osgood, N. (April 1988). Suicide in the elderly: Clues and prevention. Carrier Letter #133.

Ouslander, J. G. (1982). Physical illness and depression in the elderly. *Journal of the American Geriatrics Society, 30,* 593–599.

Parmelee, P. A., Katz, I. R., & Lawton, M. P. (1991). The relationship of pain to depression among institutionized aged. *Journal of Gerontology Psychological Sciences, 46*(1), 15–21.

Robinson, R. G., & Szetela, B. (1981). Mood changes following left hemisphere brain injury. *Annals of Neurology, 9,* 447–452.

Rovner, B. W., German, P. S., Broadhead, J., Morriss, R. K., Brant, L. J., Blaustein, J., & Folstein, M. (1990). The prevalence and management of dementia and other psychiatric disorders in nursing homes. *International Psychogeriatrics, 2*(1), 13–24.

Rovner, B. W., German, P. S., Grant, L. J., Clark, R., Burton, L., & Folstein, M. F. (1991). Depression and mortality in nursing homes. *Journal of American Medical Association, 265,* 993-996.

Rovner, B. W., Broadhead, J., Spencer, M., Carson, K., Folstein, M. (1989). Depression and Alzheimer's disease. *American Journal Psychiatry, 146*(3), 350–353.

Snowdon, J. (1990). The prevalence of depression in old age. *International Journal of Geriatric Psychiatry, 5,* 141–144.

Sunderland, T., Molchan, S. E., Martinez, R. A., & Vitiello, B. (1990). Treatment approaches to atypical depression in the elderly. *Psychiatric Annals, 20*(8), 474–478.

Wood, K. A., Rizos, A., & Harris, M. J. (1988). Drug-induced psychosis and depression in the elderly. *Psychiatric Clin North Am, 11,* 167–194.

Yesavage, J. A., & Brink, T. L. (1983). Development and validation of a geriatric screening scale: A preliminary report. *Journal of Psychiatry Residents, 17*(1), 37–49.

Young, R. C., & Meyers, B. S. (1991). Psychopharmacology. In J. Sadavoy, L. Lazarus, L. Jarvick (Eds.), *In comprehensive review of geriatric psychiatry.* APA/AAGP—Washington, DC: Chapter 22, 435–467.

Zweig, R. M., Ross, C. A., Hedrien, J. C., Steele, C., Cardillo, J. E., Whitehouse, P. J., Folstein, M. F., & Price, D. L. (1988). The neuropathology of aminergic nuclei in Alzheimer's disease. *Annals of Neurology, 24,* 233–242.

5

Impact of Personality and Personality Disorders in the Elderly

Peggy A. Szwabo
Karen R. Boesch

PERSONALITY DISORDERS

This chapter begins with an overview of personality in the elderly as it relates to assessment and diagnosis of personality disorders. The stressors of living in a nursing home and their impact on the personality-disordered resident will be emphasized. Finally, common personality disorders calling for specific interventions which nursing home staff can integrate into their treatment plans will be highlighted.

PERSONALITY AND AGING

Personality refers to an individual's lifelong style of interacting with people and the environment. There is a paucity of literature relative to personality and aging which may reflect difficulties inherent in assessing personality over the age of 65. Psychologists describe personality by using both self-report testing as well as structured and semi-structured interviews. Perhaps the most well-known self-report test is the Minnesota Multiphasic Personality Inventory (MMPI) (Hathaway & McKinley, 1943/1982). Five hundred and fifty statements are posed to the patient which are rated as either true or false. Nine clinical scales have been empirically developed and compared to abnormal personality traits. The MMPI can be administered to all age groups. At present, modifications do not exist for the geriatric population. Therefore, the validity of this common and well-respected test in the elderly is questionable (Woods & Britton, 1985). This shortcoming has been recognized, and attempts have been made to investigate the impact of aging on objective personality tests. For example, higher scores on the Hypochondriac, Depression, and Social Interaction Scales have been shown in MMPI results for some elderly subjects (Woods & Britton, 1985). Cummings and Henry (1961) described the elderly as being more "interior" and "self-engaged" compared to younger populations. These findings show older adults to be different from younger adults, but this does not mean that all old people are alike.

As nursing home staff well know, there are more differences among residents than similarities. Costa, McCrae and Arenburg (1980) conducted a longitudinal study to determine whether personality remained constant with aging. They assessed the personalities of approximately 2,000 veterans in the mid-1960s and then retested 10 years later. Surprisingly, they observed few differences and concluded that stability rather than change is the rule. The authors noted that "the degree of stability and consistency within the personality of the same person over time seems more powerful than age related changes." According to Neugarten (1977), personality is a reliable predictor of adaptation or coping style. For example, if one has a strong, dominant personality as a young person, one will most likely remain strong and dominant in later life.

ASSESSMENT AND DIAGNOSIS

Since personality remains relatively constant, a resident's past history is much more than history; it is a predictor of future behavior. During the initial interviews with residents and their families, reports of the quality of prior interpersonal relationships and reactions to stress should assist staff in anticipating potential difficulties at the nursing home. Residents with a personality disorder can be expected to have greater difficulty in a congregate living environment.

A personality "disorder" is a lifelong pattern of maladaptive behavior.

Behavior exists in a continuum. The disorder reflects the extremes. For example, dependency is a commonly observed trait. Dependency which is exaggerated is considered a disorder. The maladaptive nature of the disorder is reflected by conflicted, stormy interpersonal relationships which precipitate poor functioning in school, work, and social activities. While the behavior may be maladaptive, it is not necessarily uncomfortable to the individual (Simon, 1980). In addition, these individuals are fraught with internal complaints of anxiety, depression, loneliness, and of being misunderstood. Page (1971) describes these disorders as an aggregation of mild defects manifested by changes in affect, cognition, perceptions of self or others, and responses to life situations.

The Diagnostic and Statistical Manual (3rd ed., rev.) of the American Psychiatric Association groups personality disorders into three main groups, adapted in Table 5.1. A complete description of each type is beyond the scope of this chapter, but one can appreciate that these descriptors are commonly used and do not always indicate pathology.

Estimates of the prevalence of personality disorders in the elderly range from 2.2% to 12.6% (Kroessler, 1990). Simon (1980) noted that there have been no detailed studies of the effects of aging on personality disorders (or vice versa) that have been present since adolescence or early adulthood. In fact, specialists in geriatric psychiatry, social work, and psychology currently debate the significance of personality disorders in the elderly. Some authors believe strongly that personality disorders are identifiable in the geriatric population (George, 1978; Neugarten, 1977) and that the understanding of personality style and identification of personality disorders can affect treatment approaches and the quality of staff/patient interaction. A correct diagnosis of personality disorder can impact favorably on treatment and management of some behavior problems encountered in long-term care.

TABLE 5.1 Grouping Personality Disorders

Odd, eccentric Cluster A	Dramatic, emotional Cluster B	Anxious, fearful Cluster C
Paranoid	Antisocial	Avoidant
Schizoid	Borderline	Dependent
Schizotypal	Histrionic	Obsessive-compulsive
	Narcissistic	Passive-Aggressive

Note. From *Diagnostic and Statistical Manual of Mental Disorders* (3rd. ed., rev.) by the American Psychiatric Association, 1987, *Washington, D.C. pp. 335–358.* Copyright 1987 by *The American Psychiatric Association.* Adapted by permission.

STRESSORS OF NURSING HOME LIFE

Nursing homes are prime settings to trigger personality-disordered behavior, since the disorder is more often manifested under stressful conditions. Despite excellent staff and administrators, nursing homes are stressful environments (Beaver & Miller, 1985; Sancier, 1984; Montgomery, 1983). For most residents, families, and staff, feelings of powerlessness, dependency, uselessness, and even death are associated with nursing homes. The realities of nursing home life must be accepted, and previous levels of physical, social, and emotional functioning must be grieved. Time, support, and reassurance make the adjustment easier, so that many residents bloom in this structured care setting.

For the personality-disordered elderly, the task of adjustment to the nursing home may be monumental. Nursing homes resonate with and magnify their internal conflicts regarding control, independence, and trust. Behavior problems arise but may be attributed to old age itself and not to previous long-standing behavior patterns. Professionals working with older adults need to look for and suspect personality disorders. An understanding of personality disorders will give nursing home caregivers confidence in treatment planning. Incorporating such knowledge early in a resident's treatment plan should decrease staff's helplessness and frustration. To clarify these concepts, the common personality disorders—paranoid, obsessive–compulsive, and dependent types—will be discussed. The following cases and discussion will illustrate frequently encountered difficulties in the nursing home and appropriate interventions.

COMMON PERSONALITY DISORDERS

Paranoid Personality Disorder

Mrs. S., an 89-year-old widow, was placed in the nursing home six months ago after a hip replacement following a fall at home. She is now ambulating with the aid of a walker but is resistant to help or direction. She accuses the staff of taking her things and feels people are watching her. Frequently she refuses to take her medication. She does not go to activities and refuses to leave her room.

Treatment Considerations

Paranoid personality disorder is characterized by a history of mistrust of others. A constant sense of humiliation and shame plagues such individuals (MacKinnon & Michels, 1971). Staff may note that paranoid complaints and suspicions may decrease as self-esteem rises.

Treatment involves: (1) investigating the presence of paranoia versus reality—are the complaints based in fact?; (2) establishing a trusting relationship with resident; (3) reducing anxiety by giving information before beginning any action; (4) providing opportunities for decision making to increase self-esteem; (5) focusing on Mrs. S.'s small gains; (6) avoiding engaging in competitive activities; (7) helping to establish a daily schedule and following it; and (8) reinforcing daily coping skills (Ebersole, 1989; Sadavoy, 1987; Hyer & Harrison, 1986).

Residents like Mrs. S., who exhibit features of paranoid personality disorder, are suspicious, cautious, unwilling to share emotions, and wary of caretakers' motives. These qualities deliberately keep staff at a distance, and meaningful empathic responses are rare. The challenge for staff in caring for such residents is to recognize their own vulnerability and to always be attuned to angry feelings, which these residents most certainly will provoke. These residents are likely to view nursing home life and their debilitating illness as personal attacks. Their response is usually anger disproportionate to the situation. Invasive procedures such as venipuncture, catheterization, and feeding tube placements are especially feared. Anxiety can be decreased by explaining indications for such procedures as well as by giving a detailed description of the procedures. If staff anticipates the typical angry, threatened response, they will be less flustered and distressed when it occurs (Schultz & Dark, 1986).

Treatment plans for paranoid-personality-disordered residents should identify interventions which encourage resident involvement. The likelihood of mistrust and suspicious reactions decreases if the resident contributes to decisions regarding his/her care. Consistency and honesty among caregivers are essential. Staff indecisiveness and ambiguity will fuel paranoid responses. A firm but kind attitude, rather than a warm friendly one, will be better tolerated by such residents. This may cause frustration among staff. Nursing home health professionals often choose their careers based on the desire to empathically help alleviate suffering and gain personal and professional satisfaction in developing relationships. Not only do paranoid residents reveal little emotion to empathize with, they view staff's helpful interventions as threatening assaults. Reassuring support from colleagues and supervisors can reduce the staff caregivers' doubt of their ability to "care" for such residents (Ebersole, 1989; Hyer & Harrison, 1986; Schultz & Dark, 1986).

Obsessive-Compulsive Personality Disorder

Mr. J., an 83-year-old widowed male, was admitted to an extended care facility five years ago with arthritis, cardiac problems, and increasing self-care deficits. Mr. J., a proud, self-made man, ran his own business as an accountant. He is alert and oriented but is in considerable pain. He continually uses his call light or yells for the nurses. He has high expectations and demands that his meals, medicines, and bath be done on time. He has a precise routine for bathing, requiring 1½ hours, a routine from which he will not deviate. When things are late or not done as he wishes, he yells, complains, calls the administrator, and accuses the staff of neglect.

Treatment Considerations

Individuals with this disorder are perfectionistic, inflexible, and unable to express warm, tender feelings. They are preoccupied with trivial details and rules and dislike changes in routine. Illness may be perceived by obsessive-compulsive individuals as a threat to their control over impulses. Generally, stress intensifies compulsive and obstinate behavior. Residents may become more inflexible than before, which may lead to complaints about the sloppiness of the facility and imprecision of the care being given. When these residents complain of the staff's failure to meet their standards, the staff should avoid defensive, authoritarian rebuttal. These residents have a fear of losing control, which may lead to a struggle for control with staff. Control should be shared with residents in as many ways as possible, with residents being allowed to actively participate in the decisions and details of their actual care.

An obsessive-compulsive individual may exhibit the following characteristics: perfectionism interfering with completion of tasks; preoccupation with rules, lists, and details to such an extreme that the focus of the activity is lost; insistence on doing tasks his/her way and display of an unreasonable reluctance to change; a tendency to get lost in rules and details, leading to an inability to make decisions; inflexibility and scrupulousness about issues of ethics or morality; stinginess with both compliments and gifts; and inability to discard worn-out or useless objects despite lack of sentimental value.

The medical and psychiatric illnesses requiring nursing home placement are conditions that compromise the independence which these residents so highly value. Nursing home placement is not seen as beneficial but is viewed as a loss of order and self-control. This is compounded by the fact that aging, with its inherent losses of both a physical and emotional nature, seems to worsen the obsessive-compulsive pathology (Solomon, 1981). These multiple insults to a previously effective, orderly lifestyle will be met with an increase in rigidity and control.

Obsessive–compulsive-personality-disordered older adults will also test the patience of nursing home staff. Individuals like Mr. J. are overly concerned with details, control, rules, organization, and schedules. Their rules are inflexible, and they insist that others conform to their high standards.

Preoccupation with minutiae leads to poor appreciation of the overall picture, so that one cannot see the forest for the trees.

Management is similar to that of the paranoid resident. Staff should provide detailed instructions about any procedures and daily activities. One should expect that disruptions, (commonplace in a busy, possibly understaffed facility) will yield vociferous, angry complaints and anxious, demanding behavior. Anticipating alterations from normal routines and keeping residents apprised of them are helpful. If at all possible, staff should attempt to stimulate the resident to use his/her organizational skills in a more productive manner. Unlike the paranoid type, obsessive-compulsives who are physically able will be flattered if asked to organize activities and take on volunteer work assignments in the facility. This individual needs some latitude, but the staff should not relinquish total control and responsibility, but rather recognize their need for lists and details, and provide an outlet for these needs which is acceptable to staff (and resident). This will hopefully decrease the amount of control the resident tries to exert on staff. Again, a concentrated effort by all caregivers and mustering of peer support are essential in developing an individualized care plan for this resident.

Gradually reducing the frequency of compulsive behaviors and replacing them with new, healthier behaviors will minimize the resident's anxiety in the transition, encourage success and independence, and promote self-esteem. Participation in activities, treatment, and interactions should be promoted by staff. To ensure success, these activities should be enjoyed by the resident and generate a high degree of success in accomplishment.The resident may need to learn ways to manage anxiety so the he/she can deal with it directly. This will increase confidence in managing anxiety and other feelings. Staff need to encourage the resident to decrease the frequency of compulsive behaviors in a gradual manner. The resident and staff may identify a baseline frequency and then keep a record of the decrease. After the behavior has been identified and charted for frequency, occurrence, and responses, specific time periods can be allotted, such as 10 minutes every hour when the resident can focus on his/her obsessive thoughts or rituals. The staff would require the resident to attend to other behaviors, thoughts, or feelings for the remainder of the hour. As the resident's anxiety decreases and as the trusting relationship with the staff builds, alternative behaviors and ways of dealing with anxiety can be introduced to assist the resident in taking more responsibility for his/her behavior and actions.

Passive Dependent Personality Disorder

Mrs. F., a 73-year-old female living in the extended care facility for two years, has a history of coronary artery bypass graft, chronic obstructive pulmonary disease, anxiety, and recurrent depression. Her depression is in remission. She is social, active, ambulatory, alert, and cognitively intact. Unexpectedly, Mrs. F. becomes easily excited and begins to beg the nurses to help her. She cries "Help me, help me" and gets on her knees, begging them not to let her suffer like this. She cries for relief. She has these episodes three to four times a day. Medication such as anxiolytics has been ineffective.

Treatment Considerations

Residents who are very dependent lack adequate skills to deal effectively with daily life. These individuals may survive adequately on their own until faced with change or a crisis. Passive dependent residents may rely on significant others in their lives (see Table 5.2 for elaboration of behaviors). Loss of this person can precipitate a crisis. Residents then may transfer their dependency needs to the facility's staff members.

Being sick usually means being taken care of, and one might expect that dependent individuals would be good residents. However, illness may stir up intolerable feelings of fear of abandonment and helplessness for these residents. There is a pull to regress to an earlier state of dependency, which may frighten the resident because of its intensity. Feelings of dependency increase. Generally, these residents become demanding and complaining when sick. It is important for staff to come together to plan, and identify with the resident, which types of care are going to be given. For instance, it should be clear to the resident how often the staff caregiver will come by to check on him/her. If this is not done early, the negative reactions that these residents stir up can lead to punitive behaviors on the part of caregivers.

TABLE 5.2 Passive Dependent Personality Disorder Behavioral Characteristics

Inability to make decisions without excessive reasurances
Being overly agreeable with opinions of others, even when he/she disagrees
Inability to initiate things by oneself
Agreeing to do tasks just to be liked
Inability to tolerate being alone and going to great lengths to avoid it
Exhibiting extreme reactions to ending relationships
Worries or fears abandonment
Being hurt by criticism or disapproval
Feeling helpless

Note. Clinical Gerontology (pp. 399–415) adapted from L. Hyer and W. Harrison, 1986, New York: Haworth Press, and from *Clinical Social Work Practice with the Elderly* (pp. 202–203) by M. *Beaver* and D. Miller, 1985, Homewood, IL: The Dorsey Press.

Effective interventions in this type of resident include: (1) encouraging development of a trusting relationship with staff with appropriate limit-setting; (2) providing a safe, structured environment; (3) decreasing attention to inappropriate or acting-out behaviors and increasing attention to appropriate behaviors; (4) encouraging the expression of feelings verbally or in other ways such as through physical activity or in writing. This helps the resident to learn acceptable ways of expressing their feelings; (5) giving positive feedback to encourage self-confidence; (6) providing opportunities to increase independence, insight, and self-esteem. One should structure simple tasks and activities to ensure success and pride in accomplishment; (7) encouraging independent action and problem-solving skills. One can help the resident anticipate situations by asking: "What would you do if. . . ."; (8) and helping to establish support systems without fostering undue dependence.

In sharp contrast to the obsessive–compulsive personality, the dependent-personality-disordered resident exerts control by demanding that others fulfill their needs. These residents seek excessive encouragement and reassurance for seemingly minor endeavors. Self-initiative is low. They long for direction and prodding and fear being alone or being abandoned, since this would force them to make independent decisions.

Nursing homes and chronic disabling illnesses pose a unique challenge for these individuals. On the one hand, they welcome the opportunity to be cared for and pampered, but on the other hand, their feelings of abandonment and loneliness are triggered. Their family may not visit as frequently as they would like, and their loneliness increases. This heightens their frustration which is likely to be directed toward staff (Sancier, 1984; Pinkston & Link, 1984). Encouraging independence will only trigger more anxiety. However, staff cannot devote 100% of their time to one demanding, dependent resident. Agreeing to comply with more appropriate demands can occur if accompanied by firm limit-setting. Specifying exactly how much time a particular activity requires and not straying from that limit are important. Scheduling of daily activities can be helpful for the dependent individual. Knowing when, where, and what they will be doing, and that they will not be abandoned, may be reassuring. Helping to develop their schedule of care and keeping copies of their own schedule may subtly encourage independent behaviors (Ebersole, 1989; Hyer & Harrison, 1986).

An appreciation of personality style and disorder can also assist in unit management. Assigning two very dependent, needy residents to one room will certainly frustrate staff and influence their attitude upon entering that room. However, placing an obsessive personality with a dependent personality will be complementary. The controlling obsessional can assist the passive dependent, thereby meeting both their needs.

SUMMARY

Recognizing personality disorders in nursing home residents not only assists in day-to-day management but also may help to decrease other psychiatric morbidity. Since personality-disordered residents are so very sensitive to interpersonal conflicts, their incidence of major psychiatric disorders is high. If those at risk are identified, staff can be attuned to early changes consistent with major psychiatric illness described elsewhere in this text. Appropriate psychiatric treatment can begin, and the resident's recovery thus hastened.

The key to successfully treating the personality-disordered older adult is to recognize their illness and to accept that the individual is unlikely to change but that staff can make an impact on their behaviors through staff's approaches. On occasion, residents may be referred for therapy and may indeed incorporate lasting personality changes. More often than not, however, residents will continue their maladaptive ways for the duration of their life. Staff members can assess personal and outside resources to adapt to their residents' personality disorders. Insight into a resident's personality style or disorder will help explain his/her behavior and thereby facilitate more empathic caregiving. Anger, mistrust, and demandingness are not solely and intentionally directed at staff. These have been lifelong reactions used by such residents. Recognizing these behaviors as reflections of much deeper, painful, and lifelong psychological conflicts can make care of personality-disordered elderly more challenging and rewarding.

This chapter addressed assessing personality and personality disorders in the institutionalized elderly. These conditions may manifest differently in older adults than in younger individuals and are often overlooked in attempting to understand a resident's behavior and symptomology. Personality is a central dimension along which staff can understand problems and provide treatment. As part of the admission assessment, personality, usual coping styles, and family and resident's perceptions of lifestyle need to be evaluated.

REFERENCES

Beaver, M., & Miller, D. (1985). Clinical social work practice with the institutionalized elderly. In *Clinical social work practice with the elderly* (pp. 202–203). Homewood, IL: The Dorsey Press.

Costa, P. T., McCrae, R. R., & Arenburg, D. (1980). Enduring dispositions in adult males. *Journal of Personality and Social Psychology, 38*, 793–800.

Cummings, E., & Henry, W. (1961). *Growing old: The process of disengagement.* New York: Basic Books.

Ebersole, P. (1989). *Caring for the psychogeriatric client* (pp.101–126). New York: Springer Publishing Co.

George, L. (1978). The impact of personality and social status factor upon levels of activity and psychological well-being. *Journal of Gerontology, 38,* 840–847.

Hathaway, S. R., & McKinley, J. C. (1943/1982). *Minnesota multiphasic personality inventory.* Minneapolis, MN: The University of Minnesota Press.

Hyer, L., & Harrison, W. (1986). Later life personality model diagnosis and treatment (pp. 399–415). In *Clinical gerontology.* New York: Haworth Press.

Kroessler, D. (1990). Personality disorder in the elderly. *Hospital and Community Psychiatry,* 1325–1329.

MacKinnon, R. A., & Michels, R. (1971). *The psychiatric interview in clinical practice* (pp. 260–262). Philadelphia, PA: W. B. Saunders.

Montgomery, R. J. V. (1983). Staff family relations and institutional care policies. *Journal Gerontol Social Work, 5,* 83.

Neugarten, B. (1977). Personality and aging. In J. Birren & K. Schaie (Eds.), *Handbook of the psychology of aging* (pp. 626–644). New York: Van Nostrand Reinhold.

Page, J. D. (1971). *Psychopathology: The science of understanding deviance* (pp. 303–305). New York: Aldine.

Pinkston, E., & Link, N. (1984). *Intervention procedures and guidelines in care of the elderly: A family approach* (pp. 33–49). New York: Pergamon Press.

Rovner, B. W., Kafonek, S., Filipp, L., Lucas, M. J., & Folstein, M. F. (1986). Prevalence of mental illness in a community nursing home. *American Journal Psychiatry, 143,* 1446–1449.

Sadavoy, J. (1987). Character disorders in the elderly: An overview. In J. Sadavoy & M. Leszcz (Eds.), *Treating the elderly with psychotherapy* (pp 175–229). Madison, CT: International Universities Press.

Sancier, B. (1984). A model for linking families to their institutionalized relative. *Social Work, 29,* 63.

Schultz, J. M., & Dark, S. L. (1986). *Manual of psychiatric nursing care plans* (2nd ed.). Boston: Little, Brown & Company.

Simon, A. (1980). The neuroses, personality disorders, alcoholism, drug use and misuse, and crime in the aged. In J. E. Borren & R. B. Sloane (Eds.), *Handbook of mental health and aging.* Englewood Cliffs, NJ: Prentice-Hall.

Solomon, K. (1981). Personality disorders in the elderly. In E. Lion, Jr. (Ed.), *Personality disorders: Diagnosis and management* (2nd ed., pp. 310–338). Baltimore: Williams & Wilkins.

Woods, R. T., & Britton, P. C. (1985). *Clinical psychology with the elderly* (pp. 59–79). Rockville, MD: Aspen Systems Corp.

Whanger, A. (1984). Paranoid and schizophrenia disorders. In A. Whanger & A. Meyers (Eds.), *Mental health and therapeutic intervention with older adults* (pp. 96–97). Rockville, MD Aspen Systems Corp.

6

Interrelationship of Anxiety and Sleep Disorders in the Elderly

Pamela J. Swales
Leah F. Friedman
Javaid I. Sheikh

INTRODUCTION

Surveys suggest that both anxiety and sleep disorders are quite common in the elderly. For example, a review of the literature (Sheikh, 1991) finds that various epidemiological studies over the last three decades estimate 10% to 20% of older adults experience significant symptoms of anxiety. The Epidemiological Catchment Area (ECA) investigators (Myers, Weissman, Tischler, Holzer, Leaf, Orvaschel et al., 1984) found phobias to be the most common psychiatric syndrome in elderly women and the second most common in elderly men. In the same vein, a recent analysis of the ECA data in the Duke County sample (Blazer, George, & Hughes, 1991) reported that

Supported by NIMH Training Grant MH16744 (Dr. Swales). Supported by NIMH Grant MH45143 (Dr. Friedman) and a grant from the Teaching Nursing Home Project at Stanford, (Dr. Sheikh).

both the six-month and lifetime prevalence of all anxiety disorders combined stand at a prevalence of 19.70% and 34.05%, respectively. It thus appears that anxiety symptoms and disorders are among the most common psychiatric ailments experienced by older adults.

About five million elderly patients in this country have a severe sleep disorder (Dement, Miles, & Carskadon, 1982; Mellinger, Balter, & Uhlenhuth, 1985; Zorick, Roth, Hartze, Piccione, & Stepanski, 1981). In the United States, the elderly currently represent about 10% to 12% of the population but they are prescribed about 25% to 40% of the sedative-hypnotics (Regestein, 1980; U.S. Department of Health, Education and Welfare, 1976). Women consistently complain more about changes in their sleep and notice these changes earlier than do men (Karacan, Thornby, & Anch, 1976).

Thus, anxiety and sleep problems are commonly found in older adults. In this chapter, we will describe normal sleep, the various commonly reported age-related changes in sleep architecture, and the association of various anxiety disorders with sleep disturbances. We will then present preliminary findings from our own research, looking at the association of anxiety and insomnia, and provide general guidelines for management of anxiety and sleep problems.

AGE-RELATED CHANGES IN SLEEP PATTERNS

Normal sleep may be understood to consist of five distinctly different electroencephalographic (EEG) conditions (stages), nonrapid eye movement sleep (NREM), Stages 1 through 4, and rapid eye movement sleep (REM). These levels of brain activity alternate in a cyclical pattern, five to seven times during the course of a night's sleep (Kelly, 1985). A progression of increasingly slower EEG frequencies with parasympathetic activity characterizes Stages 1-4 sleep. In adulthood, 75% of the sleep time is spent in Stages 2 through 4, and REM sleep periods occur about every 90 minutes.

REM sleep is the deepest stage of sleep. Visual dreaming usually takes place in REM sleep and is characterized by a high degree of brain activity (desynchronized, low-voltage and fast) and is similar to that of Stage 1. Broad sympathetic arousal also accompanies this stage, however, voluntary muscle activity is suppressed.

With aging, changes occur in the duration, quality, and cycles of sleep. Older people complain frequently about their sleep-wake disturbances, and this has been well documented (Carskadon, 1976; Miles & Dement, 1980). Naturally, medical illness (Reynolds, Coble, Black, Holzer, Carroll, & Kupfer, 1980) and environmental and social factors may contribute to such problems.

Several researchers have described a variety of age-related changes with respect to the architecture of sleep (Bixler, Kales, Jacoby, Soldatos, & Vela-Bueno, 1984; Williams, Webb, 1982; Karacan, & Hursch, 1974; Tune, 1969). The mean time of sleep onset and of awakening becomes progressively earlier with advancing age (Tune, 1969; McGhie & Russell, 1962). However, sleep latency (the time it takes to actually fall asleep) does not change substantially with age (Moran, Thompson, & Nies, 1988).

Generally, there is an increase in the number and duration of nocturnal awakenings (Kelly, 1985; Bixler et al., 1984) and once awakened, many older individuals find it difficult to return to sleep (Kales, Wilson, Kales, Jacobsen, Paulson, Kollar et al., 1967; Wiliams et al., 1974). Many elders return to a polyphasic cycle of sleep and wakefulness during each day (Lewis, 1969; Tune, 1969; Webb, 1969; Miles & Dement, 1980). This pattern, resembling that of infants, is quite possibly an artifact of environment rather than a true age-related biological change.

Apparently, age-related changes occur in REM sleep. There appears to be an increase in the length of the first REM period (Kales, 1975) and the first non-REM to REM cycle is shortened from the average 90 minutes to a 60-minute interval (Feinberg, 1974; Kales & Kales, 1974). The total duration of REM sleep decreases because total sleep time is less in advancing years. However, normally, the proportion of overall sleep time spent in REM sleep remains stable until about the seventh or eighth decade (Kelly, 1985). In addition, Kahn and Fisher (1969) found that REM sleep is often interrupted by spindles that are characteristic of Stage 2 sleep.

ANXIETY AND SLEEP DISORDERS

Clinical experience suggests that disturbances of sleep are commonly found in patients with anxiety disorders. Evidence from the literature seems to support this impression. For example, Mathew and colleagues (1982) found in a sample of anxious patients that restless sleep was the only vegetative symptom consistently related to anxiety. On the other hand, anxiety appears to be a rather common occurrence in patients with chronic insomnia (Kales & Kales, 1984; Reynolds, Shaw, Newton, Coble, & Kupfer, 1983).

In the following, we will present a review of the literature regarding comorbidity of sleep disorders in various anxiety disorders. It is important to keep in mind that most of the studies looking at this issue have been conducted in younger people, and in the absence of specific empirical research, one can only infer their applicability to the elderly.

PANIC DISORDER

Difficulties initiating and maintaining sleep are common complaints of patients with panic attacks (Sheehan, Ballenger, & Jacobsen, 1980). However, the sleep of panic patients is remarkably normal with respect to total sleep time, sleep latency, and sleep efficiency (Uhde, Roy-Byrne, Gillin, Mendelson, Boulenger, & Vittone, 1984). Of note, the only real abnormality found between panickers and normals was that of an increase in large body movement time in individuals who experience panic compared to normal controls (Hauri, Friedman, & Ravaris, 1989).

Panic attacks can occur during sleep. Nocturnal panic attacks are likely to be preceded by non-REM sleep at the transition from Stage 2 to Stage 3 sleep (Hauri et al., 1989; Roy-Byrne, Mellman, & Uhde, 1988). Additionally, nocturnal panic events occur relatively proximal (prior or post) to the first REM period. Roy-Byrne and co-workers (1988) also found a significant increase in REM latency associated with panicking versus nonpanicking nights. Interestingly, movement time is most prominent on nonpanic nights. When panickers are deprived of sleep for a night, there is often an exacerbation of attacks the following day (Roy-Byrne et al., 1988).

GENERALIZED ANXIETY DISORDER

The individual with generalized anxiety disorder (GAD) has difficulty initiating and maintaining sleep and therefore displays increased sleep latency, decreased sleep efficiency, and more awakenings than normal. The sleep characteristics associated with generalized anxiety include relatively normal REM measures, increased Stage 1 and 2 sleep, and possibly, a reduction in the amount of REM sleep (Reynolds et al., 1983; Rosa, Bonnett, & Kramer, 1983). In addition, possibly because of sleep fragmentation, GAD sufferers show less delta sleep than do normal individuals (Hauri et al., 1989).

OBSESSIVE–COMPULSIVE DISORDER

Many patients with obsessive–compulsive disorder (OCD) find they have sleep difficulties. Investigators have found that the sleep of their OCD patients (age range 18 to 71 years) is restless, fragmented with awakenings, and is of shorter duration than that of matched control subjects (Insel, Gillin, Moore, Mendelson, Loewenstein, & Murphy, 1982). In addition, shortened REM latency (up to 50%), less Stage 4 sleep, decreased REM sleep, and shallower sleep (decreased delta sleep) are also characteristic of the sleep of individuals with OCD (Insel et al., 1982; Insel, Mueller, Gillin, Siever, & Murphy, 1984).

These same authors (Insel et al., 1982; Insel et al., 1984) comment on the similarity of OCD subjects' sleep architecture and characteristics to those of depressives. Of seventeen sleep variables, significant differences were found on just two. Patients with OCD evidenced more Stage 1 and Stage 3 sleep than depressives. In addition, there was a tendency for lowered REM density in the OCD patients.

POST-TRAUMATIC STRESS DISORDER

Difficulty falling and staying asleep and recurrent distressing dreams are prominent symptoms of post-traumatic stress disorder (PTSD). Recurrent nightmares and a lower percentage of REM sleep in post-traumatic stress patients were reported by Ross, Ball, Sullivan, & Caroff, 1989). An absence of Stage 4 sleep, numerous body movements (in Stage 2) and periodic tachycardia during the night's sleep also characterize the sleep of these individuals (Schlosberg & Benjamin, 1978).

Other researchers (Kales, Soldatos, Caldwell, Charney, Kales, Markel et al., 1980) found that in these patients, nightmares occur early in the sleep period. The often repeated contents of the dreams (with accompanying body movements) are likely to portray re-enactments of actual events (Van der Kolk, Blitz, Burr, Sherry & Hartmann, 1984). There is some evidence (Carlson & White, 1982; Kales et al., 1980; Schlosberg et al., 1978) that PTSD nightmares occur in both REM and non-REM sleep. By way of contrast, common nightmares are more likely to occur later in the sleep period, are rarely repetitive, appear with no concomitant body movements, and occur out of REM sleep.

OTHER ANXIETY DISORDERS

Published research literature is scant regarding sleep problems experienced in simple phobia and in social phobia. The nature of these disorders allows for avoidance of phobic situations; therefore, problems with sleep may be less likely than in other anxiety disorders. However, social phobia does tend to be chronic, and depending upon the extent and degree of anxiety, individuals may experience concomitant sleep problems. Individuals with simple or social phobia, in periods of exacerbation, would be expected to have difficulty initiating and maintaining sleep.

Little research has targeted specific sleep problems associated with organic anxiety syndromes. Underlying medical conditions and their treatment course may dictate which sleep problems, if any, will be associated with organic anxiety.

PRELIMINARY FINDINGS

In a preliminary study, we found some support for the relationship between poor sleep and anxiety among the elderly. Thirty-three community-residing older adults (11 men and 22 women with a mean age of 68.8 years) were recruited for participation in an insomnia treatment program through presentations at senior organizations and residences, articles in senior newsletters, and from among subjects who completed participation in studies of cognitive treatments for benign memory complaints.

In an initial telephone interview, subjects were given a brief description of the study and were screened for interest in participation and for disqualifying medical conditions. (For a detailed description of the methodology, see Friedman, Bliwise, Yesavage, & Salom, 1991.) As part of a more extensive in-person evaluation session, subjects were administered the Spielberger State Anxiety Scale (Spielberger, 1983) and the NEO Personality Inventory (Costa & McRae, 1985b), a personality measurement which has been validated in older populations (Costa & McRae, 1985a).

As the final stage in the evaluation process, subjects were given instructions for reporting information about their sleep-related behavior (using standardized sleep logs) to a telephone answering machine twice daily for two weeks. These self-report data formed the baseline measure for the study. Analysis of baseline sleep data for these insomniac subjects indicated a significant relationship ($r=.46$, $p <.01$) between time to sleep onset and scores on the Spielberger Anxiety Scale. This suggests that subjects who had higher anxiety scores took longer to fall asleep than less anxious subjects. Given this finding, it is perhaps not surprising that there was also a trend (statistically nonsignificant) for those subjects scoring as more anxious on the Spielberger measure to report shorter total sleep time during the two weeks of baseline.

Parallel findings were noted when scores on the Anxiety subscale of the NEO Personality Inventory were compared with baseline data. Thus, subjects scoring higher on the anxiety dimension of the personality measure had significantly less total sleep time during baseline ($r= -.37$, $p <.05$) than those with lower scores. Furthermore, anxious subjects tend to have longer sleep latencies when initiating sleep at the beginning of the night, though the trend was not statistically significant. These results seem to support the earlier suggestions of comorbidity of sleep problems and anxiety.

MANAGING ANXIETY AND SLEEP PROBLEMS IN THE ELDERLY

Clinicians working with the elderly must possess a comprehensive understanding of age-related physical changes and characteristic presentations of physical and emotional disorders common to the elderly. In addition, an understanding of such complexities as the individual patient's environmental and social life is crucial to appropriate treatment. In the following section, we address the general principles of management of anxiety and of sleep disorders.

GENERAL PRINCIPLES FOR MANAGEMENT OF ANXIETY DISORDERS

Though specific management of various anxiety syndromes and sleep problems will differ according to the diagnosis, certain guidelines can be useful in most situations. A calm, reassuring manner, combined with a supportive interaction, can be very comforting to an anxious patient. Before prescribing any anxiolytic medications, the clinician needs to be fully aware of the common older-age-related changes in absorption, distribution, protein binding, metabolism, and excretion of drugs which may lead to a relatively higher level of active medication or its metabolites compared to those in younger people. For illustration, an increase in proportion of body fat with aging may mean that a strongly lipophilic medication (for example, the benzodiazepine, diazepam) will lead to a high accumulation in the tissues (Ouslander, 1981). Practitioners thus need to practice caution when prescribing medications to the elderly.

As with pharmacological interventions for anxiety and sleep problems, psychologically based interventions need to be considerate of the complex nature of these conditions in order to provide the most appropriate treatment. Cognitive-behavioral principles are very effective in the management of anxiety and other psychiatric symptoms (Beck & Emery, 1985; Black & Bruce, 1989) as well as in sleep disorders (Borkovec, 1982; Morin & Azrin, 1988; Morin & Rapp, 1987).

GENERAL PRINCIPLES OF MANAGEMENT FOR SLEEP PROBLEMS

A careful evaluation of sleep problems is important before proceeding with management. Specific management of sleep disorders requires individually

Table 6.1 Aids to Sleep for the Elderly

Schedule regular hours for bedtime and for waking up.
Do not nap during the day.
Light exercise daily can keep one physically fit and improve the quality of sleep.
Do not exercise within a few hours of going to sleep.
Take dinner at least two hours before going to bed.
Keep the bedroom clean and quiet, with a comfortable bed, and use it for primarily for sleeping.
Caffeine, nicotine, and any medications with stimulants should be avoided several hours before going to sleep.
Avoid anxiety-producing situations (e.g., tense family interaction) before going to bed.
A warm bath, a glass of milk, and light reading can help induce sleep.

Note: From "Anxiety Disorders in the Elderly" by J. I. Sheikh, 1991, *Current Problems in Geriatrics*, pp 1–26. Copyrighted 1991 by *J. Sheikh, M.D.* Mosby *Year Book Inc.* Littleton, Mass. Adopted by permission.

tailored interventions, discussion of which is beyond the scope of this chapter. However, general guidelines to improve the quality of sleep in the elderly are presented in Table 6.1.

CONCLUSION

Our review of the literature indicates that anxiety and sleep problems are inter-related. Specifically, anxiety disorders can create problems in initiating and maintaining sleep as well as significantly affecting its quality. Further, anxious patients manifest frequent awakenings and state changes, and very commonly complain of insomnia.

These findings suggest a need for paying careful attention to sleep characteristics and problems in anxious patients as well as the experience and symptoms of anxiety in patients with sleep disorders. This is important since effective management strategies, pharmacological and non-pharmacological, exist for both anxiety and for sleep disorders.

REFERENCES

Black, J. L., & Bruce, B. K. (1989). Behavior therapy: A clinical update. *Hospital and Community Psychiatry*, 40, 1152–1158.

Beck, A. T., & Emery, G. (1985). *Anxiety disorders and phobias: A cognitive perspective*. New York: Basic Books.

Bixler, E. O., Kales, A., Jacoby, J A., Soldatos, C. R., & Vela-Bueno, A. (1984). Nocturnal sleep and wakefulness: Effects of age and sex in normal sleepers. *International Journal of Neuroscience, 23*, 33–42.

Blazer, D., George, L., & Hughes, D. (1991). The epidemiology of anxiety disorders: An age comparison. In C. Salzman & B. Liebowitz (Eds.), *Anxiety disorders in the elderly*. Hillsdale, NJ: Lawrence Erlbaum.

Borkovec, T. D. (1982). Insomnia. *Journal of Consulting and Clinical Psychology, 50*, 880–895.

Carlson, C. R., & White, D. K. (1982). Night terrors: A clinical and empirical review. *Clinical Psychology Review*, 2, 455–468.

Carskadon, M. A. (1976). Self-reports versus sleep laboratory findings in 122 drug-free subjects with complaints of chronic insomnia. *American Journal of Psychiatry*, 133, 1382–1388.

Costa, P. T., & McRae, R. R. (1985a). Concurrent validation after 20 years: Implications of personality and stability for its assessment. In N. J. Butcher & C. D. Spielberger (Eds.), *Advances in personality assessment* (Volume 4, pp. 31–54). Hillsdale, NJ: Lawrence Erlbaum.

Costa, P. T., & McRae, R. R. (1985b). *NEO Personality Inventory*. Baltimore: Psychological Assessment Resources.

Dement, W. C., Miles, L. E., & Carskadon, M. A. (1982). "White paper" on sleep and aging. *Journal of the American Geriatrics Society*, 30, 25–50.

Feinberg, I. (1974). Changes in sleep cycle patterns with age. *Journal of Psychiatric Research*, 10, 293–305.

Friedman, L. F., Bliwise, D., Yesavage, J. A., & Salom, S. R. (1991). A preliminary study comparing sleep restriction and relaxation treatments for insomnia in older adults. *Journal of Gerontology*, 46, 1–8.

Hauri, P. J., Friedman, M., & Ravaris, C. L. (1988). Sleep in patients with spontaneous panic attacks. *Sleep*, 12, 323–337.

Insel, T. R., Gillin, J. C., Moore,. A., Mendelson, W. B., Loewenstein, R. J., & Murphy, D. L. (1982). The sleep of patients with obsessive-compulsive disorder. *Archives of General Psychiatry*, 39, 1372–1377.

Insel, T. R., Mueller, E. A., Gillin, J. C., Siever, L. J., & Murphy, D. L. (1984). Biological markers in obsessive-compulsive disorders. *Journal of Psychiatric Research*, 4, 407–423.

Kahn, E., & Fisher, C. (1969). The sleep characteristics of the normal aged male. *Journal of Nervous and Mental Disorders*, 148, 477–494.

Kales, J. D. (1975). Aging and sleep. In R. Goldman & M. Rockstein (Eds.), *The physiology and pathology of human aging* (pp. 187–202). New York: Academic Press.

Kales, A., & Kales, J. D. (1974). Sleep disorders: Recent findings in the diagnosis and treatment of disturbed sleep. *New England Journal of Medicine*, 290, 487–499.

Kales, A., & Kales, J. D. (1984). *Evaluation and treatment of insomnia* (pp. 61–86). New York: Oxford University Press.

Kales, A., Soldatos, C. R., Caldwell, A. B., Charney, D.S., Kales, J. D., Markel, D. & Cadieux, R. (1980). Nightmares: Clinical characteristics and personality patterns. *American Journal of Psychiatry*, 137, 1197–1201.

Kales, A., Wilson, T., & Kales, J., Jacobsen, M. S., Paulson, M. J., Kollar, E., & Walter, R. D. (1967). Measurements of all-night sleep in normal elderly persons: Effects of aging. *Journal of the American Geriatrics Society*, 15, 405–414.

Karacan, I., Thornby, J., & Anch, M. (1976). Prevalence of sleep disturbance in a primarily urban Florida county. *Social Science Medicine*, 10, 239–244.

Kelly, D. D. (1985). Sleep and dreaming. In E. R. Kandel, & J. H. Schwartz (Eds.), *Principles of neural science* (2nd ed, pp. 648–658). New York: Elsevier.

Lewis, S. (1969). Sleep patterns during afternoon naps in the young and elderly. *British Journal of Psychiatry*, 115, 107–108.

Mathew, R. J., Swihart, A. A., & Weinman, M. L. (1982). Vegetative symptoms in anxiety and depression. *British Journal of Psychiatry*, 141, 162–165.

McGhie, A., & Russell, S. (1962). The subjective assessment of normal sleep patterns. *Journal of Mental Science*, 108, 642–654.

Mellinger, G. D., Balter, M. B. & Uhlenhuth, E. H. (1985). Insomnia and its treatment: Prevalence and correlates. *Archives of General Psychiatry*, 42, 225–232.

Meyers, J. K., Weissman, M. M., Tischler, G. L., Holzer, C. E., Leaf, P. J., Orvaschel, H., Anthony, J. C., Boyd, J. H., Burker, J. D. Jr., Kramer, M., & Stoltzman, R. (1984). Six-month prevalence of psychiatric disorders in three communities, 1980–1982. *Archives of General Psychiatry*, 41, 959–967.

Miles, L. E., & Dement, W. C. (1980). Sleep and aging. *Sleep*, 3, 119–120.

Moran, M. D., Thompson, T. L., & Nies, A. S. (1988). Sleep disorders in the elderly. *American Journal of Psychiatry*, 145, 1369–1378.

Morin, C. M., & Azrin, N. H. (1988). Behavioral and cognitive treatments of geriatric insomnia. *Journal of Consulting and Clinical Psychology*, 56, 748–753.

Morin, C. M., & Rapp, S. R. (1987). Behavioral management of geriatric insomnia. *Clinical Gerontologist*, 6, 15–23.

Ouslander, J. G. (1981). Drug therapy in the elderly. *Annals of Internal Medicine*, 94, 711–722.

Regestein, Q. R. (1980). Insomnia and sleep disturbances in the aged: Sleep and insomnia in the elderly. *Journal of Geriatric Psychiatry*, 13, 153–171.

Reynolds, C. F., Coble, P. A., Black, R. S., Holzer, B., Carroll, R., & Kupfer, D. J. (1980). Sleep disturbances in a series of elderly patients: Polysomnographic findings. *Journal of the American Geriatrics Society*, 28, 164–170.

Reynolds, C. F., Shaw, D. H., Newton, T. F., Coble, P. A., & Kupfer, D. J. (1983). EEG in sleep in outpatients with generalized anxiety: A preliminary comparison with depressed outpatients. *Psychiatry Research*, 8, 81–89.

Rosa, R. R., Bonnett, M. M., & Kramer, M. (1983). The relationship of sleep and anxiety in anxious subjects. *Biological Psychology*, 16, 119–126.

Ross, R., Ball, W., Sullivan, K., & Caroff, S. (1989). Sleep disturbance as the hallmark of post-traumatic stress disorder. *American Journal of Psychiatry*, 146, 697–707.

Roy-Byrne, P. P., Mellman, T. A., & Uhde, T. W. (1988). Biologic findings in panic disorder: Neuroendocrine and sleep-related abnormalities. *Journal of Anxiety Disorders*, 2, 17–29.

Schlosberg, A., & Benjamin, M. (1978). Sleep patterns in three acute combat fatigue cases. *Journal of Clinical Psychiatry*, 39, 546–549.

Sheehan, D. V., Ballenger, J., & Jacobsen, G. (1980). Treatment of endogenous anxiety with phobic, hysterical, and hypochondriacal symptoms. *Archives of General Psychiatry*, 37, 51–59.

Sheikh, J. I. (1991). Anxiety disorders in the elderly. *Current Problems in Geriatrics*, 1, 1–26.

Spielberger, C. D. (1983). *State-trait anxiety inventory*. Palo Alto, CA: Consulting Psychologists Press.

Tune, G. (1969). Sleep and wakefulness in 509 normal adults. *British Journal of Medical Psychology*, 42, 75–80.

Uhde, T. W., Roy-Byrne, P., Gillin, J. C., Mendelson, W. B., Boulenger, J. P., & Vittone, B. J. (1984). The sleep of patients with panic disorders: A preliminary report. *Psychiatric Research*, 12, 251–259.

U. S. Department of Health, Education, and Welfare. (1976). *Physicians' drug prescribing patterns in skilled nursing facilities*. (DHEW Publication No. OS 76-50050). Bethesda MD.

Van der Kolk, B., Blitz, R., Burr, W., Sherry, M. A., & Hartmann, E. (1984). Nightmares and trauma: A comparison of nightmares after combat with lifelong nightmares in veterans. *American Journal of Psychiatry*, 141, 187–190.

Webb, W. (1969). Twenty-four-hour sleep cycling. In A. Kales (Ed.), *Sleep physiology and pathology* (p. 53). Philadelphia: J. B. Lippincott.

Webb, W. B. (1982). Sleep in older persons: Sleep structure of 50 to 60-year-old men and women. *Journal of Gerontology*, 37, 581–586.

Williams, R. L., Karacan, I., & Hursch, C. J. (1974). *Electroencephalography (EEG) of human sleep: Clinical applications*. New York: John Wiley & Sons.

Zorick, F. J., Roth, T., Hartze, K. M., Piccione, P. M., & Stepanski, E. J. (1981). Evaluation and diagnosis of persistent insomnia. *American Journal of Psychiatry*, 138, 769–773.

7

Psychotropics in the Extended Care Facility

Barnett S. Meyers
Christopher T. Cahenzli

INTRODUCTION

An overview of disordered behaviors encountered in nursing home settings was provided in Chapter 3. Dysfunctional behavior resulting as a consequence of dementia can lead to excessive disability or danger to other residents, staff, or self. In these instances, the use of psychotropic medication may be necessary for the delivery of basic care and can lead to improvement in the quality of a resident's life. The administration of psychotropic agents for therapeutic effect must be distinguished from use of their sedative side effects to "chemically restrain" disruptive behavior.

Behavioral disturbances can also result from a primary psychiatric illness. Despite recent Federal regulations, nursing homes are often the repositories for elders with mental health problems (Birkett, 1991); the mental health consultant must, therefore, consider whether disordered behavior results from a primary psychiatric diagnosis. In this chapter we will review the epidemiology of primary psychiatric disorders in late life that are frequently associated with behavioral disturbance. We will then discuss relevant classes of psychotropic agents and their usage in long-term-care settings.

EPIDEMIOLOGY OF PSYCHIATRIC DISORDERS IN THE NURSING HOME

Studies carried out before the use of modern diagnostic instruments or nomenclature reported an 80% to 90% percent prevalence of mental illness in nursing homes. In a larger study of newly admitted nursing home residents, Rovner, et al., (1990) identified a diagnosable psychiatric disorder in 80% of 454 cases. Again, dementia was the most common diagnosis, occurring in 67.4% of admissions; in 40% of the cases dementia was complicated by depression, psychosis, or delirium; furthermore, residents with psychiatric complications of dementia were significantly more likely to receive neuroleptics (44.4%) and spend most of their time in restraints (47.9%) than nondemented residents suffering from another primary psychiatric disorder. Individuals with confused and disturbed behavior cause difficulties for caregivers, which may explain the high comorbidity noted in nursing home studies. Thus, disruptive behavior was the most common reason cited (37% of admissions) for seeking nursing home placement in the study by Rovner et al. (1990).

Despite the use of nursing homes to provide custodial care for older patients with a primary psychiatric disorder, behavioral complications of dementia are the most frequently encountered problem requiring psychiatric intervention. Consideration of the appropriate use of psychotropic medications to manage complicated dementia requires a discussion of agitation, a generic term commonly used to describe disordered behaviors associated with psychiatric disturbance.

AGITATION AND OTHER PSYCHIATRIC DISTURBANCES SECONDARY TO DEMENTIA

Definitions of disruptive behavior and agitation noted in residents with organic brain disorder vary widely. Behaviors ranging from incontinence (Swearer et al., 1988) and wandering to assaultiveness have been included in studies of disordered behavior (Teri, Larson, & Reifler, 1988). Variability in definitions and criteria for agitation among different studies confound our ability to appropriately diagnose and pharmacologically treat these patients. Further discussion of agitation is found elsewhere in this text.

APPLIED PSYCHOPHARMACOLOGY IN THE NURSING HOME

Multiple large-scale studies have demonstrated that 50% to 70% of residents in long-term-care facilities are receiving psychotropic drugs (Beers,

Avorn, & Soumerai, 1988; Buck, 1988; Ray, Federspiel, & Schaffner, 1980). Antipsychotic drugs, the most frequently used agents, are prescribed to 45% of elderly residents, followed by anxiolytic drugs in 21%, and sedative/ hypnotic drugs in 20% (Beardsley et al., 1989). Not surprisingly, over 50% of residents who are prescribed psychotropic drugs receive them to treat agitation (Cohen-Mansfield, 1986). The high frequency of disturbed behaviors in nursing homes and the use of psychiatric medications to treat them require careful consideration of data bearing on the effectiveness of psychopharmacologic approaches to this problem.

PSYCHOTROPICS FOR DISTURBED BEHAVIOR: CHEMICAL RESTRAINT VERSUS THERAPEUTIC EFFECT

Recent public debates over the use of psychotropics in extended care facilities reflect a long-standing controversy in the scientific community. Marked variability in psychotropic drug use in different Tennessee nursing homes, serving similar clinical populations, is interpreted as evidence that physician rather than resident characteristics determine the use of these agents. The finding that a small proportion of family practitioners with the largest nursing home practices were the heaviest prescribers supports this impression (Ray et al., 1980). The central question is whether psychotropics are prescribed for a putative therapeutic activity or as a means of managing unacceptable behavior by sedation. Are medications administered to chemically restrain and thereby control nursing home residents or to treat disorders?

The mechanisms by which medications produce therapeutic versus putative restraining effects are thought to differ. The antipsychotic activity of neuroleptics occurs through their ability to block central nervous system dopamine receptors, and antidepressants improve mood by downregulating postsynaptic beta adrenergic and serotinergic receptors (Richelson, 1991). However, psychotropic agents are "dirty drugs"; that is, they act on multiple neurotransmitter systems, including many unrelated to their mode of therapeutic action. Side effects are generally the pharmacological consequences of medications that extend beyond their primary therapeutic mode of action. Thus, sedation results from the antihistaminic properties of psychotropics and their ability to block alpha-one noradrenergic receptors (Richelson, 1991). Bradykinesia and akinesia, specific extrapyramidal side effects, are caused by blockade of dopamine receptors in the nigral-striatal pathway that controls muscle movement (Peroutka & Snyder, 1980). Chemical restraint can be considered as the use of side effects caused by psychotropic agents to manage a resident's behavior.

The high prevalence of agitation in residents with dementia and our limited understanding of both the pathogenesis and treatment of disruptive behavior in residents with organic brain disease have fueled the controversy about use of psychotropics in nursing home settings. The demonstrated association between adverse health consequences and psychotropic use in older individuals heightens the importance of this issue. Use of sedatives increases the frequency of falls in the community-residing elderly (Tinetti, Speechley, & Ginter, 1988), and antipsychotics, tricyclic antidepressants, and long-acting benzodiazepines have been found to increase the frequency of hospitalization for hip fracture among nursing home residents; furthermore, the increased risk occurs in a dose-dependent fashion (Ray et al., 1987).

Federal regulations, written into Omnibus Budget Reconciliation Act of 1987 (OBRA) legislation, are designed to control the use of psychopharmacologic agents in nursing homes accredited by Medicare. The concept of "unnecessary drugs" has been introduced and applies to the use of medications "in excessive dosage" or for "excessive durations" (Health Care Financing Administration, 1991); guidelines are being drafted to help nursing home surveyors determine whether use of prescribed medications is "unnecessary." Although the goal of federal regulations is to prevent the overutilization of medications to manage behavior, data is lacking on the mechanisms of action, appropriate dosages, and risks versus benefits of the pharmacotherapy of disturbed behavior. Nearly all medications have side effects, and untreated behavioral disturbances can lead to excess disability and diminished quality of life. Without controlled studies, we cannot determine the extent to which the risks of falls is truly increased by psychotropic medications or determine the adverse life consequences of limiting medication use. Guidelines for appropriate pharmacotherapeutic treatment have been developed (American Association for Geriatric Psychiatry, 1991).

CHOICE OF AGENT

Surprisingly little is known about the specificity of various psychotropic medications to treat subtypes of behavioral disturbances. The multidimensional approach for classifying agitation has been discussed above; however, pharmacologic trials for particular syndromes of behavioral disturbance have not been carried out; furthermore, the development of pharmacologic treatment studies is hindered by our lack of understanding of the pathogenesis of agitated behaviors (Wragg & Jeste, 1988).

Leibovici and Tariot (1988) recommend applying a systematic approach to treatment based on identifying the drug-responsive syndrome that a

TABLE 7.1 Hypothesized Types of Drug-Responsive Syndromes

Syndrome	Medication(s)
Psychosis	Neuroleptics
Generalized anxiety	Benzodiazepines
Panic	Antidepressants, alprazolam
Affective lability	Carbamazepine, lithium
Irritable depression	Antidepressants
Rage attacks	Beta blockers

patient's pattern of agitation most closely resembles. Applying this approach, use of neuroleptics would be appropriate for agitation due to hallucinations or delusions, lithium and carbamazepine for agitated syndromes marked by profound mood fluctuations, beta-blockers for episodic outbursts of aggression, benzodiazepines for agitation caused by anxiety, and antidepressants for syndromes resembling an irritable depression.

Hypothetical clinical syndromes corresponding to phenomenologic types of agitation are listed in Table 7.1. Although the general effectiveness of this approach remains unstudied, open studies have supported the use of particular agents to treat specific target symptoms. These will be discussed below. Nevertheless, the reader should keep in mind that studies reporting positive findings are far more likely to be published; thus, in the absence of controlled studies the import of case reports and open trials should be considered limited.

NEUROLEPTICS

Although neuroleptics are the most widely used agents to treat agitation secondary to organic brain disease (Beardsley, 1989; Wragg & Jeste, 1988), information about their effectiveness is inadequate. Our knowledge is limited regarding the small number of controlled studies, the heterogeneity of subject samples, and inadequate classification and measurement of behavioral target symptoms. However, as summarized in recent reviews (Devanand, Sackheim, & Mayeux, 1988; Sunderland & Silver, 1988; Wragg & Jeste, 1988; Salzman, 1987; Risse & Barnes, 1986), most studies do indicate that neuroleptics have a real, though modest, role in the treatment of dementia patients with secondary agitation.

Choice of a particular neuroleptic is generally made by balancing the medication's side effect profile with a specific patient's vulnerability to different adverse reactions. This principle is applied because of the absence of data demonstrating the superiority of one neuroleptic or class of agents over another (Helms, 1985; Risse & Barnes, 1986; Salzman, 1987; Schneider, Pollack, & Lyness, 1990) and the heightened vulnerability of elderly patients to adverse reactions and their consequences.

Recognizing how different neuroleptics affect neurotransmitter systems and the relationship of these actions to resulting side effects is crucial to minimizing risks. Low-potency neuroleptics (e.g., thirodazine and chlor-promazine) block alpha adrenergic and histaminergic receptors, while high-potency agents (e.g., haloperidol and fluphenazine) produce relatively specific blockade of dopamine receptors (Peroutka & Snyder, 1980).

Sedation was the most commonly reported side effect in Sunderland and Silver's (1988) review of 20 systematically carried out investigations. Although sedation occurred in 22% of the 1,207 study subjects, attrition due to intolerable side effects was only 6.6%. Thus, sedation was generally tolerated and could have contributed to improvement in target symptoms, perhaps by producing chemical restraint. Devanand, et al., (1989), using a single high-potency neuroleptic, haloperidol, demonstrated that patients receiving higher dosages (over 4 mg) had greater decreases in agitation measures but greater extrapyramidal side effects than those given low-intensity (close to 1 mg) treatment. Thus, both the class of agent and dose contribute to the frequency, severity, and type of side effects associated with neuroleptic treatment.

The increased association between neuroleptic use and tardive dys-kinesia that occurs with aging (Jeste & Wyatt, 1987) is of special concern. The increased frequency of spontaneously occurring dyskinesias reported in patients with Alzheimer's disease (O'Keane & Dinan, 1991) and the apparently increased risk for neuroleptic-induced tardive dyskinesia in this population (Wragg & Jeste, 1988) militates for minimizing both dosage and duration of neuroleptics in treating agitation in patients with dementia.

BENZODIAZEPINES

Apparent similarities between the fearful expression and increased psy-chomotor activity of agitation and states of severe anxiety suggest a potential use of benzodiazepines to treat nonpsychotic behavioral dis-turbance. Although a small number of pre-1975 studies demonstrated beneficial effects (Kirven & Montero, 1973; Beber, 1965; Chesrow et al., 1965), the use of benzodiazepines to treat agitation has fallen into disfavor. Early studies were flawed by the absence of placebo-controlled designs and/or the use of clinically heterogeneous and imprecisely diagnosed subject samples; furthermore, aging-related alternations in pharmacoki-netics and pharmacodynamics were not considered.

Aging is now known to increase benzodiazepine concentrations achieved at a given dose (Greenblatt, Seller, & Shador, 1982), particularly when medications with multiple metabolites (e.g., diazepam, flurazepam, and chlordiazepoxide) are administered (Greenblatt & Shader, 1981); furthermore, age is known to exaggerate and decrease in memory consolidation caused by benzodiazepines (Pomara et al., 1984). The ability of benzodiazepines to further compromise cognitive function in patients with dementia and the risk of accumulating toxic concentrations due to injudicious use have led the Health Care Financing Administration (HCFA) to include proposals to severely restrict benzodiazepine use in the proposed surveyor guidelines; the regular use of long-acting agents could be essentially precluded.

A recent double-blind study comparing haloperidol, oxazepam and diphenhydramine—an antihistamine with anticholinergic properties—to treat behavioral disturbances associated with moderate to severe dementia found the three medications produced comparable levels of improvement in behavioral rating scales (Coccaro et al., 1990). Average doses of haloperidol and oxazepam were 1.5 +/- 0.9 mg and 30 +/- 19.4 mg a day, respectively. Although standardized psychometric testing was not carried out, none of the 19 subjects receiving oxazepam developed a toxic confusional syndrome.

These results raise important questions. The three medications studied have different pharmacodynamic profiles, but all produce sedation. To what extent did the measurable decreases in behavioral disturbance result from sedation? Did the improvement, therefore, occur through a form of chemical restraint? How do we weight the multiple and different dimensions of functioning and quality of life? Finally, ethical issues must be considered; for example, who gives and should give consent for these decisions? Although the principal issues addressed by these questions apply to other pharmacotherapeutic approaches to agitation, they are especially relevant to benzodiazepines, because some of the improved behavior these agents produce could well result from sedation rather than a primary anxiolytic effect.

Some residents of extended care facilities do suffer from life-long anxiety disorders or anxiety syndromes that have developed in the institutional setting. The diagnosis is often rendered difficult by an inadequate history and a confounding dementia. A confused resident may be calling out for a number of reasons, including the need for attention, physical distress that cannot be articulated, and anxiety. As noted above, the clinician should examine the resident's phenomenology and communications to achieve a best judgment of whether significant anxiety is present, but the reader should note that criteria for making such judgments and methods for assessing their accuracy have not been developed. Pharmacologic studies of specific agents to treat well-defined behavioral syndromes are needed to improve our diagnostic acumen.

Individuals with panic disorder should not be deprived of adequate treatment because of entry into an extended care facility. Many of these individuals received pharmacotherapy prior to placement or previously arranged their living situations to avoid being left alone. These approaches to control panic disorder can be lost upon entering a nursing home, because a confused resident may be unable to articulate panic symptoms and cannot control being alone. Restrictions on type and dosage of available pharmacotherapeutic agents become an additional barrier to effective treatment. The presence of panic disorder should be considered for residents suffering recurrent episodes of spontaneously calling out which are relieved when a familiar resident or staff member is present. An appearance of severe apprehension is consistent with this diagnostic impression. Applying the conceptual approach described above, such residents warrant treatment with a standard antipanic medication, including alprazolam. The application of such conceptual approaches to diagnosis and treatment through controlled studies is warranted.

MOOD STABILIZERS: LITHIUM AND CARBAMAZEPINE

These agents are described together because of data indicating their usefulness in patients with primary bipolar disorder; whether they have similar modes of action or comparable efficacy in the treatment of subtypes of agitation remains to be clarified.

Despite a report that lithium reverses affective lability, including hypomania, in secondary organic affective syndromes (Williams & Goldstein, 1979), and a case of lithium-responsive agitation in a patient with Alzheimer's disease (Havens & Cole, 1982), there is little evidence that lithium reduces emotional disinhibition occurring secondary to late-life dementia. Schneider and Sobin's review reports a response rate of 17% in open studies that included Alzheimer's patients with agitated affective syndromes (1991). The report that late-onset manic patients, many of whom have organic brain disease, respond to lithium is encouraging (Schulman & Post, 1980), but the patients studied did not have dementia. Data demonstrating an increased risk of adverse central nervous system reactions to lithium, particularly extrapyramidal effects, in residents with dementia (Himmelhoch et al., 1980); the apparent lack of efficacy would mitigate against use of lithium to treat agitation secondary to dementia; and patients whose phenomenology closely resembles that of a classical bipolar disorder would be an exception to this.

Carbamazepine has been effective in decreasing affective lability in patients with organic brain disorders. In one study, eight patients, five with head trauma and three with Alzheimer's disease, demonstrated reduced aggressivity in response to levels of carbamazepine comparable to those used to treat temporal lobe epilepsy (Patterson, 1988). A similar response has been reported in nine Alzheimer's patients with agitation (Gleason & Schneider, 1990). Although the only controlled study of carbamazepine in behaviorally disturbed Alzheimer's patients failed to demonstrate a drug-placebo difference (Chambers et al., 1982), these patients were not selected on the basis of having affective lability or aggressivity. The principal side effects of carbamazepine reported in studies of organically impaired patients are sedation and ataxia; these tend to be dose related (Schneider & Sobin, 1991). Thus, carbamazepine continues to hold promise as a pharmacologic approach to affectively labile and aggressive syndromes of agitation in patients with dementia.

ANTIDEPRESSANTS

Post-stroke depression responds to standard concentrations of the secondary amine tricyclic antidepressant, nortriptyline (Lipsey, Robinson, & Pearlson, 1984). Data on the frequency and treatment-responsiveness of post-stroke depression may be relevant to states of affective lability that occur in the absence of a fully developed depressive disorder. Residents demonstrating agitated behavior that is associated with irritability and other depressive symptoms warrant consideration for a trial of antidepressants, whether organic brain damage is due to Alzheimer's disease or multiple cerebral infarcts. Again, controlled studies of a particular subtype of agitation to a specific class of psychotherapeutic medication are needed.

L DEPRENYL AND AGENTS AFFECTING CNS MONOAMINES

L deprenyl is a selective inhibitor of monoamine oxidase B (MAO B) at low doses (10 mg/day); at higher doses, L deprenyl inhibits both MAO A and MAO B (Elswoth et al., 1978). L deprenyl has been shown to slow the progression of Parkinson's disease, presumably by inhibiting MAO B, the catabolic enzyme for dopamine (Parkinson's Study Group, 1989). Metabolism of tyramine, norepinephrine, and serotonin occurs through MAO A and would presumably be unaffected by doses in the 10 mg area. A controlled study of L deprenyl to treat cognitive deficits in residents with Alzheimer's disease produced significant improvement on objective measures of agitation, mood, and physical tension on a 10 mg/day regimen that would inhibit MAO B, but not MAO A (Tariot et al., 1987). Although the results are surprising and unexplained, the possibility of improving agitation by altering monamine neurotransmitters is intriguing.

Successful trials of alaprocloate and citalopram, inhibitors of serotonin reuptake, have also been reported (Schneider & Sobin, 1991). These data are consistent with a hypothesis that diminished serotonin contributes to agitation in some patients with Alzheimer's disease (Schneider et al., 1988). Consistent with this, diminished platelet 3H-imipramine binding (a marker for serotonin uptake) and increased MAO activity have been identified in a subgroup of Alzheimer's disease patients with behavioral disturbance.

SUMMARY

Residents with behavioral disturbances secondary to primary major psychiatric disorders should be treated accordingly, regardless of whether dementia is present or the place of residence. Disturbed behavior secondary to dementia is especially prevalent in extended care facilities. Treatment studies in these settings demonstrate that a wide range of pharmacotherapeutic agents can reduce agitation associated with chronic organic brain diseases, including dementia. Further research is needed to clarify the subtypes of agitation associated with dementia and the specificity of pharmacologic approaches to these behavioral syndromes. A treatment strategy that considers similarities between a resident's phenomenology and the clinical picture of classical psychiatric disorders is suggested (Leibovici & Tariot, 1988); however, this conceptualization is preliminary and requires substantiation by empirical data.

Lack of knowledge about the pharmacotherapeutics of agitation has led to concerns about undue use of medication. The concept of chemical restraint is clearly pejorative and implies that improving behavior through sedative side effects is bad medical practice. Without additional information about the pharmacodynamics of reducing behavioral disturbance due to organic brain disease, practitioners are in a defensive position. Additional data about the benefits and adverse consequences of specific pharmacotherapies must be obtained in placebo-controlled trials. Psychiatrists must practice with the information provided by clinical studies and within regulatory guidelines to maximize positive outcomes in behaviorally disturbed patients. Behavioral treatment strategies, as described in other chapters, should be considered as alternatives to pharmacotherapy and are always an integral part of a comprehensive approach to the agitated resident.

REFERENCES

American Association for Geriatric Psychiatry (1991). Medical principles for use of psychotherapeutic medications in the nursing home.

Bearsdley, R. S., Larson, D. B., Burns, B. J., Thompson, J. W., & Kamerow, D. B. (1989). Prescribing of psychotropics in elderly nursing home patients. *Journal of the American Geriatrics Society, 37*, 327–330.

Beber, C. (1965). Management of behavior in the institutionalized aged. *Diseases of the Nervous System, 26*, 591–595.

Beers, M., Avorn, J., Soumerai, S. B., Everitt, D. E., Sherman, D. S., & Salem, S. (1988). Psychoactive medication use in intermediate-care facility residents. *Journal of the American Medical Association, 260*(20), 3016–3020.

Birkett, P. (1991). *Psychiatry in the nursing home.* Binghamton, NY: The Haworth Press.

Buck, J. A. (1988). Psychotropic drug practice in nursing homes. *Journal of the American Geriatrics Society, 36*(5), 409–418.

Chambers, C. A., Bain, J., Rosbottom, R., Ballinger, B. R., & McLaren, S. (1982). Carbamazepine in senile dementia and overactivity—placebo-controlled double-blind trial. *International Research Community System Medical Science Library Compendium. 10*, 505–506.

Chesrow, E. J., Kaplitz, S. E., Vetra, H. (1965). Double-blind study of exazepan in the management of geriatric patients with behavioral problems. *Clinical Medicine, 72*, 1001–1005.

Coccaro, E. F., Kramer, E., Zemishlany, Z., Thorne, A., Rice III, C. M., Giordani, B., Duvvi, K., Patel, B. M., Torres, J., Nora, R., Neufeld, R., Mohs, R. C., & Davis, K. L. (1990). Pharmacologic treatment of noncognitive behavioral disturbances in elderly demented patients. *American Journal of Psychiatry, 147*, 1640–1645.

Cohen-Mansfield, J. (1986). Agitated behaviors in the elderly: Preliminary results in the cognitively deteriorated. *Journal of the American Geriatrics Society, 34*, 722–727.

Devanand, D. P., Sackheim, H., Brown, R. P., Mayeux, R. (1989). A pilot study of haloperidol treatment of psychoses and behavioral disturbance in Alzheimer's disease. *Archives of Neurology, 46*, 854–857.

Devanand, D. P., Sackheim, H. A., & Mayeux, R. (1988). Psychosis, behavioral disturbance, and the use of neuroleptics in dementia. *Comprehensive Psychiatry, 29*, 387–401.

Elswoth, J. D., Glover, V., Reynolds, G. P., Sandler, M., Lees, A. J., Phuapradit, P., Shaw, K. W., Stern, G. M., & Kumar, P. (1978). Deprenyl administration in man: A selective monamine oxidase B inhibitor without the "cheese effect." *Psychopharmacology, 57*, 33–38.

Gleason, R. P., & Schneider, L. S. (1990). Carbamazepine treatment of agitation in Alzheimer's outpatients refractory to neuroleptics. *Journal of Clinical Psychiatry, 15*(3), 115–117.

Greenblatt, D. J., Seller, E. M., & Shader, R. I. (1982). Drug disposition in old age. *New England Journal of Medicine, 306*, 1081–1088.

Greenblatt, D. J., & Shader, R. J. (1981). Benzodiazepine kinetics in the elderly. In E. Usdin (Ed.) *Clinical pharmacology in psychiatry.* New York: Elsevier.

Havens, W. W., & Cole, J. (1982). Successful treatment of dementia with lithium. *Journal of Clinical Psychopharmocology, 2,* 71–72.

Health Care Financing Administration (1991). U.S. Department of Health and Human Services. *Federal Register, 56, 48,* 826–48, 879.

Helms, P. (1985). Efficacy of antipsychotics in the treatment of behavioral complications of dementia: A review of the literature. *Journal of the American Geriatrics Society, 33*(3), 206–209.

Himmelhoch, J. M., Neil, J. F., May, S. J., Fuchs, C. Z., & Licata, S. M. (1980). Age, dementia, dyskinesias and lithium response. *American Journal of Psychiatry, 137,* 941–944.

Jeste, D. V., & Wyatt, R. J. (1987). Aging and tardive dyskinesia. In N. E. Miller & G. D. Cohen (Eds.), *Schizophrenia and aging.* New York: Guilford.

Kirven, L. E., & Montero, E. F. (1973). Comparison of thioridazine and diazepam in the control of nonpsychotic symptoms associated with senility: Double-blind controlled study. *Journal of the American Geriatrics Society, 21,* 545–551.

Leibovici, A., & Tariot, P. N. (1988). Agitation associated with dementia: A systematic approach to treatment. *Psychopharmacology Bulletin, 24,* 49–53.

Lipsey, J. R., Robinson, R. G., & Pearlson, G. D. (1984). Nortriptyline treatment of post-stroke depression: A double-blind study. *Lancet, 1,* 297–300.

O'Keane, V., & Dinan, T. G. (1991). Orofacial dyskinesia and senile dementia of the Alzheimer's type. *International Journal of Geriatric Psychiatry, 6,* 41–44.

Parkinson's Study Group (1989). Effect of deprenyl on the progression of the disability in early Parkinson's disease. *New England Journal of Medicine, 321,* 1364–1371.

Patterson, J. F. (1988). A preliminary study of carbamazepine in the treatment of assaultive patients with dementia. *Journal of Geriatric Psychiatric Neurology, 1,* 21–21.

Peroutka, S. J., & Snyder, S. H. (1980). Relationship of neuroleptic drug effects at brain dopamine, serotonin, alpha adrenergic and histamine receptors in clinical potency. *American Journal of Psychiatry, 137,* 1518–1522.

Pomara, N., Stanley, B., Block, R., Guido, J., Ross, D., Berchou, R., Greenblatt, D. J., Newton, R. F., & Gershon, S. (1984). Adverse effects of single therapeutic doses of diazepam on performance in normal geriatric subjects: Relationship to plasma concentrations. *Psychopharmacology, 84,* 342–346.

Ray, W. A., Federspiel, C. F., & Schaffner, W. (1980). A study of antipsychotic drug use in nursing homes: Epidemiologic evidence suggesting misuse. *American Journal of Public Health, 70*(5), 485–491.

Ray, W. A., Griffin, M. R., Schaffner, W., Baugh, D. K., & Melton, J. L. (1987). Psychotropic drug use and the risk of hip fracture. *New England Journal of Medicine, 316*(7), 363–369.

Richelson, E. (1991). Biological basis of depression and therapeutic relevance. *Journal of Clinical Psychiatry, 52*(s), 4–10.

Risse, S. C., & Barnes, R. (1986). Pharmacologic treatment of agitation associated with dementia. *Journal of the American Geriatrics Society, 34,* 368–376.

Rosen, H. J. (1979). Double-blind comparison of haloperidol and thioridazine in geriatric outpatients. *Journal of Clinical Psychiatry, 40,* 24–31.

Rovner, B. W., German, P. S., Broadhead, J., Morriss, R. K., Brant, L. J., Blaustein, J., & Folstein, M. F. (1990). The prevalence and management of dementia and other psychiatric disorders in nursing homes. *International Psychogeriatrics, 2*(1), 13–24.

Rovner, B. W., Kafonek, S., Filipp, L., Lucas, J. M., & Folstein, M. F. (1986). Prevalence of mental illness in a community nursing home. *American Journal of Psychiatry, 143,* 1446–49.

Salzman, C. (1987). Treatment of agitation in the elderly. In H. Y. Meltzer (Ed.) *Psychopharmacology: A generation of progress.* New York: Raven Press.

Schneider, L. S., Pollack, V. E., & Lyness, M. A. (1990). A meta analysis of controlled trials of neuroleptic treatment in dementia. *Journal of the American Geriatrics Society, 38,* 553–563.

Schneider, L. S., Severson, J. A., Chui, H. C., & Sloan, R. B. (1988). Platelet tritiated imipramine binding and MAO activity in Alzheimer's disease patients with agitation and delusions. *Psychiatric Resident, 25,* 311–322.

Schneider, L. S., & Sobin, P. B. (1991). Non-neuroleptic medications in the management of agitation in Alzheimer's disease and other dementia: A selective review. *International Journal of Geriatric Psychiatry, 6,* 691–708.

Schulman, K., & Post, F. (1980). Bipolar affective disorders in old age. *British Journal of Psychiatry, 136,* 26–32.

Sunderland, T., & Silver, M. A. (1988). Neuroleptics in the treatment of dementia. *International Journal of Geriatric Psychiatry, 3,* 79–88.

Swearer, M. A., Drachman, D. A., O'Donnell, B. F., et al (1988). Troublesome and disruptive behaviors in dementia: Relationships to diagnosis and disease severity. *Journal of the American Geriatrics Society, 36,* 784–789.

Tariot, P. N., Cohen, R. M., Sunderland, T., Newhouse, P. A., Yount, D., Mellow, A. M., Weingartner, H., Mueller, E. A., & Murphy, D. L. (1987). L-deprenyl in Alzheimer's disease: Preliminary evidence for behavior change with monamine oxidase B inhibition. *Archives of General Psychiatry, 44,* 427–433.

Teri, L., Larson, E. B., & Reifler, B. B. (1988). Behavioral disturbance in dementia of the Alzheimer type. *Journal of the American Geriatrics Society, 26,* 1–6.

Tinetti, M. E., Speechley, M., & Ginter, S. F. (1988). Risk factors for falls among elderly persons living in the community. *New England Journal of Medicine, 319*(26), 1701–1707.

Williams, K. H., & Goldstein, G. (1979). Cognitive and affective response to lithium in patients with organic brain syndrome. *American Journal of Psychiatry, 136,* 800–803.

Wragg, R. E., & Jeste, D. V. (1988). Neuroleptics and alternative treatments: Management of behavioral symptoms and psychosis in Alzheimer's disease and related conditions. *Psychiatric Clinics of North America, 11*(1), 195–213.

PART II
Medical Disorders

8

Behavioral Concomitants of Common Medical Disorders

John E. Morley
Douglas K. Miller

Behavioral disorders occur in 68% to 94% of all residents in a long-term-care facility. In some of these cases, the behavioral disorder is a direct result of the underlying disease (e.g., delirium), while in other cases the medical disease may aggravate the underlying behavioral disorder (e.g., a depressive episode worsened by disease or by medications). Medical disease may lead to a loss of a locus of control which, in turn, may lead to aggressive or manipulative behavior by the resident in an attempt to regain control of the situation. Disorders of vision and hearing can result in sensory deprivation and the behavioral concomitants associated with it. Medical diseases and the medications used to treat them can result in sleep disorders. Both medical and psychiatric disorders can lead to protein energy malnutrition which, in turn, can result in or aggravate delirium, dementia or depression.

DELIRIUM

Delirium is the classical behavioral problem caused by medical disorders. Delirium exists when there is global cognitive impairment associated with an attention deficit. The attention deficit can be quite subtle and may be manifested by either loss of attention on a difficult task or overattention to any minor stimulus (denoted "stimulus-bound"). It usually has an acute onset (hours to days), and symptoms tend to fluctuate over the course of the day. Patients with delirium often have a reduced level of consciousness, altered psychomotor activity, a disorganized sleep-wake cycle, illusions and/or hallucinations, and are usually disorientated. Generally, delirium symptoms are present for less than one month.

The first known statement about delirium was presented by Celsus in the first century A.D. who stated ". . . during the paroxysms of fever, patients are delirious and talk nonsense (desipere et loqui aliena)." In 1870, Hood reported some cases of "senile delirium" that occurred in older persons who had no previous "mental debility." He stressed that this condition was potentially reversible but could lead to death. In 1904, Pickett distinguished between "confusion" which he believed resulted from an underlying psychological condition, (e.g., bereavement) and "delirium" which was due to an organic cause. Lipowski (1989) recently suggested that the term "pseudodelirium" (acute functional psychosis) be utilized to describe states that superficially look like delirium due to the patient's bizarre behavior, but appear to be caused by mechanisms different from delirium. The most common causes of pseudodelirium are depression, schizophrenia, or mania. Careful mental status testing will usually differentiate pseudodelirium from true delirium. Often a clue is the absence of any evident medical etiology in the case of pseudodelirium.

The prevalence of delirium ranges from 15% to 40% in acutely hospitalized older persons (Johnson, 1990). No studies have defined the prevalence of delirium in long-term-care settings. A number of factors appear to put persons particularly at risk for developing delirium (see Table 8.1). Up to one quarter of persons developing delirium have their acute symptoms superimposed on an underlying dementia (Lipowski, 1983). This is particularly important in nursing homes where the earliest signs of a delirium in a patient with dementia may be minor behavioral changes recognizable only to the staff providing regular care for the resident.

Delirium is commonly precipitated by the occurrence of an additional, acute event in a patient with one or more risk factors. The most consistent underlying mechanism appears to be central nervous system acetylcholine deficiency. Infections are particularly likely to precipitate delirium. This is presumably secondary to the release of cytokines such as tumor necrosis factor (cachectin) and interleukins. These cytokines are known to produce cognitive dysfunction, possibly by decreasing acetylcholine release in the hippocampus (Rada et al., 1991). Medications, particularly those with anticholinergic activity, are potent precipitators of delirium. Delirium has been demonstrated to occur more commonly in persons with high anti-

Table 8.1 Risk Factors for Delirium

Underlying structural brain disease (e.g. dementia)
Infection
Medications: Polypharmacy
            Psychoactive drugs
            Any drug
Malnutrition
Dehydration
Hyponatremia
Hypoxia

cholinergic activity in their serum (Golinger, Peet. & Tune, 1987). Hypoalbuminemia (albumin <3.0g/dl) is extremely common in persons developing delirium (Dickson, 1991; Levkoff, Safran, Cleary, Gallop, & Phillips, 1988), probably by decreasing drug binding. Dehydration and electrolyte disturbances are also often demonstrated as precipitants of a delirious episode. Acute urinary retention and bowel impaction have also been identified as a precipitant of delirium. Although they are not as common as the previously discussed conditions, it is essential to remember that an acute myocardial infarction can present with delirium as its only overt manifestation in an older patient, and an acute or chronic subdural commonly presents as delirium.

Almost every metabolic disorder has been associated with delirium. Historically, the classic example of a metabolic disturbance causing delirium is that of Mad King George of England (Sier, Hartnell, Morley, Giuliano, & Kaiser, 1988). George III reigned over Britain for 60 years from when it went from "a few islands, hardly visible on the face of the globe" to "an extent of territory unequalled in the history of nations" and a time that included the humiliating loss of the American colonies. His reign was punctuated by five episodes of major illness; with the second bout of illness he had an associated delirium. Mental disturbance was a prominent feature of his physical illnesses at 63 and 67 years of age, and he had mental abnormalities almost continually for the last 10 years of his life until his death at 82. King George's "madness" was caused by porphyria. This condition is characterized by intermittent abdominal pain, peripheral neuropathy, a photosensitive skin rash and intermittently port-wine-colored urine. The diagnosis is made by the identification of phorphobilinogen in the urine.

The metabolic conditions associated with delirium are listed in Table 8.2. Hypercalemia, particularly when due to hyperparathyroidism, is commonly associated with delirium. Psychiatric syndromes have been reported to occur in between 1% and 25% of patients with hyperparathyroid-

Table 8.2 Metabolic Causes of Delirium

Hypoxemia
Hypothermia
Hyponatremia
Dehydration
Acid base abnormalities
Uremia
Hepatic failure
Hypercalcemia/hyperparathyroidism
Hypoparathyroidism
Thyroid disorders
Hypoadrenalism
Hypopituitarism
Exogenous corticosteroids
Thiamine deficiency (Wernicke's encephalopathy)
Pellagra
Porphyria

ism and, besides delirium, include depression, memory disturbance, paranoia, delusions, and hallucinations (Alarcon & Franceschini, 1984). The
psychiatric symptoms have been reversed in 30% to 100% of cases of
hyperparathyroidism, though in some cases the reversal had taken a number of months to occur (Sier et al., 1988). Neuropsychological symptoms,
such as impairment of short-term verbal memory, cognition and verbal
reasoning, have all been objectively demonstrated to improve after surgery
(Numan, Torppa, & Bumeti, 1984) as have electroencephalographic findings (Cogan et al., 1978). There is some evidence that the neuropsychiatric
symptoms in hyperparathyroidism are related to the elevated parathor-
mone levels as much as to the elevated calcium levels (Sier et al., 1988). If
this is the case, it may be particularly important for nursing home residents, where secondary hyperparathyroidism is a common finding. These
findings suggest that careful attention should be paid to calcium levels in
all persons in nursing homes. Because calcium is bound to albumin and
albumin levels are often decreased in the long-term-care situation, a corrected calcium should be calculated utilizing the formula: corrected
calcium=total calcium (mg/dl)-albumin (mg/dl)+4.0. If the corrected
serum calcium is near the upper limits of normal and delirium is evident or
suspected, an ionized calcium should be obtained.

The approach to the management of delirium is outlined in Table 8.3. It
is extremely important to suspect the presence of infection in any resident
with an acute mental change, and empirical treatment with broad-
spectrum antibiotics is recommended if no obvious cause is present. Most
nursing home residents with infection will have at least one of hyper- or
hypothermia, elevated white cell count or a left shift. While the commonest

Table 8.3 Management of Delirium

Treat underlying illness
  Exclude infection
  Exclude urinary retention
  Exclude myocardial infarction
  Exclude hypoglycemia/if in doubt give 1 to 2 mg glucagon intramuscularly
  (IM) or oral glucose
  Exclude metabolic disorders (Table 8.2)
Provide appropriate fluid and electrolytes
Discontinue drugs (unless absolutely necessary)
Provide adequate calories and reverse hypoalbuminemia
Keep room well lighted. Provide gentle, dependable lighting and sound
Allay fears and agitation/orient
Avoid physical restraints
Provide a sitter
Only when all else fails-try haloperidol

infections in nursing home residents are urinary tract infections and lung infections, other sites to be considered include intra-abdominal, mouth, sinuses, skin (decubitus), and bone (osteomyelitis). Myocardial infarction and pulmonary embolism, both of which result in decreased cerebral perfusion, are other medical causes of acute delirium that are often missed. Discontinuing all drugs, especially those with anticholinergic activity (unless the drugs are absolutely necessary), is an important part of the acute management of delirium. Correcting fluid and electrolyte abnormalities and providing nutritional support are other important management modalities. All residents with acute delirium should have a glucose checked by chemstrip and, if there is any question of hypoglycemia, should receive oral or intravenous glucose. Should this prove to be impossible, glucagon, 1 to 2 mg intramuscularly, should be administered. Physical restraints are contraindicated, as they can make the symptoms of delirium worse (Ouslander, Osterweil, & Morley, 1991). If the delirious resident is severely agitated, low-dose haloperidol (0.5 to 1 mg two or three times per day) may be helpful until the delirium clears. Resolution of all manifestations of delirium can take several weeks after successful treatment of the precipitating processes, so family and staff should be advised to be hopeful while awaiting recovery.

DEMENTIA

Dementia is the loss of intellectual abilities of sufficient severity to impair an individual's ability to carry out his/her social or work-related functions. The majority of persons with dementia have either a progressive primary dementia (e.g., Alzheimer's disease) or multi-infarct dementia secondary to multiple small strokes. The presence of protein energy malnutrition may make the underlying dementia worse in these individuals, and this may be improved by improving the person's nutritional status. Persons with multi-infarct dementia may have the course of their disease slowed by taking one aspirin a day, stopping smoking, and having hypertension adequately treated. In all nursing home residents, the medical causes of potentially reversible dementias should have been ruled out. It should be recognized that completely reversible dementias are rare in nursing home residents. Nevertheless, appropriate management of these medical conditions may improve or delay the progressive deterioration in cognitive function. A useful mnemonic for remembering the medical causes of dementia has been developed by Peter Lamy and is given in an adapted form in Table 8.4 (Lamy, 1990). Many nursing home residents may have untreated delirium for long periods that can masquerade as dementia, and thus all the medical causes of delirium should also be considered in nursing home residents with dementia.

Table 8.4 Potentially Reversible Causes of Dementia

D	Drugs	Anticholinergics
		Cimetidine, ranitidine
		Digoxin
		Narcotics
		Nonsteroidal anti-inflammatory drugs
		Psychotropics
		Alcohol
		Antihypertensives, particularly when they induce hypotension
E	Emotional	Depression
M	Metabolic	Thyroid disease
		Hyperparathyroidism
		Hypoadrenalism
		Diabetes mellitus
		Porphyria
		Wilson's disease
E	Ear and eye impairment (sensory deprivation)	
N	Normal pressure hydrocephalus	
T	Tumors and other space-occupying lesions, e.g., subdural hematoma	
I	Infection	
A	Anemia	vitamin B_{12} deficiency
		folate deficiency

Hypothyroidism was found to be associated with decreased short-term memory in 64% of all patients in a classic study undertaken by the Clinical Society of London in 1988 (Bauer, Droba, & Whybrow, 1987). More recent studies have continued to confirm cognitive dysfunction in persons with hypothyroidism, though not all subjects improved after successful treatment of hypothyroidism. Older persons were particularly unlikely to show major improvement.

Hyperglycemia has been shown to produce a deficit in memory function in older persons with Type II diabetes mellitus (Mooradian et al., 1989; Morley & Flood, 1990). Animal studies have confirmed that hyperglycemia can both interfere with learning and retention of new facts (Flood, 1990). In noninstitutionalized subjects, the memory deficits associated with hyperglycemia appear to interfere with compliance (Rost et al., 1989).

Pernicious anemia (vitamin B_{12} deficiency) is well recognized to be associated with cognitive impairment. B_{12} deficiency has been reported to result in cognitive impairment in the absence of typical macrocytic changes in the peripheral blood smear (Strachan & Henderson, 1965). Low levels of vitamin B_{12} are also often reported in persons with Alzheimer's disease. Residents with pernicious anemia are at increased risk of developing polyglandular failure and, as such, if their cognitive impairment fails to improve after treatment with vitamin B_{12}, they should be screened for thyroid disease, hypoadrenalism, diabetes mellitus, and coeliac disease (Trence, Morley, & Handwerger, 1984). Pure folate deficiency can also result in dementia (Strachen & Henderson, 1967).

DEPRESSION

A variety of medical disorders can result in potentially curable depression (see Table 8.5). In particular, nearly one third of nursing home residents who have had a stroke will develop depression within the next two years (Fitten, Morley, Gross, Petry, & Cole, 1989). These nursing home residents need to be screened every three months for the two years following a stroke. Persons with diabetes mellitus are particularly prone to develop depression, possibly secondary to multiple small strokes and also due to the demands placed on the person to adequately manage his/her disease.

Corticotropin releasing factor (CRF) levels are increased in the cerebrospinal fluid of persons with depression (Morley, 1986). CRF appears to produce a number of the vegetative symptoms seen in persons with depression, such as anorexia, sexual dysfunction, and psychomotor retardation. Thus, it is not surprising that persons in whom CRF levels are elevated, such as those with Cushing's syndrome (in which CRF drives the release of adrenocorticotrophic hormone, or ACTH, and cortisol) and

Addison's disease (in which CRF is elevated secondary to a lack of corti-sol), tend to have a higher prevalence of depression. Addison's disease is particularly easy to miss in nursing home residents and should be sus-pected in any resident with depression or dysphoria in association with postural hypotension, blood glucose levels between 50 and 90 mg/dl, hyperkalemia, and/or hyponatremia. The diagnosis of Addison's disease can be made by administering synthetic corticotropin and then measuring the cortisol level between 30 and 60 minutes later.

A nonagitated depression occurs in approximately 9% of older persons with hyperthyroidism (Davis & Davis, 1974). These persons often have an atypical presentation of hyperthyroidism which includes weight loss, prox-imal myopathy, hooded eyes, atrial fibrillation, and heart failure. All older persons with depression should be screened for hyperthyroidism because of the difficulty in making the clinical diagnosis of apathetic hyperthyroid-ism.

SLEEP DISTURBANCES

Between 15% and 75% of older persons are unhappy with the quality and/or quantity of their sleep. Objectively, older persons tend to have more Stage 1 and Stage 2 sleep and less Stage 3 and 4 sleep. There is a reduction in rapid eye movement sleep with advancing age (Kales & Kales, 1974). Overall, older persons spend more time in bed but have less total sleep time. Older persons tend to take longer falling asleep and are more likely to have episodes of wakefulness after falling asleep. Sleep disturbances may result in psychological disturbances, or, alternatively, they may signal the onset of psychological disease (e.g., depression).

Sleep apnea is the major medical sleep disorder (Ouslander et al., 1991). It is defined as the cessation of airflow at the nose and mouth for at least a 10-second duration. Sleep apnea is more commonly observed with advanc-ing age and is commoner in residents with Alzheimer's disease, multi-infarct dementia, and depression. Sleep apnea can either be due to a central disturbance of breathing rhythm or due to occlusion of the upper airways producing obstruction or a combination of both. Sleep apnea is a potentially curable disorder whose diagnosis should not be missed.

Residents with Parkinson's disease often wake up two to three hours after going to sleep. Nocturia is an important cause of disrupted sleep. A variety of medical disorders that may alter sleeping patterns are outlined in Table 8.6. Sleep disorders may present as daytime fatigue, irritability, anxiety, difficulty concentrating, or enuresis, or may come into considera-tion in the differential diagnosis of depression.

Table 8.5 Medical Causes of Depression

Metabolic
  Hyperthyroidism (especially the apathetic form)
  Hypothyroidism
  Hyperparathyroidism
  Diabetes mellitus
  Addison's disease
  Cushing's disease
Chronic Infections
Malnutrition
Tumors
  Central nervous system
  Pancreatic carcinoma
  Other
Electrolyte imbalance/dehydration
Medications
  Propranolol
  Methyldopa
  Indomethacin
  Narcotics
  Digoxin
  Amantadine
  Neuroleptics
  Benzodiazepines

ANXIETY AND PANIC DISORDERS

Anxiety and panic disorder are not rare in older persons. There is a marked increase in the prevalence of both of these disorders in females over 80 years of age.

  Pheochromocytoma is a tumor of the adrenal medulla or sympathetic ganglia that produces catecholamines (Krahn & Morley, 1987). The syndrome produced by pheochromocytomas has been characterized as the panic syndrome. These persons present with anxiety, hyperventilation, tachycardia, palpitations, paroxysmal or sustained hypertension, excessive sweating, and occasionally elevated glucose levels. The diagnosis of pheochromocytoma is made by obtaining three 24-hour urine specimens for metanephrines, vanillylmandelic acid, or normetanephrines. An elevated level of catecholamines or their metabolites makes the diagnosis likely. At this stage a computerized tomography (CT) scan should be obtained in an attempt to localize the tumor. Recently, it has been reported that pheochromocytoma occurs as commonly in older persons as in young persons but that the diagnosis is rarely made (Stenstrom & Svardsudd, 1986). In any nursing home resident with weight loss and failure of his/her

Table 8.6 Medical Conditions that May Interfere with Sleep in Older Persons

A. Difficulty in falling asleep or maintaining sleep

1. Iatrogenesis:
    Resident being awakened after falling asleep at night (e.g., for medication dosage)
    Drugs   caffeine
            theophylline
            corticosteroids
            beta-blockers
            alcohol or sedative/hypnotic withdrawal
            diuretics
2. Heart failure
            paroxsymal nocturnal dyspnea
            orthopnea
            nocturia
3. Pain
4. Esophageal reflux
5. Hyperthyroidism
6. Parkinson's disease
7. Venous insufficiency causing nocturia
8. Exacerbation of chronic obstructive pulmonary disease

B. Hypersomnolence

1. Sleep apnea
2. Nocturnal myoclonus
3. Drugs   sedative/hypnotics
            antihistamines
            methyldopa
            trazadone

hypertension to improve in association with the weight loss, the diagnosis of pheochromocytoma should be entertained.

Hyperthyroidism is classically associated with anxiety, nervousness, irritability, palpitations, tachycardia and, increased sweating. With advancing age most of these symptoms become less common; for example, irritability occurs in 47% of hyperthyroid persons in the second decade and only in 18% of those in the eighth decade (Nordyke, Gilbert & Harada, 1988). On the other hand, nervousness remains as common up to the end of the seventh decade, and this symptom is only slightly decreased in the eighth decade.

Numerous other medical disorders have been associated with either anxiety or panic disorders in older persons (Grossberg et al., 1990). These include cardiovascular and respiratory disorders and anemia. Of the drug-induced causes, theophylline is one of the commonest observed in the long-term-care setting.

SENSORY DEPRIVATION SYNDROME

Our senses are constantly bombarded by a series of stimuli. When college students were deprived of sensory stimuli in their environment, they had a deterioration of cognitive abilities within 24 hours, and by 48 hours they developed hallucinations and perceptual disorders. A sensory deprivation syndrome commonly occurs in persons in the long-term-care setting. Features of this syndrome include decreased quality of life, decreased cognition, hallucinations, perceptual distortions, delusions, emotional lability, passive behavior, altered body image, and in some instances, agitation (Ouslander, et al., 1991). Even good long-term-care institutions tend to promote states of inactivity that interact with age-related perceptual changes to result in the development of a sensory deprivation syndrome.

Approximately 46% of nursing home residents have hearing impairment, and 25% of nursing home residents are legally blind. Besides the general sensory deprivation syndrome that occurs when there is decreased sensory stimuli, there are also a number of specific behavioral syndromes that have been described. Older residents with deteriorating hearing have been reported to develop musical hallucinations (Gilchrist & Kalucy, 1983). Residents with age-related macular degeneration may develop a series of visual hallucinations or delusions that can masquerade as psychosis or result in altered behavior and the development of a neurosis (Casey & Wandzilak, 1988). Finally, the isolation produced by deteriorating hearing and vision can lead to a form of depression, similar to the anaclitic depression seen in infants when they are deprived of the attention of a suitable mother figure (Keckich & Young, 1983).

It is particularly important that physicians recognize that nearly a quarter of nursing home residents with hearing impairment have cerumen impaction as a cause. Following well-established guidelines for improving communication for hearing-impaired nursing home residents (Vocks, Gallagher, Langer, & Drinka, 1990) and adaptive strategies to compensate for visual problems (Hooyman & Lustbader, 1986) will decrease the possibility of the sensory deprivation syndromes developing.

CONCLUSION

Medical disorders commonly result in behavioral disorders in long-term-care settings. The physician needs to carefully search for medical triggers of these behavioral disorders before treating the condition as a psychiatric disorder. Certain relatively common medical disorders, such as occult infections, thyroid disorders, protein energy malnutrition, and hypercalcemia, appear to be capable of generating a variety of behavioral patterns and should be carefully screened for in nursing home residents. Medications commonly produce behavioral disorders in nursing home residents and should be discontinued whenever possible when a resident develops an unusual behavior.

REFERENCES

Alarcon, R., & Franceschini, J. (1984). Hyperparathyroidism and paranoid psychoses: Case report and review of the literature. *British Journal of Psychiatry*, *145*, 479–484.

Bauer, M. S., Droba, M., & Whybrow, P. C. (1987). Disorders of the thyroid and parathyroid. In C. B. Nemeroff & P. T. Loosen (Eds.), *Handbook of clinical psychoneuroendocrinology* (pp. 41–70). New York: Guilford Press.

Casey, D. A., & Wandzilak, T. (1988). Senile macular degeneration and psychosis. *Journal of Geriatric Psychiatry*, *1*, 108–109.

Cogan, M., Corey, C., Arieff, A., Wisnewski, A., & Clark O. H. (1978). Central nervous system manifestations of hyperparathyroidism. *American Journal of Medicine*, *65*, 963–967.

Davis, P. J., & Davis, F. B. (1974). Hyperthyroidism in patients over the age of 60 years. *Medicine*, *53*, 161–181.

Dickson, L. R. (1991). Hypoalbuminemia in delirium. *Psychosomatics*, *32*, 317–322.

Fitten, L. J., Morley, J. E., Gross, P. L., Petry, S. D., & Cole, K. D. (1989). Depression. *Journal of the American Geriatrics Society*, *37*, 459–472.

Flood, J. F., Mooradian, A. D., & Morley, J. E. (1990). Characteristics of learning and memory in streptozotocin-induced diabetic mice. *Diabetes*, *39*, 1391–1398.

Gilchrist, P. N., & Kalucy, R. S. (1983). Musical hallucinations in the elderly: A variation on the theme. *Australian and New Zealand Journal of Medicine*, *17*, 286–291.

Golinger, R. C., Peet, T., & Tune, L. E. (1987). Association of elevated plasma anticholinergic activity with delirium in surgical patients. *American Journal of Psychiatry*, *144*, 1218–1220.

Grossberg, G. T., Hassan, R., Szwabo, P. A., Morley, J. E., Nakra, B. R. S., Bretscher, C. W., Zimny, G. H., & Solomon, K. (1990). Psychiatric problems in the nursing home. *Journal of the American Geriatrics Society*, *38*, 907–917.

Hood, P. (1970). On senile delirium. *The Practitioner*, *5*, 279–289,

Hooyman, N. R., & Lustbader, W. (1986). *Taking care of your aging family members*. New York: The Free Press.

Johnson, J. C. (1990). Delirium in the elderly. *Emergency Medicine Clinics of North America*, *8*, 255–265.

Kales, A., & Kales, J. (1974). Sleep disorders: Recent findings in the diagnosis and treatment of disturbed sleep. *New England Journal of Medicine*, *290*, 487–491.

Keckich, W. A., & Young, M. (1983). Anaclitic depression in the elderly. *Psychiatric Annals*, *13*, 691–696.

Krahn, D. D., & Morley, J. E. (1987). Endocrinology for the psychiatrist. In C. B. Nemeroff, P. T. Loosen (Eds) *Handbook of clinical psychoneuroendocrinology*, pp. 3–40, New York: Guilford Press.

Lamy, P. P. (1990). *Prescribing for the elderly*. Littleton Mass: PSG Publishing.

Levkoff, S. E., Safran, C., Cleary, P. D., Gallop, J., & Phillips, R. S. (1988). Identification of factors associated with the diagnosis of delirium in elderly hospitalized patients. *Journal of the American Geriatrics Society, 36*, 1099–1104.

Lipowski, Z. J. (1989). Delirium in the elderly patient. *New England Journal of Medicine, 320*, 578–582.

Lipowski, Z. J. (1983). Transient cognitive disorders (delirium, acute confusional states) in the elderly. *American Journal of Psychiatry, 140*, 1426–1436.

Mooradian, A. D., Perryman, K., Fitten, J., Kovonian, G. D., & Morley, J. E. (1984). Cortical function in elderly non-insulin-dependent diabetic patients. *American Journal of Medicine, 77*, 1043–1048.

Morley, J. E., & Flood, J. F. (1990). Psychosocial aspects of diabetes mellitus in older persons. *Journal of the American Geriatrics Society, 38*, 605–606.

Morley, J. E. (1986). Neuropeptides, behavior and aging. *Journal of the American Geriatrics Society, 34*, 52–61.

Nordyke, R. A., Gilbert, F. I., & Harada, A. S. M. (1988). Graves' disease: Influence of age on clinical findings. *Archives of Internal Medicine, 148*, 626–631.

Numan, P., Torppa, A., & Blumeti, A. (1984). Neuropsychologic deficits associated with primary hyperparathyroidism. *Surgery, 96*, 1119–1123.

Ouslander, J. G., Osterweil, D., Morley, J. E. (1991). *Medical care in the nursing home*, New York: McGraw-Hill Inc.

Pickett, W. (1904). Senile dementia: A clinical study of two hundred cases with particular regard to types of the disease. *Journal of Nervous and Mental Disorders, 31*, 81–88.

Rada, P., Mark, G. P., Vitek, M. P., Magano, R. M., Blume, A. J., Beer, B., & Itopbel, B. G. (1991). Interleukin-1B decreases acetylcholine measured by microdialyses in the hippocampus of freely moving rats. *Brain Research, 550*, 287–290.

Rost, K., Rotter, D., & Quill, T. (1989). Recall of prescription medication changes. *Diabetes, 38*(Suppl 2), 40.

Sier, H. C., Hartnell, J., Morley, J. E., Giuliano, A. E., & Kaiser, F. E. (1988). Primary hyperparathyroidism and delirium in the elderly. *Journal of the American Geriatrics Society, 36*, 157–170.

Stenstrom, G., & Svardsudd, K. (1986). Pheochromocytoma in Sweden 1958–1981: An analysis of the national cancer registry data. *ACTA Medica Scandanavia, 220*, 225–232.

Strachan, R. W., & Henderson, J. G. (1965). Psychiatric syndromes due to avitaminosis B[12] with normal blood and marrow. *Quarterly Journal of Medicine, 34*, 303–325.

Strachen, R. W., & Henderson, J. G. (1967). Dementia and folate deficiency. *Quarterly Journal Medicine, 36*, 189–198.

Trence, D. L., Morley, J. E., & Handwerger, B. S. (1984). Polyglandular autoimmune syndromes. *American Journal of Medicine, 77*, 107–115.

Vocks, S. V., Gallagher, C. M., Langer, E. M., & Drinka, P. J. (1990). Hearing loss in the nursing home. *Journal of the American Geriatrics Society, 38*, 141–144.

9

Diagnosis and Treatment of Delirium in the Nursing Home

Sanford I. Finkel

WHAT IS DELIRIUM?

The concept of delirium dates back to the Greek and Roman medical writers, 2,500 years ago (Lipowski, 1980, 1990). The specific term *delirium* was elaborated by Celsus almost 2,000 years ago. In the intervening millennium, almost two dozen terms have been used to describe the syndrome of delirium, including "acute confusional state," "acute organic brain syndrome," "acute brain failure," "toxic confusion," "acute organic psychosis," "reversible brain disorder," and "metabolic encephalopathy" (Conn, 1991; Lindesay, MacDonald, & Starke, 1990; Listen, 1982). Delirium emanates from the Latin, "away from" and lira, "off a track in the fields." Thus, delirium is to "be off the track" (Henderson, 1991).

Medical writers of the 18th century described and elaborated the clinical presentations of delirium (Hartley, 1966). Delirium has been described as a reduction in consciousness. The concept of "clouding of consciousness" consolidated in the 19th century. The term *confusion* began to be utilized in that century and is still used in clinical practice, in spite of its vagueness (Lipowski, 1990; Simpson, 1984). Doctors and nurses often use the word *confused* when describing delirium patients (Lipowski, 1990).

A major breakthrough in the understanding of delirium occurred in the 1940s (Engel & Romano, 1959). Their clinical and experimental work demonstrated that delirium was characterized by both attention and cognitive disturbances. Further, they demonstrated that there was a slowing of EEG background activity, thereby demonstrating a reduction in the brain metabolic rate. Finally, they demonstrated that the greater the EEG slowing, the greater the deficits. Attention, memory, and thinking were all correlated with EEG slowing. Lass, Gibson, Duffy, and Plum (1981), hypothesized a reduced synthesis of acetylcholine and other neurotransmitters as a result of a reduction of oxydated metabolism in the brain.

In the 1980s, delirium was classified in DSM-III (American Psychiatric Association, 1980) and DSM-III-R (American Psychiatric Association, 1987) as an organic mental disorder whose essential feature is a psychological or behavioral abnormality associated with transient or permanent dysfunction of the brain. Delirium can occur secondary to many causes. Thus, it is described as the syndrome, rather than a specific organic mental disorder.

The DSM-III-R diagnostic criteria for delirium are as follows:

1. Reduced ability to maintain attention to external stimuli (e.g., questions must be repeated because attention wanders) and to appropriately shift attention to new external stimuli (e.g., perseverates answer to a previous question).
2. Disorganized thinking, as indicated by rambling, irrelevant, or incoherent speech.
3. At least two of the following:
    (a) reduced level of consciousness, e.g., difficulty keeping awake during examination;
    (b) perceptual disturbances: misinterpretations, illusions, or hallucinations;
    (c) disturbance of sleep-wake cycle with insomnia or daytime sleepiness;
    (d) increased or decreased psychomotor activity;
    (e) disorientation to time, place, or person;
    (f) memory impairment, e.g., inability to learn new material, such as the names of several unrelated objects after five minutes, or to remember past events, such as history of current episode or illness;
4. Clinical features develop over a short period of time (usually hours to days) and tend to fluctuate over the course of a day.
5. Either (a) or (b):
    (a) evidence from their history, physical examination, or laboratory tests of a specific organic factor (or factors) judged to be etiologically related to the disturbance;

(b) in the absence of such evidence, an etiologic organic factor can be presumed if the disturbance cannot be accounted for by any nonorganic mental disorder, e.g., manic episode accounting for agitation and sleep disturbance.

HOW COMMON IS DELIRIUM IN THE NURSING HOME?

Epidemiological data on delirium in late life are sparse. Gillick (Gillick, Serrell, & Gillick, 1982) reported an incidence of delirium of at least 30% in medical and surgical patients in a general hospital. Yet Henker (1979) in a retrospective review of hospital charts, found that fewer than 1% of all patients had a diagnosis of delirium. This strongly suggests that delirium is overlooked.

There is ample evidence that delirium occurs more commonly in older patients than in younger ones, but this may be a result of sensory impairment, brain disease, or toxicity secondary to medication. Old age itself does not directly predispose to delirium (Davison, 1989; Folstein, Bassett, Romanski, Anthony, & Nestadt, 1991; Lipowski, 1980) examined the prevalence of delirium in the general adult population from 3,841 households in the 1981 East Baltimore Mental Health Survey, which was part of the Epidemiological Catchment Area (ECA) program. For those over 55 years of age, the prevalence of delirium was 1.1%. This compares with 0.4% for the population as a whole. Those with a diagnosis of delirium had a greater number of medical illnesses, took more prescription medications, and had a higher level of physical disability.

Rovner and his colleagues, in their classic studies on psychiatric illness in nursing homes (Rovner, Kafonek, Philipp, Luckes, & Folstein, 1986; Rovner, et al., 1990), determine prevalence of DSM-III-R delirium. In one study (1986), three of fifty residents (6%) were diagnosed as having delirium as a result of drug intoxication. Another study (1990) revealed that 7.3% (33 of 454 patients) from eight different nursing homes had a diagnosis of delirium, often secondary to complications of dementia. Bienenfeld and Wheeler (1989) studied a consecutive series of referrals to a psychiatric consultation-liaison nursing home service and found that 6% of residents were diagnosed as delirious. Katz, Parmalee, and Brubacker (1991) found that of 157 patients followed for one year, that 6% to 12% had a reversible component of their cognitive impairment. Review of records indicates that six suffered from adverse drug effects, two were depressed, and three demonstrated impairment secondary to metabolic encephalopathies.

Katz emphasizes that although reversible cognitive impairment occurs commonly in long-term-care residents, the sensitivity and specificity of the symptoms of delirium as markers for reversible forms of cognitive impairment have not been established. False positives may occur on a resident with irreversible dementia who presents with apathetic withdrawal, sleep disturbance, and anxiety. False negatives will occur when reversible cognitive disorders may be manifested by symptoms of dementia.

Katz's sample revealed that not only psychotropic medications, such as Diazepam and Flurazepam, contributed or caused delirium, but drugs utilized for the treatment of physical illnesses, for example, Cimetidine, Amantadine, Digoxin, and Alpha-Methyldopa, may be causal. There are many explanations for the prevalence of delirium in at least 6% in this nursing home survey: vulnerability of residents who have multiple chronic illnesses and disability, extreme old age, and increased sensitivity to medication. Further, case identification is more difficult in a population in which 75% demonstrate cognitive deterioration, many from Alzheimer's disease or multi-infarct dementia.

Larson, Kukall, Buchner, & Reiffler (1987) discovered that 10% of patients who were evaluated for dementia experienced toxic effects to medication that either caused or contributed to cognitive impairment. This included nonpsychotropic medication as well as psychotropic medication. Katz (1991) calls our attention to the fact that in 1989, 72 of the 200 most prescribed medications have confusion or disorientation listed as adverse side effects in the Physician's Desk Reference (1990).

WHAT CAUSES DELIRIUM IN NURSING HOME RESIDENTS?

The factors which contribute to delirium can be divided into two types: predisposing or precipitating. The predisposing factors increase the person's vulnerability to an actual precipitating cause. Thus, factors such as sensory impairment, psychiatric disorders, and bereavement are contributing, but not causal, factors. On the other hand, physical illness and/or toxic reactions to medication are considered precipitants (Grimley, 1982; Lipowski, 1980a; Lindesay, McDonald, & Starke, 1990).

Yet, in as many as 41% of cases, no obvious causal factor may be determined (Sirois, 1988). Further, Koponen (1989) attributed 9% of cases of delirium to psychological and environmental stress caused by a major life change in a demented patient. Moreover, 4% of his sample of delirious patients were attributed to affective psychosis.

Medication is believed to be a major causative factor of delirium in late life. Sixteen percent of Cutting's population had delirium secondary to medication (Cutting, 1980). In an additional 27% medication was thought to be a contributory factor. Tune and Bylsma (1991) reviewed the role of benzodiazepines and anticholinergic medication in the elderly and found them to be a significant contributing factor. Pomara, et al., (1985) demonstrated that even in healthy elderly subjects, there is delayed visual memory recall, delayed verbal learning, and decreased reaction time, compared to younger subjects.

It is well known that elderly persons are particularly at risk for cognitive deficits in response to anticholinergic medication. Blazer, Federspiel, & Ray (1983) studied 5,902 nursing home residents and found that 60% were receiving an anticholinergic medication. This compared to 23% of elderly controls. Further, 10% to 17% of the nursing home residents received three or more anticholinergic medications in a single year. Moreover, 5% received five or more anticholinergic medications.

There is a significant correlation between elevated serum levels of anticholinergic medication, as measured by radioreceptorassay, and cognitive impairment, which includes delirium. Tune and Coyle (1981) noted that seven of eight delirious patients had significantly elevated serum anticholinergic drug levels which correlated highly with the decline in the Mini Mental State Examination (MMSE).

Dopamine agonists, such as levodopa and bromocriptine, are also known to produce hallucinations in elderly patients with Parkinson's disease. Certain antihypertensive medication may cause hypercalemia and thus delirium. Medications that may produce arrythmia also contribute to delirium.

Infection is a common cause of delirium in nursing home elderly, but it may be more difficult to diagnose. One does not always find fever in conjunction with infection, and white blood cell count may not be as high as it would be with a younger individual with infection. However, viral gastroenteritis (which contributes to electrolyte imbalance and dehydration), urinary tract infection, and pneumonia are all common causes of delirium in nursing home elderly. Other less common infections include septicemia, meningitis, encephalitis, and infections secondary to gangrene.

Metabolic etiologies include uncontrolled diabetes mellitus, hypercalcemia, and dehydration. Hypothyroidism, hyperthyroidism, Addison's disease, and hypopituitarism also cause delirium. Hypothermia, vitamin deficiencies—especially thiamine—renal failure, hepatic failure, and malnutrition are other metabolic causes.

Congestive heart failure was found to account for 24% of all cases of delirium in Hodkinson's sample (1973). Cerebral vascular accidents, pulmonary emboli, and anemia are additional causes. In one sample, (Dunne, Leedman, & Edis, 1986) 13% of major strokes presented as delirium. Brain tumors and intra-abdominal pathology are other causes. Alcohol and drug abuse are generally not looked for in a nursing home setting.

Psychiatric and neurologic disorders predispose to delirium. Kopone and colleagues have demonstrated a greater frequency of dementia and Parkinson's disease in patients with delirium (Kopone, Hurrill, Stenback et al., 1989). Some clinicians believe that depression and anxiety also predispose to delirium. Others have hypothesized that impaired vision and hearing may do so as well (Lipowski, 1983).

Kennedy (1959) hypothesized that bereavement and relocation—such as to a nursing home—predisposes to delirium in vulnerable elderly. Rabins (1991), in his review of psychosocial contributants to delirium, concludes that there is empiric evidence that psychosocial factors contribute to the precipitation to delirium, though scientific support for this belief is lacking.

CLINICAL FEATURES

Because the delirious resident may have a rapidly changing level of attention and may demonstrate symptoms of memory impairment, it is critical to obtain a collateral history from the nursing staff and family members. A review of the chart with particular attention to medications is mandatory. So are the results of a physical examination, as well as basic laboratory tests which would include a complete blood count (CBC), erythrocyte sedimentation rate, blood chemistry, urinalysis, chest X-ray, and electrocardiogram.

Other laboratory studies which may be helpful include an electroencephalogram, computerized tomography (CT) scan or magnetic resonance imaging (MRI) scan of the head, tests for syphilis, toxicology screen of blood/urine, thyroid function studies, vitamin B_{12} and folate levels, cerebrospinal fluid examination, and urine test for porphobilinogen. Chedru and Geschwind (1972) describe major abnormalities in writing ability in patients with delirium. Tests for visual/spatial ability and motor fluency show that these are invariably impaired.

The DSM-III-R criteria for diagnosing delirium have been previously described. It is important to note that the clinical picture often denotes widespread abnormalities in brain functioning.

Gottlieb, Johnson, Wanich, & Sullivan (1991) operationalized definitions for the following DSM-III criteria, including both presence and severity:

1. Clouding of consciousness
2. Perceptual disturbances
3. Coherence
4. Disturbances of the sleep/wake cycle

5. Increased psychomotor activity
6. Ratings of disorientation and memory impairment
7. Acuity of onset
8. Fluctuation

Their data analysis revealed that the DSM-III criteria described a discrete, recognizable syndrome.

Ross and colleagues (1991) categorized patients with delirium as "activator" (relatively alert, despite clouding of consciousness) or "somnolent" (relatively stuporous along with clouding of consciousness). They determined that the activated patients were more likely to have delusions, hallucinations, illusions, and agitated behavior compared to somnolent patients. Patients with alcohol withdrawal were more likely to have activated delirium, whereas patients with hepatic encephalopathy were more likely to have somnolent delirium. These different subtypes suggest different pathophysiology, and perhaps different management and treatment.

A variety of evaluation screenings has been utilized, although many are unable to consistently differentiate delirium from dementia. These include the Mini Mental State Evaluation (Folstein, Folstein, & McHugh, 1975), the Short Portable Mental Status Questionnaire (Pfeiffer, 1975), and the Cognitive Capacity Examination (Jacobs, Bernhard, Delgado, & Strain, 1977).

A variety of symptom-rating scales have attempted to operationalize delirium. These include the Confusion Rating Scale (Williams, 1991; Williams, Ward, & Campbell, 1986), the NEECHAM Confusion Scale (Champaign, Neelon, McConnell, & Funk, 1987; Lowy, Engelsmann, & Lipowski, 1973) and the Delirium Rating Scale (Trzepacz, Baker, & Greenhouse, 1988). Cognitive screening is underutilized in clinical practice, despite its helpfulness in establishing the presence of cognitive impairment. It is not clear that any one test is more useful than others in detecting delirium for either clinical or research purposes. At the same time, they may be used in combination with each other and with clinical interviews and review of medical records to establish a diagnosis of delirium. Fogel and Faust have devised a High Sensitivity Cognitive Screen (HSCS) to more accurately test for delirium (Fogel, 1991; Fogel & Faust, 1989). This test takes 25 minutes and consists of a series of moderately difficult items testing memory, language, attention/concentration, visual/motor skills, spatial awareness, and self-regulation and planning.

TREATMENT AND MANAGEMENT

Two goals toward managing delirium are the treatment of the causes of the delirium, as well as a reduction in the resident's symptoms and suffering.

Supportive care is essential (Conn, 1991). This would include appropriate nutrition, fluids, sedation, and nursing care. There must be careful attention to the environment, which would include a well-lit room, photographs of the family, familiar personal possessions, and rapid availability of communication, reassurance, and social contact for the resident with delirium. Contact with caregivers may be critical, both in alleviating their anxiety and facilitating their communication with the resident. Psychiatric consultation is often necessary and useful.

It is imperative to treat the underlying medical disorder—such as infection, acute myocardial infarction, malnutrition, and other medical etiologies.

Medications are an extremely common cause of potentially reversible cognitive impairment, although it should be noted that residents may refuse to have their medications reduced, and, in fact, may seek out another physician's care if their own physician insists on medication reduction (Kroenke & Pinholt, 1990).

Certain symptoms, such as agitation and hallucinations, may be alleviated or reversed by psychotropic medication. Small doses of short-acting benzodiazepines or neuroleptics often decrease signs of psychosis, insomnia, and anxiety. In general, it is preferable for the resident to be treated in the nursing home, as opposed to experiencing a transfer to a hospital—a new environment—with all the unfamiliarity and overstimulation that such a transfer would cause. In general, the patient is under less stress with a staff and a room that is familiar, a routine that is well known, and a minimum of disruption.

OUTCOME

The outcome for patients with delirium is typically complete recovery or death. Roth (1955) described a population with delirium where 40% were dead within six months. This was similar to results found by Rabins and Folstein (1982). One third of the population of delirious patients followed by Bedford (1959) died within a month. Bergmann and Eastham's (1974) study revealed a mortality rate of 37.5%. One quarter of Hodkinson's delirious patients died within a month (Hodkinson, 1973). On the other hand, those that survived, did well. Eighty percent of Bedford's survivals recovered within less than a month, and approximately 5% were subacutely ill. Thirty-five percent of Hodkinson's group significantly improved within a month, as did 44% in Bergmann and Eastham's group. Rockwood (1989) reported an 80% recovery rate. Lindesay et al. (1990) pointed out that "since much of the delirium experienced by elderly patients is mild, transient, and undetected, these reported recovery and discharge rates are probably underestimates." Delirium is also likely to increase the length of hospital stay and thus the cost of care (Thomas, Cameron, & Fahs, 1988).

FUTURE RESEARCH DIRECTIONS

What research questions need to be answered regarding nursing home residents? They include:

1. What percentage of residents with delirium are not diagnosed?
2. What contributes to this missed diagnosis? To what extent is it related to clinical acumen?
3. What is the role of psychosocial stress in contributing to delirium in nursing home residents?
4. What are other risk factors for nursing home residents?
5. How do we develop and validate a sound diagnostic scale for delirium?
6. How does delirium in nursing home residents differ from delirium in noninstitutionalized elderly? How does it differ from delirium in younger individuals?
7. How do we design a more effective management and treatment approach?

CONCLUSION

Delirium is a consistent finding in nursing home populations. Medications are a common etiology, but probably represent a minority of cases. Research in this area has been difficult due to the fact that the concept of delirium—though one that has been with us since ancient times—has been most difficult to operationalize. Proper diagnosis and treatment are critical; otherwise, excess disability and premature mortality are expected. The growing attention to this important syndrome bodes well for earlier diagnosis and treatment as well as for better diagnostic and management approaches.

REFERENCES

Altenberg, J., & Brockhaus, B. (1932). In J. Taylor (Ed.), *A treatise on frenzy selected writing*. London: Gardner.
American druggist, physicians desk reference. (1990, February). The top 200 drugs of 1989 (pp. 26–39), 4th Ed. Montvale, NJ: Medical Economics.

Lipowski, Z. J. (1980a). *Delirium: Acute brain failure in man.* Springfield, IL: C. C. Thomas.

Lipowski, Z. J. (1983). Transient cognitive disorders in the elderly. *American Journal of Psychiatry, 140,* 1426–1436.

Bedford, P. B. (1959). General medical aspects of confusional states in elderly people. *British Medical Journal, ii,* 185–188.

Bergmann, K., & Eastham, E. J. (1974). Psychogeriatric ascertainment and assessment for treatment in an acute medial setting. *Age and Ageing, 3,* 174–188.

Bienenfeld, D., & Wheeler, B. G. (1989). Psychiatric services to nursing homes: A liaison model. *Hospital and Community Psychiatry, 40,* 793–794.

Blazer, D. G., Federspiel, C. F., & Ray, W. A. (1983). The risk of anticholinergic toxicity in the elderly: A study of prescribing practices in two populations. *Journal of Gerontology, 38,* 31–35.

Champaign, E. T., Neelon, V. J., McConnell, E. S., & Funk, S. (1987, October special 4a). The NEECHAM Confusion Scale: Assessing acute confusion in the hospitalized and nursing home elderly. *The Gerontologist, 27.*

Chedru, F., & Geschwind, N. (1972). Writing disturbances in acute confusional states. *Neuropsychologia, 10,* 343–353.

Conn, D. K., Listen, E. H., Lindesay, J., MacDonald, A., & Starke, I. (1991). Delirium and other organic mental disorders. In J. Sadavoy, L. Lazarus, & L. Jarvik (Eds.), *Comprehensive review of geriatric psychiatry* pp. (311–321). Washington, DC: American Psychiatric Press.

Cutting, J. (1980). Physical illness and psychosis. *British Journal of Psychiatry, 136,* 109–119.

Davison, K. (1989). Acute organic brain syndromes. *British Journal of Hospital Medicine, 41,* 89–92.

American Psychiatric Association. (1980). *Diagnostic and statistical manual of mental disorders* (3rd ed.). Washington, DC: Author.

American Psychiatric Association. (1987). *Diagnostic and statistical manual of mental disorders* (3rd ed., rev.). Washington, DC: Author.

Dunne, J. W., Leedman, P. J., & Edis, R. H. (1986). In-Obvious stroke: the cause of delirium and dementia. *Australian and New Zealand Journal of Medicine, 16,* 771–778.

Engel, G. L., & Romano, J. (1959). Delirium, the syndrome of cerebral insufficiency. *Journal of Chronic Diseases, 9,* 260–277.

Fogel, B. S., & Faust, D. (1989). The development and initial validation of a sensitive bedside cognitive screening test. *Journal of Nervous and Mental Disease, 177,* 25–31.

Fogel, B. S. (1991). The high sensitivity cognitive screen. *International Psychogeriatrics. 3*(2), pp. 273–288.

Folstein, M. F., Bassett, S. S., Romanski, A. J., Anthony, J., & Nestadt, G. (1991). The epidemiology of delirium in the community: The Eastern Baltimore Mental Health Survey. *International Psychogeriatrics.* 169–176.

Folstein, M. F., Folstein, S. E., & McHugh, P. R. (1975). Mini mental state examination: A practical method for grading the cognitive state of patients for the clinician. *Journal of Psychiatric Research, 12,* 189–198.

Gillick, M. R., Serrell, N. A., & Gillick, L. S. (1982). Adverse consequences of hospitalization in the elderly. *Social Science Medicine, 16,* 133–138.

Gottlieb, G. L., Johnson, J., Wanich, C., & Sullivan, E. (1991). Delirium in the medically ill elderly: Operationalizing the DSM-III criteria. *International Psychogeriatrics.* 181–196.

Grimley, E. J. (1982). The psychiatric aspects of physical disease. In R. Levy and F. Post (Eds.), *The psychiatry of late life* (pp.114–142). Oxford, England: Blackwell Scientific Publications.

Hartley, D. (1966 reprint). *Observations on man, his frame, his duty, and his expectations* (Vols. 1–2). In History of Psychiatry—Series, 6th Ed. Delmar, NY: Ibis Publishers School of Facsimilies & reprints.

Henderson, A. S. (1991). Delirium. *International Psychogeriatrics.* 349–352.

Henker, F. O. (1979). Acute brain syndrome. *Journal of Clinical Psychiatry, 40,* 117–120.

Hodkinson, H. M. (1973). Mental impairment in the elderly. *Journal of the Royal College of Physicians, 7,* 305–317.

Jacobs, J. W., Bernhard, M. R., Delgado, A., & Strain, J. J. (1977). Screening for organic mental syndromes in the medically ill. *Annals of Internal Medicine, 86,* 40–46.

Katz, I. R., Parmalee, P., & Brubacker, K. (1991). Toxic and metabolic encephalopathies in long-term patients. *International Psychogeriatrics,* 337–348.

Kennedy, A. (1959). Psychological factors in confusional states in the elderly. *Gerontology Clinics, 1,* 71–82.

Koponen, H., Hurril, L., Stenback, U., & Riekkinen, P. J. (1987). Acute confusional states in the elderly: A radiological evaluation. *Acta Psychiatrica Scandinavia, 76,* 726–731.

Koponen, H., Hurrill, L., Stenback, U., Mattila, E., Soininen, H., & Riekkinen, P. J. (1989). Computed tomography findings in delirium. *Journal of Nervous and Mental Disease, 177,* 226–231.

Koponen, H., Stenback, U., & Mattila, E., Soininen, H., Reininkainen, K., & Riekkinen, P. J. (1989). Delirium in elderly persons admitted to a psychiatric hospital: Clinical course during the acute stage and one-year follow-up. *Acta Psychiatrica Scandinavica, 79,* 579–585.

Kroenke, L. T., & Pinholt, D. M. (1990). Reducing polypharmacy in the elderly. *Journal of the American Geriatrics Society, 38,* 31–36.

Larson, E. B., Kukall, W. A., Buchner, D., & Reiffler, B. V. (1987). Adverse drug reactions associated with global cognitive impairment of elderly persons. *Annals of Internal Medicine, 107,* 169–173.

Lass, J. P., Gibson, G. E., Duffy, T. E., & Plum, F. (1981). Cholinergic dysfunction: A common denominator in metabolic encephalopathies. In G. Pepeu & H. Ladinsky. (Eds.), *Cholinergic mechanisms,* New York: Plenum Press.

Leake. F. L., & Greiner, F. C. (1917). *Der traum und das fieberhafte irresein.* Altenberg: Brockhaus Frings.

Lindesay, J., MacDonald, A., & Starke, I. (1990). *Delirium in the elderly.* London: Oxford Medical Publications.

Lipowski, Z. J. (1989). Delirium in the elderly patient, *New England Journal of Medicine, 320,* 578–582.

Lipowski, Z. J. (1980b). Delirium updated. *Comprehensive Psychiatry, 21*, 190–6.

Lipowski, Z. J. (1990). *Delirium: Acute confusional states.* New York: Oxford University Press.

Lipowski, Z. J. (1991). How its concept has developed. *International Psychogeriatrics.* 115–120.

Listen, E. H. (1982). Delirium in the aged. *Psychiatric Clinics of North America, 5*, 49–66.

Lowy, F. H., Engelsmann, F., & Lipowski, Z. J. (1973). Study of cognitive functioning in a medical population. *Comprehensive Psychiatry, 14*, 331–338.

Pfeiffer, D. (1975). A short portable mental status questionnaire for the assessment of organic brain deficit in elderly patients. *Journal of the American Geriatrics Society, 23*, 433–441.

Pomara, N., Stanley, B., Block, R., Berchou, R. C., Greenblatt, S. M., Newton, R. E., & Dershan, S. (1985). Increased sensitivity of the elderly to the central depressant effects of diazepam. *Journal of Clinical Psychiatry, 46*, 185–187.

Rabins, P. V. (1991). Psychosocial and management aspects of delirium. *International Psychogeriatrics.* 319–324.

Rabins, P. V., & Folstein, M. F. (1982). Delirium and dementia: Diagnostic criteria and fatality rates. *British Journal of Psychiatry, 140*, 149–153.

Rockwood, K. (1989). Acute confusion in elderly medical patients. *Journal of the American Geriatrics Society, 37*, 150–154.

Ross, C. A., Peyser, C. E., Shapiro, I., & Folstein, M. F. (1991). Delirium: The phenomenologic and etiologic subtypes. *International Psychogeriatrics.* 135–148.

Roth, M. (1955). Natural history of mental disorder in old age. *Journal of Mental Science, 101*, 281–301.

Rovner, B. W., German, P. S., Broadhead, J., Morriss, R. K., Brant, L. J., Blaustein, J., & Folstein, M. F. (1990). The prevalence and management of dementia and other psychiatric disorders in nursing homes. *American Journal of Psychiatry, 2*(1), 13–24.

Rovner, B. W., Kafonek, S., Philipp, L., Luckes, M. J., & Falstein, M. F. (1986). Prevalence of mental health in a community nursing home. *American Journal of Psychiatry, 143*, 1446–1449.

Simpson, C. J. (1984). Doctor's and nurses' use of the word confused. *British Journal of Psychiatry, 148*, 441–443.

Sirois, F. (1988). Delirium: 100 cases. *Canadian Journal of Psychiatry 33*, 375–378.

Thomas, R. I., Cameron, B. J., & Fahs, M. C. (1988). A prospective study of delirium and prolonged hospital stay. *Archives of General Psychiatry, 45*, 937–940.

Trzepacz, P. T., Baker, R. W., & Greenhouse, J. (1988). A symptom rating scale for delirium. *Psychiatric Research, 23*, 89–97.

Tune, L. E., & Bylsma, F. W. (1991). Benzodiazepine and anticholinergic-induced delirium in the elderly. *International Psychogeriatrics.* 325–332.

Tune, L. E., & Coyle, J. T. (1981). Acute extrapramidal side effects: Serum levels of neuroleptics and anticholinergics. *Psychopharmacology, 95*, 9–15.

Williams, N. A., Ward, S. E., & Campbell, D. B. (1986). Confusion: Testing vs. observation. *Journal of Gerontological Nursing, 14*(1), 25–30.

Williams, N. A. (1991). Delirium/acute confusional states: Evaluation devices in nursing. *International Psychogeriatrics.* 301–308.

10

Eating and Nutritional Disorders

Andrew Jay Silver

INTRODUCTION

The maintenance of an adequate nutritional status remains the.cornerstone of preventive geriatrics. In no setting is this more true than in long-term care, because the prevalence of malnutrition in the geriatric population in this environment has been estimated to range from 25% to 60% compared to that in the ambulatory outpatient (0% to 3%) or in the homebound elderly (5% to 12%). Although in the acute hospital setting the prevalence of malnutrition is similar (35% to 65%), a significant proportion of these individuals will be transferred to a long-term-care facility with their nutritional deficiencies still not adequately worked up or treated.

Recognition of the numerous risk factors which can interfere with the nutritional status of institutionalized elderly is the most important aspect of nutritional management. In this chapter, we will explore these risk factors as well as discuss the diagnosis and treatment of this important geriatric syndrome.

RECOGNITION

Psychological, social, pathophysiological, and physiological factors can influence the intake of food and subsequently determine the nutritional status of long-term-care residents (Morley & Silver, 1988). Because of the complex nature of these patients, it is likely that more than one factor is involved and that a multidisciplinary approach (nursing, dietary, social services, rehabilitation personnel, dentistry, pharmacy, and medicine) is crucial in the overall assessment process.

PSYCHOLOGICAL FACTORS

Dementia can affect 30% of a nursing home population (Cummings & Benson, 1983) with up to 50% having protein and/or energy malnutrition (Sandman et al., 1987). Cognitive impairment represents a "double-edged sword" when it is applied to the state of nutrition in that nutritional parameters can affect memory, and a decrease in cognition can affect nutrition (Silver, in press). Aluminum toxicity as well as deficiencies of iron, niacin, thiamine, folate, and vitamin B_{12} have all been suggested as nutritional causes of memory loss (Gray, 1990). Memory loss and impairment of judgment can affect food intake directly, or it can lead to a diminished functional capacity in such tasks as food preparation and shopping. In fact, inability to self-feed accounts for 18% of the reasons for institutionalization (Chenoweth & Spencer, 1986), with the cost of managing this eating dependence estimated to be 25% of the overall care cost (Kottkee, 1974). Apraxia (the inability to carry out motor activities despite intact comprehension and motor function) and "cheeking" of food can also occur. Finally, neurotransmitter abnormalities may play a role in that neuropeptide Y and norepinephrine (potent stimulators of food intake) levels have been found to be reduced in various brain regions of patients affected with Alzheimer's disease (Morley & Silver, 1988).

In the Sandman et al. study (1987), which examined weight loss in demented patients, despite a mean dietary intake of over 2000 kilocalories (kcal)/day, the mean reference weight was 82%. Malnourished residents had four times as many infectious periods treated with antibiotics compared to nonmalnourished residents. Possible causes for this low weight include side effects of the antibiotics, protein needs not being met at a time of increased nitrogen turnover (stress), or increased release of tumor necrosis factor (cachectin) with an increase in lipoprotein lipase and subsequent weight loss.

Other potential causes for weight loss in the demented institutionalized include swallowing difficulties (especially those with multi-infarct dementia) and lack of time spent in feeding these patients. Hu, Huang, and Cartwright (1986) found that for severely demented patients, 18 minutes each day were spent feeding these patients in a long-term-care environment, compared to 99 minutes each day if the resident was being cared for in the home setting. This problem can essentially be eliminated by utilizing trained volunteers to assist with feeding.

Depression is another psychological factor which can predispose the elderly in long-term-care settings to malnutrition. Depressive symptoms which interfere with nutrient intake, such as constipation, stomach pains, and loss of appetite, are frequently reported (Kivela et al., 1986). Also, weight loss is more prevalent in older compared to younger depressed patients (Blazer, Bachar, & Hughes, 1987).

A decrease in food intake can occur because of lack of activity, or with increased isolation, loss of food's symbolism as warmth and sharing. Malabsorption with subsequent weight loss can occur with laxative and/or enema abuse in psychotically depressed residents attempting to self-purge. Also, death by starvation can be one avenue by which older depressed residents attempt suicide. Neurotransmitter alterations may also be responsible for malnutrition in these residents. Elevated levels of corticotropin releasing factor (a potent inhibitor of food intake) have been found in the cerebrospinal fluid of depressed residents (Nemeroff, Bissette, & Widerlov, 1984). Also, antidepressants which enhance the function of the catecholamine system (norepinephrine stimulates feeding) increase appetite (Zung, 1967). On the other hand, the side effects of certain antidepressants can diminish food intake either directly as an appetite suppressant such as fluoxetine (Winograd, 1991) or indirectly with orthostatic hypotension and weakness leading to overall malaise.

A final type of psychological disorder which can affect nutrition is abnormal eating attitudes (Silver, 1991). Classic anorexia nervosa has been described in older patients either as a recurrence (having appeared earlier in life) or occurring for the first time in later life, anorexia tardive (Russell, Berg, & Lawrence, 1988). Miller (1991), through the use of the Eating Attitudes Test (EAT-26) assessment instrument used to identify anorectic attitudes, has identified a group of elderly patients with low body weight, who display certain oral control patterns such as avoiding eating when hungry or cutting food into small pieces, yet at the same time exhibit less frequent dieting behavior. Although more work is needed in this area, it is important to consider abnormal eating attitudes in a patient who is losing weight and is at risk for malnutrition.

SOCIAL

Social factors which can interfere with the nutritional status of long-term-care residents include isolation and financial constraints. As a result of institutionalization, many individuals feel as if they have lost all independence as well as all familiar surroundings. They may become depressed, isolate themselves (particularly at times of meals), and may begin to lose weight or "fail to thrive." Reliance upon nursing aides and others to identify these individuals is a key to recognizing and reversing this problem.

Financial constraints often limit the type of long-term-care facility that one can afford as well as limiting how far an operator of a facility will go to ensure an adequate nutritional state among the residents. Potential areas affected include limiting the purchase of fresh fruits and vegetables, utilizing outdated preparation and storage of food techniques (resulting in folate undernutrition), and having a registered dietitian present in the facility only for as long as is mandated by law (eight hours each month, in some states). Facility administrators need to be made aware of the fact that early and rigorous intervention is the most cost-effective method to manage nutritional problems in the long-term-care setting.

PATHOPHYSIOLOGICAL

Numerous disease states or pathological processes can affect food intake. Cardiac cachexia is an entity of congestive heart failure coexisting with anorexia (gastric and hepatic congestion, digoxin effect), weight loss (aggressive use of diuretics), malabsorption (small-bowel congestion), and a protein-losing enteropathy (Gorbien, 1990). Chronic obstructive pulmonary disease patients often expend so much effort in breathing that they are unable to consume large meals at one sitting. Gastrointestinal disorders include the absence of teeth and dentures with subsequent eating dependency (Siebens et al., 1986); dysphagia secondary to stroke, Parkinson's disease, or candidial esophagitis; peptic ulcer disease, often secondary to chronic aspirin or nonsteroidal use/abuse; and malabsorption secondary to lactose intolerance or antacid overusage. Diabetics are particularly vulnerable to changes in food intake, not only because of glycemic control, but also because anorexia can increase the propensity to develop hypoglycemia (Morley & Perry, 1991). Also, alterations in the metabolism of various minerals and vitamins have been reported in diabetics (Mooradian & Morley, 1987). Patients with decubitus ulcers are at significant risk for malnutrition. Pinchcofsky-Devin and Kaminski (1986) found that 100% of patients with decubiti were malnourished, and as the stage of the decubitus worsened, the serum albumin continued to fall. Other nutritionally related disease processes to be considered (but beyond the discussion of this chapter) include osteoporosis, vitamin D deficiency, hypercholesterolemia, and obesity.

Medications are often "pathologic" in disrupting the nutritional status either by directly causing anorexia, nausea, vomiting, constipation, or diarrhea, or by indirectly causing weakness, fatigue, depression, or confusion. Medications with a direct effect include digoxin (anorexia) (Landahl et al., 1977), antibiotics such as erythromycin or nonsteroidals (nausea), narcotics (constipation), and cathartics (diarrhea). Nonsteroidals and muscle relaxants can cause weakness and fatigue, while neuroleptics used in the same dosage as in a younger population can cause excess daytime drowsiness; central-acting antihypertensive agents such as clonidine can cause depression with loss of interest in eating; and a wide variety of medications, such as metoclopramide, can cause an acute confusional state leading to a decrease in food intake, often because the individual needs to be restrained and is in an agitated state.

PHYSIOLOGICAL

Numerous physiological processes that occur during aging can affect the nutritional status of long-term patients. Early satiety, or sensation, of fullness is a frequent complaint where individuals complain of eating only a small amount before "filling up." This may be due to the enhanced sensitivity to cholecystokinin-octapeptide (CCK-8) found in an older, compared to a younger, animal model (Silver, Flood, & Morley, 1988). CCK-8 is a gastrointestinal hormone which is released during the passage of food through the gastrointestinal tract, resulting in the termination of a meal. With an enhanced sensitivity to this hormone, the meal is terminated sooner, with less food consumed and subsequently this causes weight loss and malnutrition. This finding may extend to humans, as Khalil et al., (1985) have reported levels of CCK to be elevated in older humans. There also may be a decrease in the central feeding drive in older individuals because of the finding (Gosnell, Levine, & Morley, 1983) of a decrease in the opioid-mediated feeding drive causing older rodents to consume less compared to younger rodents and lose weight.

A decrease in the basal metabolic rate as well as a decrease in activity resulting in less energy intake can also lead to less food intake and a marginal nutritional status. The recommended dietary allowance (RDA) for energy intake decreases from 2800 kilocalories (kcal)/day at age 30 to 2100 kcal/day at age 80 (Food and Nutrition Board, 1989). An increase in taste and smell thresholds (i.e., a decrease in sensitivity) is another change that occurs with aging which can affect palatability of food (Schiffman, 1979). This can be further accentuated when long-term-care residents are placed on a low-salt and cholesterol-restricted diet. Thus, it is no wonder that a frequent complaint is the blandness of institutional food!

DIAGNOSIS

The first and most important step in diagnosing malnutrition in the elderly is to assess the "at-risk" factors previously discussed. This will not only identify reversible causes of malnutrition, but will also help to "target" those high-risk individuals who may need more frequent assessment, such as weights, and who may benefit from early intervention. Factors to which dining room personnel should pay particular attention as far as nutritional assessment is concerned are listed in Table 10.1.

The assessment process should include an evaluation of functional status, mental status (including screening for cognitive impairment and depression), and dietary status (diet type, usual daily food intake). Many of these geriatric assessment tools may be found in Kane, Ouslander, & Abrass, 1984. The pharmacist should assist in identifying drug-drug, drug-nutrient, and drug-appetite interactions. In addition, an evaluation of all medications, particularly in patients taking more than four prescription/ nonprescription drugs, should be undertaken in terms of absolute need.

The physical examination should focus on: the presence/absence of orthostatic hypotension (consider dehydration); the oral cavity (rule out vitamin deficiency, candidiasis, cancer) (see Gordon & Jahnigen, 1986); the mechanisms of swallowing; and evidence of peripheral edema (consider hypoalbuminemia).

Of all the anthropometric parameters (measurements of the relative leanness or obesity of an individual) used, a loss of weight or a low age-adjusted weight-height ratio (Master, Lasser, & Beckman, 1960) is the

TABLE 10.1 Factors to be Observed in the Dining Area to Identify Patients at Risk for Malnutrition

Inability to self-feed
Inability to open containers/unwrap utensils
Difficulty in swallowing (excessive gagging/coughing during the meal)
Consuming <70% of meals provided
Certain food avoidances
Failure to wear or lack of dentures
Prefers eating alone
Altered/fluctuating mental status
Sensory loss

best detector for diagnosing malnutrition. Significant weight loss is defined as loss of 5% original weight in one month, 7.5% in three months, or 10% in six months. Also, a body mass index (weight ÷ height X height) of less than 24 denotes an individual being underweight (Lipschitz, in press). Other anthropometrics such as triceps skinfold thickness, midarm circumference, and body densitometry (underwater weighing, CT scan, electrical impedance), although of research interest, do not add greatly to the clinical assessment.

The classic marker for protein energy malnutrition is a serum albumin level of less than 3.5 gm/dl. However, it has been our experience that patients in long-term-care facilities often maintain the serum albumin "within normal limits" while continuing to lose weight (marasmic-like). Also, Rudman and Feller (1989) found that nursing home residents with a serum albumin level less than 3.5 gm/dl had similar death rates compared to those whose serum albumin ranged between 3.5–3.99 gm/dl, suggesting that perhaps, in the long-term-care setting, a serum albumin level less than 4.0 gm/dl should be used to identify those at nutritional risk.

Recently, hypocholesterolemia has been suggested as a possible marker/cause of malnutrition in the elderly. Forette, Tortrat, and Wolmark (1989) found an association between the risk of death and hypocholesterolemia in women living in a nursing home. Hypocholesterolemia (<160 mg/dl) along with the hematocrit, have been used to determine the mortality risk index in long-term-care patients (Rudman et al., 1988). Finally, hypocholesterolemia has been associated with the presence of decubiti, the use of enteral feeding, and an elevated white blood cell count, again in a nursing home environment (Vendery & Goldberg, 1991). All of these studies suggest that most residents whose serum cholesterol levels are less than 160 mg/dl are at an increased risk for malnutrition and should be considered for some sort of nutritional support intervention.

TREATMENT

Preventive strategies to be used in a dining room area within a facility are noted in Table 10.2. In particular, the use of volunteers at times of meals, to assist with feeding and to help with opening up containers, may be the best preventive measure that facilities can put into place. Various service organizations, students from local schools, spouses, and other family members have all been used to help during these crucial periods of the day.

Treatable causes of weight loss, i.e., many of the risk factors previously

TABLE 10.2 Strategies to be Used in a Long-Term-Care Dining Area to Ensure Adequate Nutrition

---

Availability of specialized utensils
  weighted spoon
  rocker bottom knife
  side-cutter fork
Availability of adequate personnel
  use of volunteers
Availability of dietitian to observe eating patterns
Separate area for disruptive patients
Sufficient financial support to prepare meals
Smaller, more frequent meals for residents with Chronic Obstructive Pulmonary Disease or early satiety
Availability of ethnic foods

---

discussed, should be the next approach in the management of malnutrition. A careful review of medications as well as screening for depression, may well identify a significant number of these residents who are losing weight or who demonstrate an abnormal nutritional parameter.

During the workup of the patient for malnutrition, one should aim for an intake of 35 kcal/kg (Morley et al., 1986). This usually cannot be accomplished by oral intake alone, necessitating a feeding tube to be placed. Although this can lead to numerous complications (Morley et al., 1986), a short course of enteral feedings can be very beneficial to the majority of residents for whom oral intake simply cannot meet their needs. Early intervention is the key to success. Of equal importance, however, is the need for the resident (or delegated individual) to participate in the treatment plan and to be able to express his or her wishes regarding the duration of tube feeding and regarding tube removal, should the disease process prove to be irreversible. Finally, the role of parenteral support in the nursing home is likely not to be warranted (in terms of cost and in terms of likelihood of reversing the malnourished state) in the majority of long-term-care patients.

Potential future modalities for the treatment of malnutrition in long-term-care patients include growth hormone, for its anabolic effect (Binnerts, Wilson, & Lamberts, 1988; Rudman et al., 1990; Kaiser, Silver, & Morley, 1991); medroxyprogesterone acetate, to enhance food intake (Nuranen, Kajanti, Tammilehto, & Mattson, 1990); and testosterone, to enhance food intake and muscle strength (Korenman et al., 1990).

REFERENCES

Binnerts, A., Wilson, J. H. P., & Lamberts, S. W. J. (1988). The effects of human growth hormone administration in elderly adults with recent weight loss. *Archives of Internal Medicine, 67*, 1312–1316.

Blazer, D., Bachar, J. R., & Hughes, D. C. (1987). Major depression with melancholia: A comparison of middle-aged and elderly adults. *Journal of the American Geriatrics Society, 35*, 927–932.

Chenoweth B., & Spencer S. (1986). Dementia: The experience of family caregivers. *The Gerontologist, 26*, 267–274.

Cummings J. L., & Benson D. F. (1983). *Dementia: A clinical approach.* Boston: Butterworths.

Food and Nutrition Board, National Research Council. (1989). *Recommended dietary allowances* (10th rev. ed.), Washington, DC: National Academy of Sciences.

Forette, B., Tortrat, D., & Wolmark, Y. (1989). Cholesterol as a risk factor for mortality in elderly women. *Lancet, 1*, 868–870.

Gorbien, M. J. (1990). Cardiac cachexia. In J. E. Morley, Z. Glick, & L. Z. Rubenstein (Eds.), *Geriatric nutrition, A comprehensive review* (pp. 315–324). New York: Raven Press.

Gordon, S. R., & Jahnigen, D. W. (1986). Oral assessment of the dentulous elderly patient. *Journal of the American Geriatrics Society, 34*, 276–281.

Gosnell, B. A., Levine, A. S., & Morley, J. E. (1983). The effects of aging on opioid modulation of feeding in rats. *Life Science, 32*, 2793–2799.

Gray, G. E. (1990). Nutrition and dementia. *Contemporary Nutrition, 15*(6).

Hu, T., Huang, L., & Cartwright, W. S. (1986). Evaluation of the costs of caring for the senile demented elderly: A pilot study. *The Gerontologist, 26*, 158–163.

Kaiser, F. E., Silver, A. J., & Morley J. E. (1991). The effect of recombinant human growth hormone on malnourished older individuals. *Journal of the American Geriatrics Society, 39*, 235–240.

Kane, R. L., Ouslander, J. G., & Abrass I. B. (1984). *Essentials of clinical geriatrics.* New York: McGraw-Hill.

Khalil, T., Walker, J. P., & Wiener, J., Fagan, C. J., Townsend, C. M., Greenley, G. H. & Thompson, J. C. (1985). Effect of aging on gallbladder contraction and release of cholecystokinin-33 in humans. *Surgery, 98*, 423–429.

Kivela, S. L., Nissin, A., Tuomilehto, J., Pekkanen, J., Punsar, S., Lammi, U. K., & Puska, P. (1986). Prevalence of depressive and other symptoms in elderly Finnish men. *Acta Psychiatrica Scandinavica, 73*, 93–100.

Korenman, S. G., Morley, J. E., Mooradian, A. D., Stanik-Davis, S., Kaiser, F. E., Silver, A. J., Viosca, S. P. & Garza, D. (1990). Secondary hypogonadism in elder men: Its relationship to impotence. *Journal of Clinical Endocrinology and Metabolism, 71*, 963–969.

Kottkee, F. J. (1974). Historia obscura hemiplegiae. *Archives of Physical Medicine and Rehabilitation, 55*, 4–13.

Landahl, S., Lindblad, B., Roupe, S., et al (1977). Digitalis therapy in a 70-year-old population. *Acta Medica Scandinavica, 202*, 437–443.

Lipschitz, D. A. (In press). The development of an approach to nutrition screening for older Americans. *Nutrition Screening Initiative.*

Master, A. H., Lasser, R. P,. & Beckman, G. (1960). Tables of average weight and height of Americans aged 65–94 years. *Journal of the American Medical Association. 172*, 658–662.

Miller, D. K., Morley, J. E., Rubenstein, L. Z., Pietruszka, F. M., & Strome, L. S. (1991). Abnormal eating attitudes and body image in older malnourished patients. *Journal of the American Geriatrics Society, 39*, 462–466.

Mooradian A. D., & Morley J. E. (1987). Micronutrient status in diabetes mellitus. *American Journal of Clinical Nutrition, 45*, 877–895.

Morley, J. E., & Perry, H. M. (1991). The management of diabetes mellitus in older individuals. *Drugs, 41*, 548–565.

Morley, J. E., Silver, A. J., Fiatarone, M., & Mooradian, D. (1986). UCLA geriatric grand rounds: Nutrition and the elderly. *Journal of the American Geriatrics Society, 34*, 823–832.

Morley, J. E., & Silver, A. J. (1988). Anorexia in the elderly. *Neurobiological Aging, 9*, 9–16.

Nemeroff, C. B., Bissette, G., & Widerlov, E. (1984). Elevated concentrations of corticotropin-releasing-factor-like immunoreactivity in depressed patients. *Science, 226*, 1342–1343.

Nuranen, A., Kajanti, M., Tammilehto, L., & Mattson, K. (1990). The clinical effect of medroxyprogesterone in elderly patients with lung cancer. *American Journal of Clinical Oncology, 13*, 113–116.

Pinchcofsky-Devin, G. D., & Kaminski, M. V. (1986). Correlation of pressure sores and nutritional status. *Journal of the American Geriatrics Society, 34*, 435–440.

Rudman, D., Dale, M. D., Mattson, E., Nagraj, H. S., Feller, A. G., Jackson, D. L., & Rudeman, I. W. (1988). Prognostic significance of serum cholesterol in nursing home men. *Journal of Parenteral and Enteral Nutrition, 12*, 155–158.

Rudman, D. & Feller, A. G. (1989). Protein-calorie undernutrition in the nursing home. *Journal of the American Geriatrics Society, 37*, 173–183.

Rudman, D., Feller, A. G., Nagraj, H. S., Gergans, G. A., Lalitha, P. Y., Goldberg, A. F., Schlenker, R. A., Cahn, L., Rudeman, I. W., & Mattson, D. E. (1990). Effects of human growth hormone in men over 60 years old. *New England Journal of Medicine, 323*, 1–6.

Russell, J. D., Berg, J., & Lawrence J. R. (1988). Anorexia tardive: A diagnosis of exclusion? *Medical Journal of Austrailia, 148*, 199–201.

Sandman, P. O., Adolfsson, R., Nygren, C., Hallman, G., & Winblad, B. (1987). Nutritional status and dietary intake in institutionalized patients with Alzheimer's disease and multi-infarct dementia. *Journal of the American Geriatric Society, 35*, 31–38.

Schiffman, S. (1979). Changes in taste and smell with age: Psychophysical aspects. In J. M. Ordy, & K. Brizzee (Eds.) *Sensory systems and communication in the elderly*. New York: Raven Press.

Siebens, H., Trupe, E., Siebens, A., Cook, F., Anshen, S., Hanaver, R., & Oster, G. (1986). Correlates and consequences of eating dependency in institutionalized elderly. *Journal of the American Geriatric Society, 34*, 192–198.

Silver, A. J. (1991). Eating disorders in the elderly. *Clinical and Applied Nutrition, 1*, 67–71.

Silver, A. J. (1992). Nutritional aspects of memory dysfunction. In J. E. Morley, R. M. Coe, R. Strong, & G. Grossberg (Eds.) *Memory function and age-related disorders*. New York: Springer Publishing Company.

Silver, A. J., Flood, J. F., & Morley, J. E. (1988). Effect of gastrointestinal peptides on ingestion in old and young mice. *Peptides*, *9*, 221–225.

Vendery, R. B., & Goldberg, A. P. (1991). Hypocholesterolemia as a predictor of death: A prospective study of 224 nursing home residents. *Journal of Gerontology*, *46*, M84–M90.

Winograd, C. (1991). *Weight loss associated with the use of fluoxetine*. Presented in a poster session, Annual Meeting of the American Geriatrics Society, Atlanta, Georgia.

Zung, W. W. (1967). Depression in the normal aged. *Psychosomatics*, *8*, 287–292.

11

Management of Pain in the Elderly

Raymond C. Tait

It is well recognized that aging is associated with numerous processes that can produce pain through degenerative conditions (osteoarthritis), pathologic conditions (cancer), and traumatic events (cerebrovascular accidents, falls). In fact, it has been estimated that pain afflicts 25% to 50% of persons aged 60 and above who live in the community (Brattberg, Mats, & Anders, 1989; Crook, Rideout, & Brown, 1984). Incidence of pain among elderly in nursing homes has been estimated to be as high as 80% (Ferrell, Ferrell, & Osterweil, 1990), with musculoskeletal factors a leading cause. Despite the prevalence of pain in the elderly, there is relatively little information available concerning the management of pain in this population, and even less has been written about pain management among the elderly in nursing homes. This chapter is intended to add to that literature.

The chapter is organized into three broad sections. The first covers general issues related to clinical pain. The second concerns assessment of pain syndromes, with attention to factors in the elderly that can complicate adequate assessment. The final section addresses treatment issues, with special attention paid to residents treated in nursing homes.

PAIN

Our understanding of pain pathways has changed dramatically since Melzack and Wall (1965) proposed a "gate" in the dorsal horn of the spine that modulated painful impulses transmitted to the brain. Pain modulation was thought to occur in several ways: (1) through stimulation of large-diameter nerve fibers ascending to the brain; (2) through stimulation of fibers descending from the brain (by cognitive and emotional activity); and (3) through activity in the autonomic nervous system. While specifics of the Gate Control model have been challenged and the model has been modified (Melzack & Wall, 1982), it is now accepted that pain is an experience modulated by physical, emotional, and environmental factors. This is reflected in the definition of pain that has been adopted by the medical community (Merskey et al., 1979): "An unpleasant sensory and emotional experience associated with actual or potential tissue damage, or described in terms of such damage."

While pain of any duration is a complex experience, it is useful to distinguish between the experiences of acute pain (duration less than three months) and chronic pain (duration greater than six months). Generally, acute pain has adaptive value, signaling tissue damage of a fairly clear origin, and its treatment has a high likelihood of success. Narcotic analgesics can be employed in treatment with little risk of addiction. Frequently, the patient with acute pain is anxious; the anxiety is part of what motivates the patient for treatment.

Chronic pain, by contrast, is often associated with depression, partly because a "cure" becomes unlikely in these conditions. Treatment is complicated by a lack of clear causation for the pain (tissue damage associated with pain onset usually has healed) and by the higher addiction potential that these patients present. Thus, chronic pain, instead of having signal value, becomes the disease itself. Because most physicians are better equipped to treat acute pain (Margolis, Zimny, Miller, & Taylor, 1984), chronic pain often presents a very frustrating picture.

Loeser (1980) has developed a conceptual model that is useful for chronic pain syndromes. He views these syndromes as composed of three parts: (1) pain sensation, a sensory component; (2) suffering, an emotional component; and (3) pain behavior, a disability component (reflecting the degree to which pain and suffering impact behavior). Clinical research also has found pain, distress, and disability to be stable factors among patients at chronic pain treatment facilities (Tait, Chibnall, Duckro, & Deshields, 1989). Because the three-dimensional model has considerable heuristic value, the following sections are organized along these dimensions as they apply to the elderly population.

Assessment and treatment also will be broken down along medical and psychological dimensions. While this division is used for purposes of organization, the reader should understand that medical/psychological variables are not dichotomous in patients with chronic pain. That is, it is incorrect to ask whether patients have either medical or psychological pain. Instead, as suggested by Brena and Chapman (1982), it is more useful to ask questions regarding the degree to which medical and/or psychological factors contribute to the pain experience. Because all patients react psychologically to protracted pain, the crucial question is how the reaction affects the pain syndrome, not whether there is a psychological reaction.

ASSESSMENT

Pain

Medical Factors
The utility of sophisticated diagnostics in evaluating patients with intractable pain has been subject to considerable discussion. Often diagnostics (e.g., X-ray, CAT scan) are necessary in order to rule out a lesion requiring surgical intervention. When these findings are positive, more aggressive investigation can be warranted. When these findings are negative or ambiguous, however, the value of further testing has been called into question. Rudy, Turk, and Brena (1988) surveyed 80 physicians who worked with chronic pain patients, asking them to rank the utility of various diagnostic procedures. The rankings showed that neurologic examination, observation of gait and posture, assessment of muscle function, and other data available from a thorough history and physical had greater utility for planning treatment than did the sophisticated diagnostic studies.

Because degenerative changes are common in the elderly, diagnostic tests show structural problems even in patients without symptoms (Hadler, 1984). Clearly, evidence of structural problems does not mandate surgical intervention with these patients. Instead, a thorough history and physical is needed to evaluate the significance of the diagnostic results. Thus, interpretation of diagnostic results/physical findings is a complicated process, requiring a thorough history and physical and knowledge of syndromes common in the elderly. Several excellent articles have been written that provide information about such syndromes: neck pain (Moskovich, 1988), back pain (Gandy & Payne, 1986), headache (Rapoport, Sheftell, & Baskin, 1983), fibromyalgia (Wolfe, 1988), postherpetic neuralgia (Portenoy, 1986).

Although the value of the physical examination has already been discussed, the pain history is of equal importance in treatment planning. A number of areas should be examined in order to construct a reasonable treatment plan.

(1) Location: Evaluation of pain location generally involves two related questions: (a) what is the pain distribution, (b) how does the distribution change? While acquiring information about pain distribution can be time-consuming, it is essential to discover whether the pain follows a nerve pathway (dermatome) or not. Similarly, changes in pain location also can be diagnostic (changes are common in myofascial pain). Finally, obtaining information about the extent of pain is valuable. There is evidence that patients with widespread pain are likely to demonstrate distress and disability that require attention in their own right (Tait, Chibnall, & Margolis, 1990).

(2) Pain Onset: Pain of acute onset clearly requires careful evaluation to rule out a surgical lesion. Pain of gradual onset is more common in the elderly as it is characteristic of degenerative changes. In such cases, it is important to evaluate the body mechanics that patients have adopted in accommodating to pain; dysfunctional body mechanics actually can contribute to severe musculoskeletal pain.

(3) Pain intensity: Pain intensity is related to both distress and disability. There are numerous rating scales available to assess pain intensity (Ferrell, 1991). It is often useful to obtain estimates of both worst and least pain. Pain conditions with considerable variability in pain levels are often responsive to coordinated pain management approaches.

(4) Factors that affect pain: For patients who report variability in pain, it is important to assess factors associated with pain increases and decreases. Musculoskeletal pain, very common in nursing home residents, is often responsive to many factors. By careful balancing of factors affecting pain, effective pain control often can be achieved.

(5) Treatments for pain: Detailed information about previous treatments can be of great importance in constructing a treatment plan. While it is clearly important to ascertain information about previous surgeries, it also can be useful to obtain information about prior experience with physical therapy, especially if musculoskeletal factors contribute significantly to pain. Previous and present drugs used to treat pain also should be assessed thoroughly. Many patients are poor historians where medications are involved, especially if the medications have affected them cognitively. Among the elderly, such ripple effects are quite common, greatly complicating the assessment.

(6) Effects of pain: It is critical to assess interference of pain in daily activities. Disabling effects of pain are especially important to assess among the elderly, as disability can lead to social isolation, depression,

and a general decline in health if it is not detected in a timely manner. While there are rating scales available to facilitate such assessment, nursing home staff are well placed to obtain this information through direct observation.

Behavioral factors

Because evaluation of pain relies heavily on self-report data, behavioral factors that compromise communication also complicate assessment. In the elderly, especially those confined to nursing homes, communication deficits are common (Haley & Dolce, 1986).

There are several reasons for communication difficulties. The most obvious involves the loss of cognitive abilities, associated either with Alzheimer's disease or the natural aging process. Cognitive decline can interfere with retrieval of information from memory, with concentration/ attention, and with abstract reasoning. Loss of memory obviously interferes with taking a thorough history; impaired concentration/attention can lead to poor tracking/inappropriate responses to interrogatories; impaired abstract reasoning is a less obvious problem, but it can lead to significant difficulties in responding to rating scales used to assess pain severity. Cognitively impaired patients often do better when words are used to assess pain severity (0 = none, 1 = mild, 2 = moderate, 3 = severe, 4 = horrible, 5 = intolerable/excruciating).

There also are other factors associated with aging that can compromise effective communication. Many older patients under-report physical symptoms, including pain (Levkoff, Cloary, Wetle, & Besdine, 1988). Several explanations have been advanced for this phenomenon, including the possibility that sensitivity to pain decreases with aging. Recent research examining pain threshold and tolerance in the elderly, however, has failed to demonstrate a significant decrease in sensitivity to pain among the aged (Kwentus, Harkins, Lognon, & Silverman, 1985).

A second explanation for under-reporting has proposed that the elderly tend to attribute symptoms to the aging process when symptom onset has been gradual (Leventhal & Prohaskas, 1990). This makes them less likely to report symptoms, undermining a thorough assessment. Staff also can attribute symptoms to aging, making them less likely to investigate symptoms that are reported. Patients whose reports are ignored are likely to respond in one of two ways. They escalate their complaints or they cease reporting. In the first case, an adversarial interaction is likely to ensue. In the second, treatment is likely to miss a significant part of the clinical problem. In either case, effective treatment can be jeopardized.

A third explanation for the reporting deficit involves the comparison group that the aged use to evaluate their health status (Levkoff et al., 1988). It is thought that the elderly use same-aged peers as a comparison group, leading to the discounting of symptoms ("I'm feeling pretty good for 80 years old"). Clearly, the comparison group in a nursing home could lead to even further symptom under-reporting.

While most elderly patients minimize their symptoms, others magnify them. These patients seem to channel distress/discomfort into somatic concerns, possibly because physical concerns are thought to be more acceptable than emotional or psychological concerns (Roy, 1986). Clearly, these patients may require a psychiatric/psychological evaluation if symptomatic treatment is unsuccessful.

Several strategies are available to enhance the accuracy of information available on nursing home residents. Interviews with family members can provide valuable historical information. Communication with nursing staff can provide information about current functioning. In addition, in a controlled setting, it is possible to collect information regarding relations between pain and activity through the use of monitoring forms. Usually, this requires staff oversight; otherwise, resident compliance with pain/ activity monitoring can be poor. This information can be captured not only on monitoring forms, but also in the progress notes maintained on these residents.

Distress

Medical

Health professionals who evaluate elderly residents with intractable pain must be sensitive to signs of distress, especially depression. The depression may have vegetative, agitative, or mixed qualities. Frequently, either the resident's family or staff at a nursing home can provide useful information regarding the emotional state of residents being evaluated.

In the face of pain complaints and psychological distress, it can be tempting to label residents as psychosomatic. Unfortunately, residents diagnosed with psychogenic pain often have their symptoms discounted, and the symptoms can go untreated. Residents whose symptoms are untreated can go into a downward spiral with worsening symptoms and increasing disability, a pattern that can be devastating for the elderly (Ferrell, 1991).

Instead of discounting physical complaints voiced by distressed residents as psychosomatic, it has been recommended that the distress be viewed as a somato-psychic, a consequence of the physical symptoms (Deshields, Jenkins, & Tait, 1989). According to this viewpoint, treatment efforts should be directed at symptom control; effective symptom control can greatly reduce emotional distress. When distress interferes with successful symptom control, of course, psychiatric/psychological treatment can be required.

Psychological

Psychological assessment of depression should examine the possible contributors to depression. Pain generally limits activities that already have been limited by age; the experience of loss is a prime contributor to depression in any age group. Another contributor to depression involves loss of self-esteem, a common phenomenon when the elderly have reached the point that they no longer are capable of independent function (Kane, Ouslander, & Abrass, 1989); pain can further compromise independence.

Many residents also feel helpless as they are frustrated in their efforts to manage pain. Such learned helplessness (Seligman, 1975) can occasion passivity and interfere with learning. Clearly, passive residents who have difficulty learning can undermine treatments that require them to be active participants.

Disability

Medical

According to the World Health Organization, disability refers to the degree to which a condition interferes with performance of accustomed roles (Osterweis, Kleinman, & Mechanic, 1987). This definition distinguishes disability from impairment, defined as the medical conditions associated with disability. While impairment and disability usually are correlated, there are many patients for whom disability can be more or less than their impairment might indicate.

Disability assessment is a complex task, especially for the elderly in whom there are multiple medical/psychiatric disorders, and even more so for those whose chief complaints are pain, an entirely subjective experience. The medical component of disability assessment must address the impairment question. Such assessment is critical to the formulation of treatment plans because it sets parameters for rehabilitation; it can define levels of activity that the patient should not exceed and levels of activity toward which treatment can reasonably aim. Medical assessment should go beyond the evaluation of pain-related symptoms (e.g., range of motion in painful joints); it should also include evaluation of cardiovascular status, neurologic status (e.g., risk of falling), etc. The physician also will want to collect information about the patient's functional status; often, this can be gleaned from family or nursing staff who interact with the patient on a daily basis.

Psychological

While impairment constitutes one component of disability, dysfunctional pain behavior represents the other aspect of pain-related disability. Keefe and Block (1982) have developed a scoring system that facilitates observer assessment of this component of disability: verbal expressions of discomfort (moaning, sighing), facial expressions (grimacing), postural demonstrations (limping, bracing), and other behaviors (guarding, rubbing). Pain behaviors are important contributors to disability for several reasons. First, they convey the resident's distress to others. Significant others tend to respond to these behaviors through caretaking (Block, Dremer, & Gaylor, 1980), a pattern that tends to further dysfunction. Second, pain behaviors contribute to poor biomechanics, adding mechanical complications that can exacerbate musculoskeletal pain. Assessment and treatment of pain behaviors can be necessary for effective rehabilitation/pain control.

TREATMENT

Several comments should be made about the general goals of treatment for residents with chronic pain. Elimination of pain is usually not a realistic goal, although reduction of both pain levels and the frequency of severe pain exacerbations often is realistic (Aronoff, Evans, & Enders, 1985; Tait, Duckro, Margolis, & Wiener, 1988). Equally important is restoration of functional capacity. With improved function and effective pain control, improved mood and quality of life also can be expected. The following sections outline some approaches that can be used to achieve these goals.

Pain

Medical

Several classes of medication have been the backbone for the treatment of pain over the years: narcotic analgesics, nonsteroidal anti-inflammatory drugs (NSAIDs), and muscle relaxants/minor tranquilizers. While general points regarding medication use will be made here, the interested reader is referred to several excellent articles for information specific to the use of these medications in the treatment of the elderly (Ferrell, 1991; Portenoy & Farkash, 1988).

Because metabolism in the elderly differs considerably from that in younger adults, medication half-life is longer, potentiating both main effects and side effects. When these are coupled with the more fragile health found in the elderly, there is increased risk of serious complications. This necessitates careful monitoring of response to medication. Similarly, the elderly are vulnerable to drug interactions, particularly when multiple medications are needed to manage multiple health problems.

When dealing with analgesic medications, it is advisable to put medications on time interval schedules (rather than PRN). PRN administration of narcotics has been shown to promote pain behavior and distress among patients with chronic pain (White & Sanders, 1985). Moreover, time interval schedules are less dependent on vagaries of patient self-reports (over/under-reporting) and/or staffing (planned medication administration can usually be handled much more efficiently than PRN administration). Finally, the efficacy of a dose/time schedule can be gauged more accurately on a time interval schedule than a PRN schedule. The latter considerations are especially valuable in a nursing home setting, where observers can manage medication administration and monitor the efficacy of the medications used.

Some comments should be made about narcotic analgesics. While narcotics have been a frontline defense for pain for many years, recent years have seen a shift away from them in the treatment of persistent pain. In fact, avoidance of long-term narcotic use has become almost dogma. Unfortunately, alternative medications such as NSAIDs also can pose serious problems, especially in the elderly (Ferrell, 1991). In response to this situation, some clinicians have argued for the long-term use of narcotics in selected cases and have spelled out guidelines for their use (Melzack, 1990; Portenoy, 1990). These ideas are still debated, and the interested reader is referred to a recent article that challenges this strategy (Turk & Brody, 1991).

While the use of narcotic analgesics is debated in patients with chronic benign pain, narcotic analgesics are the mainstay of treatment for malignant pain when surgery/chemotherapy has failed. It is beyond the scope of this chapter to discuss narcotic management of cancer pain; the interested reader is referred to an excellent book recently published on this topic (Payne & Foley, 1987). It should be noted, however, that adjuvant medications have demonstrated abilities to potentiate the therapeutic qualities of narcotics. For example, NSAIDs can be effective in the management of pain associated with bone metastases when combined with narcotics. Similarly, antidepressants have shown benefits for pain, sleep, and mood when used in combination with narcotic analgesics.

When dealing with musculoskeletal pain, physical therapy has been shown to correct deficits in range of motion, posture, and muscle tone, providing significant benefits for patients (Wells, Frampton, & Bowsher, 1988). Several readily available modalities also can be employed to supplement exercise: ice and/or heat for myofascial pain; ice for joint pain; transcutaneous electrical nerve stimulation (TENS) for peripheral nerve pain. In elderly patients, especially those with cognitive deficits, supervision is required in order to avoid problems such as superficial burns when using heat or TENS.

Psychological
Several psychological approaches have shown value with adults (e.g., hypnosis, biofeedback), and some have recommended their use in the

elderly (Sorkin, Rudy, Hanlon, Turk, & Stieg, 1990). Others are less enthusiastic, however, especially among elderly patients who demonstrate cognitive deficits (Ferrell, 1991). This author's experience suggests that these techniques are of marginal benefit in the elderly, especially those in nursing homes, although distraction (through involvement in activities) can be helpful.

Behavioral strategies can be of significant benefit in reducing the frequency of severe exacerbations. Pain- and activity-monitoring forms (compiled either by the resident or the staff) can be used to identify appropriate levels of activity. Activity monitoring is especially valuable when rehabilitation is one of the goals of treatment; through the use of pacing strategies, increases in activity are not so likely to be met with paralyzing exacerbations of pain that can interfere greatly with rehabilitation.

Distress

Medical
Clinical trials have shown that low doses of antidepressant medications (usually one quarter to one half of the dosage recommended for a major depression), especially serotonergic medications, can yield improved mood, sleep, and pain levels in patients with intractable pain (Cunha, 1986). These medications are thought to facilitate activity in neural pathways that modulate pain and mood. Some investigators, however, believe that the primary effects are on sleep quality, so that improvement in mood and pain is secondary to improved sleep (Ferrell, 1991). Whatever the mechanisms, antidepressants have a significant place in the treatment of distressing pain syndromes.

Psychological
Several behavioral interventions can be helpful in managing distress in elderly residents with intractable pain. Relaxation training can be helpful in reducing anxiety and muscle tension associated with anxiety. For the elderly, techniques such as deep breathing and progressive muscle relaxation are concrete and can be easily followed. The primary goal in the use of relaxation training is not pain reduction; rather, it is the management of distress so that the resident's tension does not contribute to further pain exacerbations (although some residents do derive actual pain reductions). While biofeedback training, a variant of relaxation training, has been recommended by some in the treatment of pain in the elderly, it is difficult for patients with cognitive deficits and, hence, may be ineffective for many nursing home residents.

Problem solving also can be helpful to reduce the distress associated with pain by enhancing feelings of control. For example, patients who learn that weather changes increase arthritic pain can implement moist heat and/or stretching exercises to keep pain at tolerable levels during these conditions. In nursing home residents, such problem solving usually requires active staff participation.

Distress, of course, also can occur for reasons other than pain exacerbations. With intractable pain, unfortunately, such distress almost certainly will compound the suffering associated with pain. For many patients, increased involvement in pleasurable activities (music, art, etc.) can be helpful for managing distress. Among residents who are depressed over significant life changes (e.g., having to abandon independent living) or whose families demonstrate dysfunctional dynamics (e.g., are overly protective), psychological counseling can be needed to reduce distress/dysfunction and facilitate effective management of pain.

Disability

Medical

An important goal of treatment of chronic pain syndromes is to increase functional capacity. Medical oversight of such rehabilitation is necessary, especially among patients who demonstrate medical complications (e.g., cardiovascular disease) that can affect rehabilitation. Similarly, medication management can be a useful adjunct to rehabilitation. Thus, muscle relaxants can be prescribed for short-term use in the treatment of patients with musculoskeletal pain whose rehabilitation includes exercise aimed at increasing range of motion.

Certainly, the most important discipline in the rehabilitation of disabled patients is physical therapy. Patients who regain functional capacity can have much-improved quality of life even when pain is persistent. Exercise programs are the most direct way of increasing functional capacity. While exercise regimens require individual tailoring, there are several considerations that apply widely:

1. Most patients have learned activity avoidance because of pain. Aggressive rehabilitation may serve to strengthen fear-avoidance behavior. Hence, exercise levels should be comfortably within the range of the patient's tolerance for activity (75% of tolerance). Once patients learn that a given level of activity can be tolerated, activity levels can be progressed.

2. Progression of exercise should not be guided by a patient's tolerance, either. Instead, patients should exercise to a criterion that the physician and/or physical therapist has identified as safe for that patient. It is common for patients to overdo when feeling good and underdo when feeling bad; exercising to criterion helps to avoid such swings.

Psychological

Behavioral interventions aimed at improved functional capacity can reinforce work done in physical therapy. For example, the patient who complains of pain increasing with exercise can be engaged in problem solving aimed at identifying problematic activities; the staff/counselor can feed that information back to the physical therapist overseeing rehabilitation. Similarly, the patient who is fearful of activity can be taught breathing techniques designed to promote muscle relaxation, diminishing excessive tension that a patient brings to the rehabilitation task.

Behavioral approaches also can enhance patient motivation. The patient who participates in exercise in order to regain the ability to engage in a pleasurable activity (e.g., walking) will collaborate more effectively in treatment than will the patient who is exercising just to follow "doctor's orders." Moreover, the patient with high levels of motivation is likely to persevere in rehabilitation when faced with frustration.

Finally, it is worth noting that residents in a nursing home can derive significant motivation from the staff who attend to their achievements, especially when the achievements are small. Attention that is paid to adaptive responses to pain tends to increase the frequency of those responses. Conversely, residents who get attention for pain behaviors and/or other dysfunctional responses to pain are likely to demonstrate continued dysfunction.

CONCLUDING REMARKS

Elderly residents who are confined to nursing homes often demonstrate pain as part of the clinical picture. Consequently, assessment of pain and its impact on functional status should be part of the routine evaluation performed at the time of a patient's admission to a nursing home. Thorough assessment of pain conditions should include attention to medical and psychological contributors to pain, distress, and disability. Adequate assessment facilitates the development of a treatment plan that addresses the range of problems frequently associated with chronic pain syndromes. Because of the complexity of these problems, a multidisciplinary approach can be necessary in order to obtain adequate pain control and enhance the resident's quality of life.

REFERENCES

Aronoff, G. M., Evans, W. O., & Enders, P. L. (1985). A review of follow-up studies of multidisciplinary pain units. In G. M. Aronoff (Ed.), *Evaluation and treatment of chronic pain* (pp. 511–522). Baltimore, Munich: Urban & Schwarzenberg.

Block, A. R., Kremer, E. F., & Gaylor, M. (1980). Behavioral treatment of chronic pain: The spouse as a discriminative cue for pain behavior. *Pain, 9,* 243–252.

Brattberg, G., Mats, T., & Anders, W. (1989). The prevalence of pain in a general population: The results of a postal survey in a county of Sweden. *Pain, 37,* 215–222.

Brena, S. F., & Chapman, S. L. (1982). The validity of the Emory pain estimate model. *Anesthesiology Review, 9,* 42–45.

Crook, J., Rideout, E., & Browne, G. (1984). The prevalence of pain complaints among a general population. *Pain, 18,* 299–314.

Cunha, V. C. (1986). Antidepressants: Their uses in nonpsychiatric disorders of aging. *Geriatrics, 41,* 63–72.

Deshields, T. L., Jenkins, J. O., & Tait, R. C. (1989). The experience of anger in chronic illness: A preliminary investigation. *International Journal of Psychiatry in Medicine, 19,* 299–309.

Ferrell, B. A. (1991). Pain management in elderly people. *Journal of the American Geriatric Society, 39,* 64–73.

Ferrell, B. A., Ferrell, B. R., & Osterweil, D. (1990). Pain in the nursing home. *Journal of the American Geriatric Society, 38,* 409–414.

Gandy, S., & Payne, R. (1986). Back pain in the elderly: Updated diagnosis and management. *Geriatrics, 41,* 59–74.

Hadler, N. M. (1984). *Medical management of the regional musculoskeletal diseases.* New York: Grune & Stratton.

Haley, W. E., & Dolce, J. J. (1986). Assessment and management of chronic pain in the elderly. *Clinical Gerontologist, 5,* 3/4, 435–455.

Kane, R. L., Ouslander, J. G., & Abrass, I. B. (1989). *Essentials of clinical geriatrics.* New York: McGraw-Hill.

Keefe, F. J., & Block, A. R. (1982). Development of an observation method for assessing pain behavior in chronic low back pain patients. *Behavior Research and Therapy, 13,* 363–375.

Kwentus, J. A., Harkins, S. W., Lognon, N., & Silverman, J. J. (1985). Current concepts of geriatric pain and its treatment. *Geriatrics, 40,* 48–57.

Leventhal, E. A., & Prohaskas, T. R. (1986). Age, symptom interpretation, and health behavior. *Journal of the American Geriatrics Society, 34,* 185–191.

Levkoff, S. E., Cloary, P. D., Wetle, T., & Besdine, R. W. (1988). Illness behavior in the aged: Implications for the clinician. *Journal of the American Geriatrics Society, 36,* 622–629.

Loeser, J. D. (1980). Perspectives on pain. *Proceedings of the first world congress on clinical pharmacology and therapeutics,* London: MacMillan, 313–316.

Margolis, R. B., Zimny, G. H., Miller, D., & Taylor, J. M. (1984). Internists and the chronic pain patient. *Pain, 20,* 151–156.

Melzack, R. (1990). The tragedy of needless pain. *Scientific American, 262,* 27–33.

Melzack, R., & Wall, P. D. (1965). Pain mechanisms: A new theory. *Science, 150,* 971–979.

Melzack, R., & Wall, P. D. (1982). *The challenge of pain.* New York: Basic Books.

Merskey, H. (Chairman) and the IASP Subcommittee on Taxonomy (1979). Pain terms: A list with definitions and notes on usage. *Pain, 6,* 249–252.

Moskovich, R. (1988). Neck pain in the elderly: Common causes and management. *Geriatrics, 4,* 65–92.

Osterweis, M., Kleinman, A., & Mechanic, D. (1987). *Pain and disability: Clinical, behavioral, and public policy perspectives*. Washington, DC: National Academy Press.

Payne, R., & Foley, K. M. (Eds.). (1987). *The medical clinics of north america: Cancer pain*. Philadelphia: W. B. Saunders.

Portenoy, R. K. (1986). Post herpetic neuralgia: A workable treatment plan. *Geriatrics, 41*, 34–48.

Portenoy, R. K. (1990). Chronic opioid therapy in nonmalignant pain. *Journal of Pain and Symptom Management, 5*, 46–62.

Portenoy, R. K., & Farkash, A. (1988). Practical management of nonmalignant pain in the elderly. *Geriatrics, 43*, 29–45.

Rapoport, A. M., Sheftell, F. D., & Baskin, S. M. (1983). Geriatric headaches. *Geriatrics, 38*(5), 81–87.

Roy, R. (1986). A psychosocial perspective on chronic pain and depression in the elderly. *Social Work in Health Care, 12*, 27–36.

Rudy, T. G., Turk, D. C., & Brena, S. F. (1988). Differential utility of medical procedures in the assessment of chronic pain patients. *Pain, 34*, 53–60.

Seligman, M. E. P. (1975). *Helplessness*. San Francisco: W. H. Freeman.

Sorkin, B. A., Rudy, T. E., Hanlon, R. B., Turk, D. C., & Stieg, R. L. (1990). Chronic pain in old and young patients: Differences appear less important than similarities. *Journal of Gerontology: Psychological Sciences, 45*, 64–68.

Tait, R. C., Chibnall, J. T., Duckro, P. N., & Deshields, T. L. (1989). Stable factors in chronic pain. *The Clinical Journal of Pain, 5*, 323–328.

Tait, R. C., Chibnall, J. T., & Margolis, R. B. (1990). Pain extent: Relations with psychological state, pain severity, pain history, and disability. *Pain, 41*, 295–301.

Tait, R. C., Duckro, P. N., Margolis, R. B., & Wiener, R. (1988). Quality of life following treatment: A preliminary study of in- and outpatients with chronic pain. *International Journal of Psychiatry in Medicine, 18*, 271–282.

Turk, D. C., & Brody, M. C. (1991). Chronic opioid therapy for persistent noncancer pain: Panacea or oxymoron? *American Pain Society Bulletin, 1*, 1–7.

Wells, P. E., Frampton, J., & Bowsher, D. (1988). *Pain management in physical therapy*. Norwalk, CT: Appleton & Lange.

White, B., & Sanders, S. H. (1985). Differential effects on pain and mood in chronic pain patients with time- versus pain-contingent medication delivery. *Behavior Therapy, 16*, 28–38.

Wolfe, F. (1988). Fibromyalgia in the elderly: Differential diagnosis and treatment. *Geriatrics, 43*(6), 57–68.

12

Behavioral and Psychotherapeutic Interventions with Residents in the Long-Term-Care Institution

Kenneth Solomon

STRESSES UNIQUE TO THE NURSING HOME RESIDENT

Older people must cope with a significant number of stressors, regardless of the setting in which they live. These have been reviewed elsewhere (Solomon, 1990; 1989; Solomon & Szwabo, 1992). In addition, there are specific stressors that affect the older person in a nursing home setting. These are stressors that can often be minimized and, to some degree, prevented by comprehensive, individualized programming and by design of an environment which is oriented toward the maximization of individuality and reinforcement of meaningful and creative behaviors.

A stressor that occurs more commonly in nursing homes than in the community is a disruption of the "self," the identity and self-image that are part of every individual's psyche. This disruption may be partially a result of brain disease, but a more important disruption of the sense of self occurs by being placed in a strange and new environment, away from family and friends. This new environment has unfamiliar surroundings, and the new resident brings only a modicum of personal belongings, remembrances, and sentimentalia with him/her when entering the institution. The resident has few reminders of the person whom she/he was, and the staff is usually uninformed as to the meaning of the few personal belongings brought by the resident. In some institutions, this disruption of the self may be compounded by the actions of staff members who may call the resident by his/her first name (usually without permission) or a nickname, and thus foster a superficial pseudointimacy with the resident that does little to reinforce a positive sense of self.

This disruption of the self is further enhanced by the vicissitudes of institutional control. The resident rarely has any say in any aspect of institutional life. This is most important in matters of daily living, which are the most personal and habitual aspects of an individual's lifestyle and which are strongly internalized into the self. The resident has limited choice or options of when she/he awakens, what she/he wears, eats, does, and where she/he goes. Usually, the resident does not choose whom will be his/her roommate and when roommates change. Although often guaranteed through "Patient Bills of Rights" and state or Federal regulations, the basic freedoms of movement, association, and interfacing with the world outside the institution are lost or are perceived to be lost. As noted with victims (Ryan, 1976), these losses become internalized perceptions within the psyche of the resident. These perceptions are frequently verbalized, even if the nursing home allows for and even encourages options, choices, and freedoms. Because these feelings are verbalized so frequently by residents, often in the face of an opposite reality, the severity of the psychic trauma caused by relocation into a long-term-care institution becomes readily apparent. To cope with the disruption of the self, many residents develop or exaggerate previously existing maladaptive behaviors or personality quirks or traits.

A second significant stressor is the disruption of the sense of personal territoriality, of personal space. Related to this stress is the loss of privacy. The loss of psychological privacy may be as important as the loss of personal privacy, if not more so. Nursing homes are very crowded, busy environments. Because of the need for care, there are continuous assaults on residents' privacy and territorial needs. Usually, the resident shares a room with a total stranger. The frequency of witnessing the death of others only adds to the unpredictability of the environment, and encroaches on the resident's psychological privacy frequently, if not daily. Many residents respond to this stress by developing exaggerated territorial behaviors, and may go so far as to physically "defend" their perceived territory.

Another significant loss is the loss of the parent image. Miesen (1990) has noted the frequency of this dynamic issue in demented residents who misidentify individuals or who wander, continuously explore the environment, or seek to "go home." Cohen-Mansfield, Werner, Marx, & Freedman (1991) have noted the frequency of a previous life-threatening event in the lives of demented nursing home residents who are "pacers." Psychodynamically, life-threatening events often trigger unresolved primitive issues, including the lack of resolution of the anxiety and terror experienced by the infant when first separating from the nurturing mother, who is experienced unconsciously as the omnipotent parent image. Entrance into a nursing home often means that the older person gives up living with a loving caregiver, who may be no longer psychologically differentiated from the primary infantile caregiver. Solomon and Szwabo (in press) have noted that agitation is the behavioral concommitant of unconscious anxiety, and the work of Miesen (1990) and Cohen-Mansfield et al., (1991) helps link this behavior to a significant psychodynamic loss in the elderly person who enters a nursing home.

Loss of self-esteem is another major loss (Lazarus, 1988). Throughout life, all people constantly seek feedback from others. This feedback relates primarily to one's self-image, sense of cognitive and interpersonal competence, body image, and self-worth. Others describe this phenomena as consensual validation (Mullahy, 1970) or self mirroring (Weiner & White, 1988). This process is a continuous one, and includes even the smallest minutiae of daily behavior and interpersonal interactions. In the long-term-care institution, this process also occurs, but unfortunately, it occasionally may be limited to that which is primarily relevant to the staff's needs. As noted by Solomon and Vickers (1979), physicians and other health care workers frequently accept the stereotype of the elderly as ill, frail, and helpless, leading to the inappropriate prescription of medications, inadequate diagnostic evaluations, and a lack of individualization of care of the elderly resident. Thus, only the sick, helpless, incompetent, and impaired parts of the self are likely to be validated in a consistent manner. As the resident internalizes this distorted self-image, she/he begins to experience guilt. This guilt is the corollary of the guilt experienced by family members. This guilt is the belief of the nursing home resident that she/he has disappointed her/his family by becoming ill, frail, or dependent. In addition, the resident experiences the shame of being and feeling helpless and the guilt of feeling as if she/he is burdening others. The resident may believe that she/he is a burden not only to her/his family, but also to the staff of the nursing home. Some residents cope with this loss by giving up any attempts to validate any aspect of themselves. They become passive "puppets," individuals who accept what is offered to them, without question. Other patients may verbalize suicidal ideation or actually attempt suicide in an attempt to unburden themselves of their guilt and shame.

The stress of feeling useless and of not being able to make a contribution to the lives of others is experienced by many residents. When coupled with a loss of status, this leads to rolelessness (Rosow, 1976). In part, this is based on the reality of being away from family and thus losing the opportunity to express certain institutionalized role behaviors, such as that of grandparent. This leads to feelings of powerlessness, anger turned against oneself (and one's self), depression, apathy, alienation, secondary psychopathology (Solomon 1990, 1989) and suicidal ideation or behaviors (Durkheim, 1987). The stress of uselessness is often exacerbated by the additional stress of boredom. Eventually, the nursing home resident may lose the desire to participate in any activity in the nursing home, even rudimentary socialization, preferring the solitude of a painful remnant of the self.

Loss of health is another stress. Very few people enter long-term care when they are both physically and mentally healthy. Rather, they are forced to make a major change in their lifestyle at a time when they are otherwise physiologically and emotionally stressed. As noted by Rovner and his colleagues (1990), individuals admitted to nursing homes are likely to suffer from dementia and frequently demonstrate major psychiatric or behavioral symptoms. With the loss of health comes the loss of activity, the loss of the ability to pursue recent interests, and a loss of energy. This is often accompanied by the additional stress of the loss of the opportunity to do what one wants to do.

A final set of stressors faced by the resident in a long-term-care institution is existential in nature. The contributions of existential theory to psychiatry and human behavior are complex and cannot be adequately discussed here. However, certain aspects are useful in examining the unique stresses faced by nursing home residents. For example, existential theory proposes that humans are temporal in nature and are always facing the future (Heidegger, 1927/1962). This future orientation is a foundation of one's weltanschauung, one's world view. It bespeaks possibility, potential, and growth (Foy, 1974). Psychopathology develops when one's world view becomes constricted, distorted, or depleted (Binswanger, 1963), all of which occur in residents in nursing homes. The nursing home resident has few goals, no raison d'être, and few opportunities to experience the world at large. Opportunities to retain a meaning for one's life in the life of the nursing home resident are few. This existential emptiness often leads to an emotional emptiness frequently seen on the faces of nursing home residents. Clinically, this is translated into depression, apathy, and alienation.

PSYCHODYNAMIC RESPONSE TO STRESS IN THE ELDERLY

There is a unique psychodynamic sequence of events experienced by an older person when experiencing stress. Much of this work is based on the pioneering work of Goldfarb (1968), upon which Solomon and his colleagues have expanded in several publications (Solomon & Ruskin, 1985; Solomon & Szwabo, 1992). When stressed, the older person initially experiences a diminished sense of mastery. These feelings are experienced as diminished mastery over internal environment (e.g., as a result of illness) and/or external environment. For the nursing home resident, this diminished mastery has a basis in reality, at least in part, because of cognitive or physical disabilities. Individuals with a personality style that emphasizes mastery over both the external and internal environments (e.g., paranoid or obsessive-compulsive individuals) may have additional difficulties with this psychological experience (Solomon, 1981b). These feelings of diminished mastery trigger feelings of helplessness. Goldfarb (1968; 1974) has noted that a "search for aid" is the usual response to internally perceived helplessness in the elderly. But because the American elderly live in a society that has valued and reinforced independence, these feelings of helplessness and associated feelings about asking for help become ambivalently experienced. The very presence of helpless feelings leads to a self-deprecatory self-commentary and a loss of self-esteem. The elderly person finds herself/himself in a no-win psychosocial situation (e.g., helpless but unable to ask for help). By not asking for help, the resident begins to feel more helpless and more inadequate. Asking for help demonstrates to others their incompetence to cope with problems, and thus, they suffer a heavy blow to their self-esteem. This psychological dilemma is generally harder for elderly men to resolve, than it is for elderly women (Solomon, 1984). Individuals with psychologic conflicts about helplessness and dependency will have further difficulties coping with these feelings (Solomon, 1981b). This helplessness is further complicated by the fact that most residents in long-term-care institutions have conditions that are associated with real helplessness. Thus, reality impinges and reinforces these uncomfortable and ambivalent feelings. At the same time, these reality situations also become stresses in and of themselves.

Helplessness and dependency are integral aspects of the sick role (Parsons, 1951). However, in long-term care, the majority of residents do not have an acute illness (except as episodic disruptions of the chronic care process). The residents in nursing home settings have combinations of chronic illness and functional disabilities. However, both staff and residents insist on a relatively rigid adherence to the sick role, in part because it is a societally acceptable institutionalized role that is unlikely to cause anxiety, whereas disabled roles are not socially acceptable and cause anxiety to the actor adopting this role (Rosow, 1976). The sick role leads to the development and reinforcement of learned helplessness, as a result of the power differential inherent in the role. The healers (e.g., the physicians, nursing staff, occupational therapists, social workers), and by extension, the institution, have all the power. When this very skewed relationship is properly used to help heal an acutely ill resident, problems are unlikely to arise.

Helplessness, dependency, and ambivalence are uncomfortable psychic phenomena. These internal experiences trigger the classic stress affects of fight (or anger) and flight (or fear), with their concomitant physiologic manifestations (Selye, 1950). In addition, as humans age, they develop a third stress affect, loss (or sadness). However, as people get older, these affects become separate from each other and have separate psychological lives. In addition, loss is often perceived as a narcissistic injury, which becomes a secondary stressor in itself.

These three stress affects are extremely uncomfortable. They disrupt psychological homeostasis. The resident experiences a secondary dysphoria which triggers a psychological response. If the resident has not allowed helplessness to take over her psychological processes, she will start a search for aid. This search may be internal (e.g., coping skills or psychodynamic defenses), supportive (e.g., family members or friends), or professional (e.g., counseling or therapy). If the search for aid is successful, psychopathology will not develop. However, if the resident does not have the ability to search for aid, if helplessness has rooted itself in the resident's psyche, or if the search for aid is unsuccessful, demoralization, and subsequent psychopathology, will develop.

There are three groups of older residents in long-term-care institutions who develop psychopathologic symptoms. The first group is those who have been able to function well throughout life, but who are now overwhelmed by the intensity, severity, and clustering of the stressor(s) that they are experiencing. The second group is those residents who may or may not have had good coping skills in the past. However, because of dementia, they are unable to utilize those coping skills, either because these skills are no longer available to them or because these skills have become an exaggerated part of their personality. The third group of residents has never been able to cope well. They may have had previous major psychiatric disorders or may have had personality disorders. They may have been individuals who had lived within a social or family environmental cocoon that protected them from having to cope with potentially overwhelming stress.

The reaction of most elderly people to stress affects falls somewhere on a continuum between pure fear and pure anger. Most elderly residents do not have a significant predominance of either fear or anger, and thus display a semiology consistent with depressive and anxious symptomatology. The experience of loss will alter the clinical manifestations of the individual's symptomatology. The more loss that is experienced, the less likely the individual will demonstrate manifest evidence of anxiety. In addition, the more somatically invested is the resident's libido, or the more narcissistic the resident, the more likely the resident will be to show evidence of somatic symptoms.

PRINCIPLES AND TECHNIQUES OF SUPPORTIVE PSYCHOTHERAPEUTIC TREATMENT OF THE NURSING HOME RESIDENT

Optimal psychiatric treatment of the elderly resident in a nursing home must have clear goals. These goals should include relief of symptoms, strengthening of coping and defense mechanisms, reduction or reversal of the severity of the triggering stresses, and prevention of future psychopathology. Treatment is most successful when done in the context of a multidisciplinary team in which different team members (these may include the resident, family members, or friends) have clear responsibilities and in which the goals of treatment are also clear. Treatment is also most successful when the plan is comprehensive and is part of a holistic orientation to the total care of the resident. Treatment is most successful when the resident is an active participant in, and not a passive recipient of, treatment.

In presenting a schema of treatment approaches, the author will be presenting a clear set of sequential steps. The reader is aware that psychiatric treatment never proceeds in such a simple, sequential manner. The first step in treatment is symptom relief. For major psychiatric symptoms, and for symptoms of severe impulse dyscontrol, psychopharmacotherapy is necessary. This is reviewed elsewhere in this book. With other kinds of symptoms, such as interpersonal behavioral difficulties, anxiety, behavioral manifestations of dementia that interfere with the care of the resident or other residents, or mildly aggressive behaviors, nonpsychopharmacologic modalities are the treatments of choice. Symptoms of anxiety may respond to relaxation techniques (Wolpe, 1969), vigorous (but not overly taxing) physical exercise, meaningful activities, meditation techniques, or diversional techniques. Simple interpersonal behavioral dysfunctions and interfering behavioral manifestations of dementia will respond to informal behavior modification techniques and other simple (and often common-sense) responses by caregivers, such as those outlined by Gwyther (1990) and Mace (1990) for demented residents. Complex or chronically maladaptive behaviors require a formal behavior modification plan. A behavior modification plan requires a detailed and formal behavior assessment, as discussed by Dye (1989), and this may be difficult to accomplish in most nursing homes. In addition, the ability to develop and successfully carry out a complex behavior modification treatment plan may be beyond the staffing availabilities of many nursing homes, although Lomranz (1991) and Santmyer and Roca (1991) have recently described successful programs in such a setting.

Ventilation of affect is the next step in the psychiatric treatment of residents in nursing homes. Residents need to express their feelings. Caregivers and therapists need to give residents explicit permission, even encouragement, to express their feelings. It is especially imperative to give men permission to express their feelings, as men in the age cohort currently institutionalized never learned how to express or label their feelings and learned that the expression of feelings is "feminine" behavior and is to be avoided (David & Brannon, 1976). Permission giving, often as simple as using the word "OK" in a validating statement, is necessary. Also, it may be necessary to express feelings for the moderately or severely demented, the inexpressive resident, or the severely depressed or psychotic but the clinician should always modify these statements so that she, and not the resident, "owns" the statement of feelings. For the resident who underexpresses feelings and overexpresses thought, a focus on both the verbal and nonverbal ventilation of feelings is necessary; Gestalt therapy techniques may be helpful. Those who overexpress feelings, often in a nonverbal way, require a focus on cognition, so that emotions and thoughts become linked to each other in a therapeutically useful manner.

The reversal of helplessness is the next therapeutic step. This almost always occurs concomitantly with the next step, the re-creation of mastery. The use of adjunctive treatment modalities and rehabilitation techniques is vital at this stage of treatment. Occupational therapists, recreation/activities therapists, and art, dance, and music therapists are necessary members of the treatment team if helplessness is to be reduced and mastery re-created.

However, all staff members can use simple behavioral reinforcement techniques to reverse helplessness. There are many behavioral techniques that can be used with nursing home residents. Many of these techniques (Shaefer & Martin, 1969), require special training. However, behavioral shaping is easily accomplished. Without realizing it, most staff members are constantly reinforcing resident behaviors. For behavioral shaping to be successful, the positive behaviors to be reinforced need to be specifically elucidated. These behaviors are broken down into its component parts. Residents should be given "homework," simple tasks related to these behaviors that the resident is capable of completing. Only one task at a time should be given. Praise is the easiest reinforcer to use, but the praise must be genuine if the behaviors and accomplishments are to be reinforced. Reinforcement should be consistently given for each positive behavior, as the clinician is attempting to break down powerful but maladaptive behavior patterns and replace them with adaptive behavior patterns. Some respond to a system of earning stars or points, which can be accumulated and subsequently used to "buy" special privileges or treats. Negative behaviors or helplessness and dependency-oriented behaviors should be extinguished by ignoring these behaviors in a matter-of-fact way. These behaviors should not be noted in interactions with the resident, as even noting them will reinforce them. Adjunctive therapists can develop more complex tasks for the resident, which, when successfully completed, will help reverse helplessness and dependency and improve self-esteem and self-confidence. As tasks are completed, increasingly complex behaviors are asked of the resident, with the same process of reinforcement and successful task completion being repeated until the resident's helplessness and dependency symptoms are reversed.

For some, a cognitive orientation to reversing helplessness can be utilized. As part of the reversal of helplessness, cognitive therapy should be considered for all depressed residents who are not significantly demented (Wright, 1988). It has been demonstrated that cognitive therapy is a beneficial therapeutic technique for the depressed elderly (DeBerry, Davis, & Reinhard, 1989). Those residents who cannot participate in formal cognitive therapy may be aided by techniques taken from that approach, including "homework assignments" that require the resident to write down positive attributes about her/himself, with a subsequent review and expansion, using supportive psychotherapeutic techniques.

The re-creation of mastery requires the development of choice. The nursing home resident with psychopathology needs to learn how to make choices. Even for demented residents, simple options in attire, foods, or activities can be developed. Many residents have a "black-and-white" cognitive set (Shapiro, 1965) and cannot develop options that are not polar opposites. Clinicians need to help them develop intermediate options, and may need to be directive and offer suggestions. As the dysfunctions improve, the level of choice can become more complex.

In the final step of the initial stage of treatment, one attempts to reverse the stressors. If this is not possible, an attempt to minimize the severity of the stress should be made. Family or marital therapy can be extremely helpful in reducing stress that emanates from interactions within the family group or the marital dyad (Goldstein, 1991). A variety of substitutive and diversional techniques, most based on common-sense responses to the source of the resident's stress, have been developed. Most of these involve programming within the nursing home environment.

The supportive psychotherapeutic techniques noted above are done by most clinicians when they interact with their resident. This is not necessarily a formal psychotherapy. More formal supportive psychotherapy is also done frequently in long-term care institutions, usually by social workers, but also by other clinicians and consultants. The informal supportive psychotherapeutic measures outlined above often take as little as 10 or 15 minutes in a "session," especially with demented residents. These "sessions" can be combined with other activities, such as meals, baths, or housekeeping activities. In supportive psychotherapy, the clinician's goals are symptom relief, allowing the resident to ventilate and clarify his/her feelings and helping the resident examine options (Lazarus, 1989). In supportive therapy, the clinician does not aim to have the resident understand her/his deep and inner psychological motivators and conflicts, although the clinician uses this understanding to help obtain the therapeutic goals.

Behavioral techniques are helpful with any resident who is demonstrating isolated types of disordered behavior. They are particularly helpful in treating dysfunctional behaviors of significantly demented residents who cannot participate in a verbal therapy. Supportive psychotherapy can be utilized with any resident who is alert, regardless of the nature of the problem. Supportive interventions also are helpful with residents who are not displaying overt behavioral or psychopathologic problems, as these techniques will help prevent the development of those problems.

INSIGHT-ORIENTED INDIVIDUAL PSYCHOTHERAPIES

Outcome studies have demonstrated that insight-oriented psychotherapeutic techniques are efficacious in the treatment of elderly psychiatric patients (Sparacino, 1978-79). Insight-oriented therapeutic techniques can benefit residents with depression, very mild dementias. episodic psychoses, and personality disorders (Hausman, in press; Lazarus, Sadavoy, & Langsley, 1991). Residents having difficulty adjusting to the institutional environment or their functional impairments may benefit from this treatment approach.

Hausman (in press) has provided an excellent summary of the goals of insight-oriented psychodynamic psychotherapy with the elderly. They are:

(1) a relationship in which the patient feels cared about; (2) emotional outlet or catharsis; (3) enhancement of self-esteem; (4) minimization of psychological and behavioral problems; (5) increase in coping skills; (6) enhancement of role functioning; (7) a sense of control; (8) the ability to grieve over losses of roles, capacities, and significant others; (9) development and maintenance of the most mature and productive defenses possible while shedding inappropriate defenses; (10) the development of insight." Similar goals have been noted by Pollock (1987) and Lazarus, Sadavoy, and Langsley (1991). The basic techniques of insight-oriented psychotherapy are generally unchanged with the elderly and include questioning, clarification, redefinition, and interpretation (Lazarus, 1989; Solomon & Ruskin, 1985). However, these techniques may need some modifications for use with some elderly.

GROUP PSYCHOTHERAPIES

Group psychotherapy is indicated for residents whose primary problems are more interpersonal than intrapsychic (Leszcz, 1991; Tross & Blum, 1988). These residents generally have difficulties with socialization, are depressed, or have personality disorders. There are many different group psychotherapies that are beneficial for the elderly (Leszcz, 1991; Solomon & Szwabo, 1992). It is important to note that not all groups can be considered group psychotherapy. To be considered a psychotherapy, a focus on changing behavior, and not maintaining behavior, supplying a recreational diversion, or preventing the development of dysfunctional behavior, must be the primary goal of the group.

Analytic or psychodynamic group psychotherapy is helpful with the same group of elderly who benefit from insight-oriented psychotherapy (Goldwasser, Auerbach & Harkins, 1987; Lazarus, 1980; Leszcz, 1991; Tross & Blum, 1988). Cognitive/behavioral therapy groups are particularly useful in the treatment of depressed elderly (Steuer et al., 1984). Groups with a supportive orientation may be helpful for those residents in institutions who cannot work at the level of abstract insight demanded by the type of group noted above. Indeed, the first psychotherapy groups for the elderly were supportive therapy groups for chronic schizophrenic and demented residents in nursing homes, and the results of these groups were quite favorable (Linden, 1953; Silver, 1950).

The primary goals of group psychotherapy are symptom reduction, a change in interpersonal behaviors, and improvement in interpersonal skills (Leszcz, 1991; Solomon & Szwabo, 1992). Other goals of group therapy include the reduction of isolation, mutual support and conflict resolution, the enhancement of communication skills, and an increase in self-esteem and self-acceptance (Solomon & Zinke, 1991). Themes expressed in group psychotherapy have some commonality with the themes of individual psychotherapy. Losses, the existential uncertainty of life and the future, and the role of medical illnesses and functional disabilities in the patients' lives are particularly common themes (Solomon & Zinke, 1991). Conflicts over dependency, interpersonal conflicts outside the group, and psychodynamic concommitants of depression are other frequent themes (Leszcz, 1991).

In developing groups, it is important to plan for residents whose level of cognitive and functional impairments is relatively homogeneous. Homogeneity allows for the development of clinical goals relevant to the specific problems of those residents and the rapid development of a group cohesiveness that enhances the efficacy of the group (Leszcz, 1991).

Reality orientation groups are probably the most common groups in nursing homes. However, there are no good data that reality orientation does anything other than provide another structured means of socialization for severely impaired patients (Solomon, 1991). There is no evidence that attendance in this kind of group improves orientation and contact with reality for severely impaired patients, although there is some evidence to suggest that social interactions improve. Other formats can be used to achieve this goal, and more cognitively intact individuals can relate to each other and to events that are going on outside the nursing home by participating in other types of groups that are appropriate for their level of intellectual functioning.

Over the past 40 years, many different kinds of groups have developed in nursing homes (Lazarus, 1989; Leszcz, 1991; Tross & Blum, 1988). These include a variety of socialization groups, including kaffee klatsches, happy hours, and sports groups. Other groups have a focus on intellectual and spiritual stimulation, and include religious groups, Bible study, book review, and current events groups. Groups with specific therapeutic goals, such as assertiveness training groups, have been developed or adapted for use in nursing homes. Groups utilizing alternatives to traditional verbal psychotherapeutic groups, such as psychodrama, art therapy, music therapy, poetry therapy, and dance/movement therapy, have also been utilized successfully. Some groups have a rehabilitative orientation, and may include budgeting and shopping groups, activities of daily living retraining groups, cooking groups, and exercise groups. Other groups emphasize physical activity and sensory-motor stimulation, and include exercise, walking, and swimming groups. Details about technical issues involved in starting and leading these varied groups are readily available in publications easily found in most professional libraries. The number and kinds of groups that one can develop for residents in long-term-care institutions are limited only by the creativity of the staff.

PREVENTION OF PSYCHIATRIC PROBLEMS IN NURSING HOMES

Most publications in psychogeriatrics focus on diagnostic and treatment issues. Prevention is rarely addressed. Although most of the stresses that may trigger psychopathology in this population cannot be prevented, a psychosocial environment can be developed in nursing homes that minimizes the negative impact of these stresses and enhances aggressive interventions that may prevent the development of major psychopathologic symptoms. A prophylactic environment requires adequate numbers of trained staff who are satisfied with their jobs. Solomon and Vickers (1979) have demonstrated that staff who work with the elderly in a growth-oriented environment are less likely to stereotype the elderly.

The psychosocial environment must create meaningful options and expect residents to make choices for themselves. By creating an environment in which residents and staff are challenged and in which they experience the rewards of their efforts on a daily basis, the chance of developing a power differential in the relationships between staff and residents is diminished.

REFERENCES

Binswanger, L. (1963). *Being-in-the-world.* New York: Basic Books.

Cohen-Mansfield, J., Werner, P., Marx, M. S., & Freedman, L. (1991). Two studies of pacing in the nursing home. *Journal of Gerontology, 46,* M77–M83.

David, D. S., & Brannon, R. (1976). The male sex role: Our culture's blueprint of manhood and what it's done for us lately. In D. S. David, & R. Brannon (Eds.), *The forty-nine percent majority: The male sex role* (pp. 1–45). Reading, PA: Addison-Wesley.

DeBerry, S., Davis, S., & Reinhard, K. E. (1989). A comparison of meditation-relaxation and cognitive/behavioral techniques for reducing anxiety and depression in a geriatric population. *Journal of Geriatric Psychiatry, 22,* 231–247.

Durkheim, E. (1987). *Le suicide* [Suicide]. Paris: R. Alcon.

Dye, C. J. (1989). Assessment in behavior management programs for older adults. In T. Hunt & C. Lindly (Eds.), *Testing older adults* (pp. 163–184). Austin, TX: Pro-Ed.

Foy, J. L. (1974). The existential school. In S. Arieti (Ed.), *American handbook of psychiatry* (2nd ed., Vol. I, pp. 926–940) New York: Basic Books.

Goldfarb, A. I. (1968). Clinical perspectives. In A. Simon; L. J. Epstein (Eds.), *Aging in Modern Society. Psychiatric Research Report No. 23.* pp. 170–178. Washington, American Psychiatric Association.

Goldfarb, A. I. (1974). Minor maladjustments of the aged. In S. Arietti & E. B. Brody (Eds.), *American handbook of psychiatry* (2nd ed., Vol. III, pp. 820–860). New York: Basic Books.

Goldstein, M. (1991). Family therapy. In J. Sadavoy, L. W. Lazarus & L. F. Jarvik (Eds.), *Comprehensive review of geriatric psychiatry* (pp. 513–525). Washington, DC: American Psychiatric Press.

Goldwasser, A. N., Auerbach, S. M., & Harkins, S. W. (1987). Cognitive, affective, and behavioral effects of reminiscence group therapy on demented elderly. *International Journal of Aging and Human Development, 25,* 209–222.

Gwyther, L. P. (1990). Clinician and family: A partnership for support. In N. L. Mace (Ed.), *Dementia care. Patient, family, and community* (pp. 193–230). Baltimore: Johns Hopkins University Press.

Hausman, C. P. (in press). Dynamic psychotherapy with elderly demented patients. In G. Jones & B. Miesen (Eds.), *Caregiving in dementia.* Amsterdam: Routledge Publishers.

Heidegger, M. (1962). *Being and time.* New York: Harper & Row. (Original work published 1927).

Lazarus, L. W. (1980). Self-psychology and psychotherapy with the elderly: Theory and practice. *Journal of Geriatric Psychiatry, 13,* 69–88.

Lazarus, L. W. (1988). Self-psychology—Its application to brief psychotherapy with the elderly. *Journal of Geriatric Psychiatry, 21,* 109–125.

Lazarus, L. W. (1989). Psychotherapy with geriatric patients in the ambulatory care setting. In E. Busse & D. Blazer (Eds.), *Geriatric psychiatry* (pp. 567–591). Washington, DC: American Psychiatric Press.

Lazarus, L. W., Sadavoy, J., & Langsley, P. R. (1991). Individual psychotherapy. In J. Sadavoy, L. W. Lazarus, & L. F. Jarvik (Eds.), *Comprehensive review of geriatric psychiatry* (pp. 487–512). Washington, DC: American Psychiatric Press.

Leszcz, M. (1991). Group therapy. In J. Sadavoy, L. W. Lazarus, & L. F. Jarvik (Eds.), *Comprehensive review of geriatric psychiatry* (pp. 527–546). Washington, DC: American Psychiatric Press.

Linden, M. (1953). Group psychotherapy with institutionalized senile women: Studies in geronotologic human relationships. *International Journal of Group Psychotherapy, 3,* 150–170.

Lomranz, J. (1991). Mental health in homes for the aged and the clinical psychology of aging: Implementation of a model service. *Clinical Gerontologist, 10*(3), 47–72.

Mace, N. L. (1990). The management of problem behaviors. In N. Mace (Ed.), *Dementia care. Patient, family, and community* (pp. 74–112). Baltimore: Johns Hopkins University Press.

Miesen, B. (1990). *Gehechtheid en dementie [Attachment and dementia]* (pp. 223–225). Nijmegen: Katholieke Universiteit Nijmegen.

Mullahy, P. (1970). *Psychoanalysis and interpersonal psychiatry: The contributions of Harry Stack Sullivan* (pp. 84–85). New York: Science House.

Parsons, T. (1951). *The social system* (pp. 428–473). New York: Free Press.

Pollock, G. H. (1987). The mourning-liberation process: Ideas on the inner life of the older adult. In J. Sadavoy, M. Leszcz, & (Eds.), *Treating the elderly with psychotherapy. The scope for change in later life* (pp. 3–29). New York: International Universities Press.

Rosow, I. (1976). Status and role change through the life span. In R. H. Binstock & E. Shanas (Eds.), *Handbook of aging and the social sciences* (pp. 457–482). New York: Van Nostrand Reinhold.

Rovner, B. W., German, P. S., Broadhead, J., Morriss, R. K., Brant, L. J., Blaustein, J., & Folstein, M. F. (1990). The prevalence and management of dementia and other psychiatric disorders in nursing homes. *International Psychogeriatrics, 2,* 13–24.

Ryan, W. (1976). *Blaming the victim* (rev. ed). New York: Vintage Books.

Santmyer, K. S., & Roca, R. P. (1991). Geropsychiatry in long-term care: A nurse-centered approach. *Journal of the American Geriatrics Society, 39,* 156–159.

Selye, H. (1950). *The physiology and pathology of exposure to stress.* Montreal: Acta.

Shaefer, H. H., & Martin, P. L. (1969). *Behavioral therapy.* New York: McGraw-Hill.

Shapiro, D. (1965). *Neurotic styles.* New York: Basic Books.

Silver, A. (1950). Group psychotherapy with senile psychotic patients. *Geriatrics, 5,* 147–150.

Solomon, K. (1981a). The elderly patient. In E. B. Brody (Ed.), *Clinical medicine: Vol. XII. Psychiatry* (pp. 1–14). Hagerstown MD: Harper & Row.

Solomon, K. (1981b). Personality disorders in the elderly. In J. R. Lion (Ed.), *Personality disorders: Diagnosis and management* (2nd ed). Baltimore: Williams & Wilkins.

Solomon, K. (1984). Psychosocial crises of older men. *Hillside Journal of Clinical Psychiatry, 6,* 123–134.

Solomon, K. (1989). Psychosocial dysfunction in the aged: Assessment and intervention. In O. L. Jackson (Ed.), *Physical therapy of the geriatric patient* (2nd ed., pp. 95–127). New York: Churchill Livingstone.

Solomon, K. (1990) Mental health and the elderly. In A. Monk (Ed.), *Handbook of gerontological services* (2nd ed., pp. 228–267) New York: Columbia University Press.

Solomon, K. (1991). Learned helplessness in the elderly: Theoretic and clinical implications. *Occupational Therapy in Mental Health, 10*(3), 31–51.

Solomon, K., & Ruskin, P. (1985). Psychodynamic psychotherapy with the elderly. In M. Bright, E. Stilwell, & M. Tayback (Eds.), *Proceedings of the Second Annual Meeting and Scientific Conference of the Maryland Gerontological Association* (pp. 17–21). Baltimore: Maryland Gerontological Association.

Solomon, K., & Szwabo, P. A. (1992). The subjective experience of and psychodynamic psychotherapies for the patient with Alzheimer's disease. In J. E. Morley, R. Coe, R. Strong, & G. T. Grossberg (Eds.). *Memory functioning and aging-related disorders.* New York: Springer.

Solomon, K., & Vickers, R. (1979). Attitudes of health care workers toward old people. *Journal of the American Geriatrics Society, 27,* 186–191.

Solomon, K., & Zinke, M. R. (1991). Group psychotherapy with the depressed elderly. *Journal of Gerontological Social Work, 17*(1/2), 47–57.

Sparacino, J. (1978–79). Individual psychotherapy with the aged: A selective review. *International Journal of Aging and Human Development, 9,* 197–220.

Steuer, J. L., Mintz, J., Hammen, C. L., Hill, M. A., Jarvik, L. F., McCarley, R., Motoike, P., & Rosen, R. (1984). Cognitive-behavioral and psychodynamic group psychotherapy in treatment of geriatric depression. *Journal of Consulting and Clinical Psychology, 52*(4), 80–189.

Tross, S., & Blum, J. E. (1988). A review of group therapy with the older adult: Practice and research. In B. W. MacLennan, S. Saul, & M. B. Weiner (Eds.), *Group psychotherapies for the elderly* (pp. 3–29). Madison CT: International Universities Press.

Weiner, M. B., & White, M. T. (1988). The third chance: Self-psychology as an effective group approach for older adults. In B. W. MacLennan, S. Saul, & M. B. Weiner (Eds.), *Group psychotherapies for the elderly* (pp. 57–66). Madison CT: International Universities Press.

Wolpe, J. (1969). *The practice of behavior therapy.* New York: Pergamon Press.

Wright, J. H. (1988). Cognitive therapy of depression. In A. J. Frances & R. E. Hales (Eds.), *Review of psychiatry* (Vol. 7, pp. 554–570). Washington, DC: American Psychiatric Press.

13

Wandering: Assessment and Intervention

Donna L. Algase

ASSESSMENT AND INTERVENTION

A growing number of studies on behavioral issues in long-term care focus on wandering behavior. Most of these studies examine the efficacy of possible interventions for wandering, while few describe or explain this puzzling behavior.

Faced with the immediate demands of caregiving, clinicians may regard a research emphasis on intervention as desirable. But emphasis on intervention without bases in description and cause is palliative, at best. Further, such emphasis reflects a view of wandering as a given in cognitively impaired persons and overlooks any meaning or purpose to the behavior in its own right. Yet not all cognitively impaired persons wander and, though hazards are associated with wandering, the behavior itself can be regarded as meaningful, rather than problematic.

In this chapter, wandering is cast as meaningful behavior. It is described and explained by existing theoretical work and research findings pertaining to its pattern and bases. Assessment and intervention protocols for the management of wandering are then developed from this foundation.

THE PHENOMENON OF WANDERING

Clinicians are imprecise in using the term wandering. To some it means a propensity to elope from the unit or facility. To others it signifies the ambulation patterns of persons with wayfinding problems. The term can also apply to the frequent and repetitive activity patterns of cognitively-impaired persons, considered remnants of earlier habits and preferences.

Among researchers, clarity on the meaning of wandering is also lacking. A variety of definitions have been proposed, but few have been operationalized in any clinically useful way. However, aimlessness (Monsour & Robb, 1982; Synder, Rupprecht, Pyrek, Brekhus, & Moss, 1978), disregard for hazards (Hussain, 1981, 1982; Robb, 1987), and a sense of dis- or misplacement (Algase, 1988; Hussain, 1981, 1982; Wolanin & Phillips, 1981) are all qualities that have been used to characterize the phenomenon. Aside from cognitive impairment, movement is the only universal in definitions of wandering.

The actual movement patterns of wanderers have received little study (Algase & Cheng, 1991; Hussain, 1981, 1982; Snyder, Rupprecht, Pyrek, Brekhus, & Moss, 1978). However, across these works, wandering is not continuous activity; rather, it consists of frequent starts and stops. Compared to nonwanderers, wanderers spend more time alone and in motion (Snyder et al., 1978). Wanderers also stop more frequently at or near other persons: 59% as compared to 41% at other locations (windows, chairs, and water fountains) (Hussain, 1981, 1982).

In a random sample of 31 wanderers from eight nursing homes observed over two 24-hour periods one week apart (Algase & Cheng, 1991), wanderers averaged 79 episodes of locomotion per day (range = 13 to 206). On average, wanderers ambulated during 14 hours of the day, but may have moved during as few as 6 or as many as 20 hours. In every hour that a person walked, they averaged about 5 episodes (range = 1.56 to 12.8).

In total, each wanderer spent a mean of 110 minutes ambulating per day, ranging from 22.8 to 257.0. They averaged 4.7 minutes in motion (range = 1.0 to 10.7) during every hour of the day, or 7.4 minutes per hour (range = 2.5 to 16.0) when ambulation was averaged only over those hours during which episodes occurred.

Figure 13.1 presents the distribution of wandering episodes and minutes in motion for this sample averaged over the two observation days. Although number of episodes, number of hours during which ambulation occurred, and minutes ambulating varied widely among subjects, a given wanderer's pattern was stable over the two-day period. Number of episodes and minutes in motion are somewhat parallel, generally increasing over the late morning hours and peaking in the late afternoon.

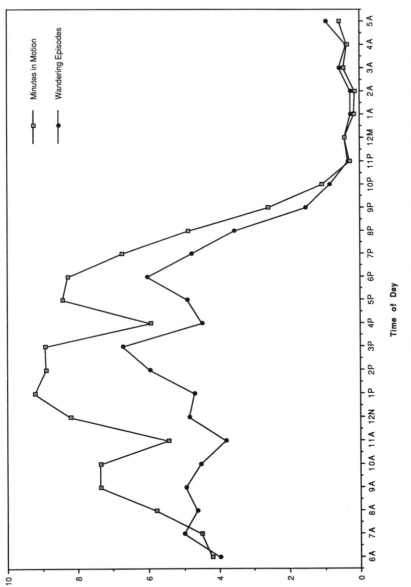

FIGURE 13.1 Two-Day Hourly Average of Wandering Episodes and Minutes in Motion (N = 31).

WANDERING TYPES

Several wandering types have been proposed, but none were derived by valid scientific methods. However, these types deserve mention because they suggest possible alternative reasons or causes for wandering. Synder et al. (1978) named three types of wandering: overtly goal-directed/searching (S), goal-directed/industrious (I), and nongoal-directed (N). An S searched almost constantly for something not attainable. An I was characterized by an inexhaustible drive to remain busy. Finally, an N was highly distractible. Hoffman and Platt (1990) expanded Snyder's types by differentiating wandering in terms of energy level and presence or absence of a goal. The four resulting types are: (1) high energy level/goal directed (wants to go home), (2) high energy/no defined goal (activity itself is the goal and movement is soothing), (3) low energy level/goal directed (unexpectedly leaves), and (4) low energy level/no defined goal (a pacer).

Clinicians have suggested several other kinds of wandering. Three are: (1) active wandering, including agitated behavior, where the wanderer is searching for something or attempting to keep busy; (2) passive or placid wandering, where ambulation is aimless and the wanderer is easily distracted; and (3) nocturnal or night-time wandering, which could be either active or passive (Hirst & Metcalf, 1989).

Finally, Hussain and Davis (1983) offered yet another categorization. Four types were named. Akathesia-induced ambulation was the term for the inability to sit still found among long-term users of neuroleptics. Exit-seeking behavior was highly motivated movement, persisting until gratification was found to reduce the desire to leave. Self-stimulatory wandering was a signal for inadequate sensory stimulation. Lastly, modeling was the term for shadowing or following someone.

WHO WANDERS?

By one estimate, one in five ambulatory, cognitively impaired nursing home residents is a wanderer (Algase, 1988). Approximately 11% of all nursing home residents wander (National Center for Health Statistics, 1979). Wanderers do not differ from other nursing home residents in age, length of residence in the facility, and gender distribution. Wanderers have been described best in terms of cognitive function, medical diagnoses, and various psychosocial dimensions.

In two studies comparing wanderers and nonwanderers within one clinical setting, wanderers compared to other residents in overall levels of impairment (Cornbleth, 1977; DeLeon, Potegal, & Gurland, 1984; Snyder et al., 1978). DeLeon and associates (1984) also showed that wanderers had poorer parietal lobe functioning than subjects with similar degrees of cognitive impairment. However, in a multisite random sample of 163 ambulatory, cognitively impaired subjects, wanderers showed significantly greater impairment in basic skills (orientation, memory, and concentration) and in the higher-order skills of language, abstract thinking, judgment, and spatial skills (Algase, 1991). Language was the higher-order skill best differentiating these two groups. Approximately 95% of nonwanderers were correctly classified based on language skills, while only 38% of wanderers were correctly grouped. Thus, nonwanderers may be a more homogenous group with regard to type of cognitive skill deficit than are wanderers. According to nurses' judgments, wanderers had more difficulty with speech and reading but better social skills, less withdrawal, and more mobility than other cognitively impaired nursing home residents. Though wanderers may have more cognitive decline, they exhibit an intact social facade which masks their deficits (Dawson & Reid, 1987).

In Snyder's (1978) sample, 54% of wanderers had organic brain syndrome (OBS), 27.3% had at least one stroke, and 63.3% suffered from heart disease. In contrast to nonwanderers, differences were highly significant for OBS. In Monsour and Robb's (1982) sample, 36 of 44 subjects had OBS, dementia or Alzheimer's disease; 8 had cerebral vascular accidents or arteriosclerosis. Comparing medical diagnoses charted in the nursing home record for 159 wanderers and nonwanderers, Algase (1991) found a significant association between medical basis of cognitive impairment and status as a wanderer or nonwanderer: wanderers were more likely to have a mixed basis of impairment (75.5% versus 54.0%) while nonwanderers were more likely to have only reversible causes documented (38.1% versus 5.1%).

Snyder and associates (1978) also identified that wanderers had a higher number of psychosocial needs than nonwanderers on the Human Development Inventory (HDI) test. As compared to nonwanderers for the period from age 40 to onset of illness, wanderers had engaged in more social and leisure activities, experienced more stressful life events, employed a more motor than emotional reaction to stress, and displayed a more motor behavioral style as reported by their significant others (Monsour & Robb, 1982).

WONDER WHY THEY WANDER?

As a behavior, wandering can be affected by factors in the person, the environment, or both. Personal bases for wandering behavior include physiological and psychological explanations.

PHYSIOLOGICAL BASES

Biochemically, the dopamine hypothesis of schizophrenia may explain wandering. Accordingly, amphetamines and dopamine agonists can cause restlessness and non goal-directed behavior (Costa & Garrattini, 1970). Thus, reduced levels of acetylcholine found in Alzheimer's disease (AD) victims could result in a relative excess of dopamine, leading to increased motor activity and restlessness (Weller, 1987). Though compatible with wandering in AD victims, this hypothesis has not been tested.

Other physiological explanations of wandering include: medication interactions, sedatives, or tranquilizers; physical discomfort due to pain, hunger, thirst, constipation, or need to urinate; and desire to exercise. Nocturnal wandering may signal cardiac decompensation or circadian rhythm disturbance (Burnside, 1980). Again, empirical testing is needed to support these claims.

PSYCHOLOGICAL BASES

Psychological causes for wandering have also been offered. Wandering has been viewed as a form of agenda behavior, aimed at meeting felt social, emotional, or physical needs (Rader, Doan, & Schwab, 1985). Through anecdotes, wandering was shown to stem from loneliness and separation. Three sources for agenda behavior were named: (1) fear engendered by separation from the people and environment to which a wanderer feels connected, (2) frustration when staff thwart agenda behavior, and (3) the need to be needed. Results of Monsour and Robb's (1982) study also suggest that wandering addresses a psychological need: it may dissipate stress.

Other untested psychological explanations for wandering include anxiety, agitation, tension, boredom with or lack of activity, living in the past and sustaining old habits, feeling useless or helpless while watching others perform tasks, depression, loneliness, separation, and perceiving caregivers' anger or impatience (Robinson, Spencer, & White, 1989).

ENVIRONMENTAL BASES

Factors in the environment may also precipitate wandering. Hussain (1981) concluded that wandering was not random; rather, episodes were terminated by reinforcing stimuli. Wanderers develop consistent geographic travel patterns, stopping at points of interest. Further, wandering patterns can be altered by using behavior modification and environmental cuing (Hussain, 1981, 1982; Hussain & Brown, 1987).

Other environmental factors thought to induce wandering include difficulty making sense of the environment (Algase, 1988), overly stimulating (Hall & Buckwalter, 1987) or nonstimulating environments, restrictive surroundings, and new or unpredictable situations (Roberts & Algase, 1988).

A poor or impoverished social environment may also play a role in wandering behavior. Compared to nonwanderers in the psychosocial areas of friendliness, communication skills, and self-control, wanderers declined over time (Cornbleth, 1977). Wanderers also spend a greater percentage of time in nonsocial behavior, like being alone or sleeping (Synder et al., 1978). Though each of these studies reflects differing views and measures of social functioning, they suggest that wandering and social interaction are inversely connected. For some persons, wandering may replace interaction, as cognitive decline affects the ability of wanderers to relate effectively.

ASSESSING THE WANDERER

An analysis of the wanderer's behavior can provide a basis for a plan to moderate or alter wandering behavior. The definitions and explanations of wandering reviewed thus far offer some direction. Outlined in Table 13.1 is a protocol for assessing wanderers. Because the use of this guide can reveal the wanderer's pattern, as well as factors contributing to wandering behavior, it provides a sound basis for intervention.

INTERVENTIONS FOR WANDERING

Though many interventions for wandering have been suggested, few have been systematically tested. Those that have been examined are generally focused on reducing the exit behavior of wanderers and not on altering the overall quantity, timing, or spatial pattern of wandering. Thus, the efficacy of most strategies for managing or reducing wandering behavior remains unknown.

Though physical or chemical restraint can be detrimental for wanderers (Miller, 1975), many other strategies are noninvasive and inexpensive, offering few risks or hazards. While further research can improve our understanding of the techniques that are most effective and efficient, lack of research should not inhibit use of common sense or trial and error with low-risk strategies.

Table 13.1 Assessment Protocol for Wandering Behavior

Aspect	Approach
Pattern	
Quantity of movement	Count and time episodes for 10 minutes/hour around the clock to establish three-day baseline (Algase & Cheng, 1991).
Frequency of movement	Graph the number of episodes and total minutes in motion per hour from observations.
Distance and direction of movement	Map pathway by tracing movements on a floor plan during each observation period (Snyder et al., 1978).
Motor output	Apply activity meters to trunk or ankle to register accumulated movement hourly over periods of 12–24 hours. (Algase, 1988).
Contributing factors	
Cognitive status	Assess level of cognitive impairment at admission and monthly using the Mini Mental Status Examination (Folstein, Folstein, & McHugh, 1975), the short memory-orientation-concentration test (Katzman, Brown, Fuld, Peck, Schecter, & Shimmel, 1983), or other valid and reliable tools.
	Assess abstract thinking, judgment, language and spatial skills (Algase & Beel-Bates, 1991).
	Determine medical rationale for cognitive impairment to identify reversible causes.
Physiologic parameters	Assess vital signs on a schedule coinciding with hours of greatest motion, longest distances, and/or largest motor output.
	Monitor patterns of elimination, exercise, and food and fluid intake. Correlate with dimensions of wandering pattern.
	Check for pain.
	Evaluate medication regimen. Retain only essential medications.
Psychological traits and needs	Get history of previous habits, interests, leisure activities (Snyder et al., 1978), and ways of coping with stress (Monsour & Robb, 1982) from family member.
	Attempt to detect motive, goal, or agenda (Rader et al., 1985) by observing for signs of fear, anxiety, boredom, loneliness.
	Distinguish apparent wandering from problems of wayfinding.
Environmental triggers	
Time of day	Review graph for times of high activity. Correlate with unit activities, care activities, change of shift, etc.
Associated activity	Monitor activity antecedent and consequent to wandering episodes to identify possible stimuli or rewards for wandering (Hirst & Metcalf, 1989; Hussain, 1981; 1982).

Sensory stimulation	Observe the effect of light, noise, and general ward activity on the pattern of wandering episodes. Observe for misperceptions of objects in the environment.
Locale	Observe the starting and stopping places of wandering episodes (Hussain, 1982).
Atmospheric conditions	Note the effect of weather and season on the frequency and pattern of wandering episodes.
Outcomes	
Weight change	Obtain weight upon admission and weekly.
Foot and leg trauma	Assess feet and legs for blisters, calluses, edema at admission and weekly.
Range of motion	Assess strength, flexibility, and range of motion of extremities at admission and monthly.
Social skills	Assess social capabilities at admission and monthly. Monitor frequency, and meaningfulness of social interactions.
Falls	Investigate all falls. Analyze contributing factors for pattern.
Elopement	Monitor the frequency, stated goals, destination, and time of day of all attempted exits. Analyze for pattern.

A number of interventions should be routinely used with wanderers in consideration of their general safety. These are listed in Table 13.2.

When aiming to modify or reduce wandering, several general concerns apply, regardless of the type or cause of wandering. First, interventions aimed at both personal and environmental factors should be considered. Second, it may be necessary to try several approaches before the best alternative for a given pattern becomes clear. To identify the most effective approach, attempt them sequentially and evaluate the effects of each systematically. Because of hazards associated with restraints, all types should be avoided whenever less restrictive alternatives are available. Based on etiology, additional interventions for wandering are summarized in Table 13.3.

SUMMARY

Current understanding of wandering behavior is limited. The behavior clearly requires further research to more fully describe and explain it, as well as to evaluate interventions for managing it. However, ideas from current research and clinical practice presented in this chapter do lend some direction in providing safe and effective care for wanderers.

Table 13.2 General Safety Considerations for Wanderers

Wear comfortable, well-fitting clothing

Wear shoes with rubber soles and good support; avoid slippers or socks

Provide yearly physical and eye exams

Provide functional eyeglasses and hearing aids

Use prosthetic walking devices appropriately

Provide frequent finger foods and liquids, within dietary limitations

Apply a wrist or ankle identification with name, address, phone number, and words "mentally impaired, prone to wander"

Monitor whereabouts every 10 to 15 minutes; observe continuously while actively wandering

Assign a room located away from stairwells or exits

Keep exit doors on units housing wanderers closed and, if not continuously visible to staff, equip with alarms

Table 13.3 Intervention Strategies for Wandering Behavior by Etiology

Etiology	Interventions
Physiological	
Medications	Gradually decrease and then stop antipsychotic and sleep medications whenever possible.
Need for exercise	Formal exercise classes (Robb, 1987). Supervised daily walks outside when feasible. Allow wanderer to push other residents in their wheelchair if resident is willing.
Exhaustion	Place chairs in strategic places in hallway. Encourage wanderer to rest with feet elevated. Distract wanderer with activities they can do while sitting. Massage/back rub. Offer food and drink.
Circadian rhythm upset or nocturnal wandering	Keep wanderer active during the day. Shorten or eliminate daytime naps (Young, Muir-Nash, & Ninos, 1988). Provide daily exercise (Robb, 1982). Expose to outdoor sunlight for at least one half-hour daily when feasible. Maintain stable daily routine.
Psychological	
Boredom or sensory stimulation seeking	Supervised structured activities such as music therapy, simple crafts, cosmetic sessions, or memory recall. Activities to stimulate senses (table with different-textured objects). Plan activities based on wanderer's past skills and interests.
Agenda behavior	Use distraction techniques. Approach by only one person. Use a soft voice. Repeat what wanderer has said. Leave and return in five minutes if wanderer is fearful or agitated. Give meaningful task that wanderer can successfully complete (fold laundry, make a bed, set table) (Rader et al., 1985).

Social environment

Limited opportunity or reduction in meaningful communication

Four interaction strategies to moderate wandering: (Algase & Struble, 1991).

(1) Affirm: Comments or questions aimed at validating the wanderer's experience (e.g., greeting, praising, thanking, complimenting, consoling, and validating the problem, need, or feeling state once it has been established).

(2) Clarify: Statements or questions aimed at finding out the problem or need (e.g., assessing, allowing for expression of feelings, or probing to gain information about the person).

(3) Direct: Statements or questions which lead a wanderer to a course of action or activity (e.g., suggesting an alternative, changing activities, issuing a directive, or providing distraction).

(4) Provide: Statements or questions which offer assistance or match a wanderer to a resource (e.g., extensions of personal support or presence or offerings of material or physical comfort.)

Physical environment

Safety hazards

Install alarm systems, locks and/or camouflage exit doors. Clear pathways of obstacles (rugs, medical equipment, or outside stones and branches on path). Enhance lighting, especially at night (leave bathroom or night light on). Lock up hazardous materials. Fence in yard for safe walking.

Unclear environment

Provide redundant cuing (Roberts & Algase, 1988) by giving more than one type of sensory cue (e.g., mealtimes: use a chime/dinner bell and food-scented air freshener; at bedtime: diminish lights, lower noise level, reproduce rhythmic sounds of nature). Decorate bulletin boards with information about upcoming holidays. Use large digital clocks in wanderer's room. Allow wanderer to explore safely. Relocate wanderer's room if continually entering another room. Decorate wanderer's door with meaningful items from their past and place a picture of the wanderer from their earlier years at eye level on their door. Attach identification symbols such as different colored awnings above the men's and women's bathroom (Coons, 1988). Use rooms for single purposes (do not interchange dining room for living room or craft area).

Overstimulating environment

Avoid intercom systems, buzzing call lights, and humming or noisy equipment. Avoid continuous use of television or radio. Utilize carpeting to reduce noise levels. Avoid busy, patterned interior. Direct wanderer to a private, quiet place when environment is noisy or busy (e.g., shift change).

Understimulating environment

Supervise access to outside. Encourage keeping meaningful possessions. Color contrast floors and walls. Vary texture of objects. Provide wall hangings, pictures, plants, fish aquarium, or pets.

REFERENCES

Algase, D. L. (1988). *Cognitive and social discriminants of wandering behavior among cognitively impaired nursing home residents.* Unpublished doctoral dissertation, Case Western Reserve University, Cleveland, OH.

Algase, D. L., (1991). *Cognitive discriminants of wandering.* Unpublished manuscript. University of Michigan, Ann Arbor, MI.

Algase, D. L., & Beel-Bates, C. (1991). *Everyday indicators of impaired cognition: Development of a new screening.* Unpublished manuscript. University of Michigan, Ann Arbor, MI.

Algase, D. L., & Cheng J. (1991). *Wandering behavior of cognitively impaired nursing home residents: A rhythm perspective.* Unpublished manuscript. University of Michigan, Ann Arbor, MI.

Algase, D. L., & Struble, L. M. (1991). *Interacting with wanderers: What experts say.* Unpublished manuscript. University of Michigan, Ann Arbor, MI.

Burnside, I. M. (1980). Wandering behavior. In I. M. Burnside (Ed.), *Psychosocial nursing care of the aged* (pp. 298-309). New York: McGraw-Hill.

Coons, D. H. (1988). Wandering. *The American Journal of Alzheimer's Care and Related Disorders and Research, 3*(1), 31–36.

Cornbleth, T. (1977). Effects of a protected hospital ward area on wandering and nonwandering geriatric patients. *Journal of Gerontology, 32*(5), 573–577.

Costa, E., & Garrattini, S. (Eds.) (1970). International Symposium on Amphetamines and Related Compounds. *Proceedings of the Mario Negri Institute for Pharamacological Research.* New York: Raven Press.

Dawson, P., & Reid, D. W. (1987). Behavioral dimension of patients at risk for wandering. *The Gerontologist, 27*(1), 104–107.

DeLeon, M. J., Potegal, M., & Gurland, B. (1984). Wandering and parietal lobe signs in senile dementia of Alzheimer's type. *Neuropsychobiology, 11*, 155–157.

Folstein, M. F., Folstein, S., & McHugh, P. R. (1975). Mini-mental state: A practical method for grading the cognitive status of patients for the clinician. *Journal of Psychiatric Research, 12*, 189–198.

Hall, G., & Buckwalter, K. (1987). Progressively lowered stress threshold: A conceptual model for care of adults with Alzheimer's disease. *Archives of Psychiatric Nursing, 1*(6), 399–406.

Hirst, S. T., & Metcalf, B. J. (1989). Whys and whats of wandering. *Geriatric Nursing, 9,* 237–238.

Hoffman, S. B., & Platt, C. A. (1990). Wandering. In S. B. Hoffman & C. A. Platt (Eds.), *Comforting the confused* (pp. 133–154). Owings, MD: National Health Publishing.

Hussain, R. A. (1981). *Geriatric psychology: A behavioral perspective.* New York: Van Nostrand Reinhold.

Hussain, R. A. (1982). Stimulus control in the modification of problematic behavior in elderly institutionalized patients. *International Journal of Behavioral Geriatrics, 1*, 33–42.

Hussain, R. A., & Brown, D. C. (1987). Use of two-dimensional grid patterns to limit hazardous ambulation in demented patients. *Journal of Gerontology, 42*(5), 558–560.

Hussain, R. A., & Davis, R. (1983). *Analysis of wandering behavior in institutionalized geriatric patients.* Paper presented at the meeting of the Association for Behavioral Analysis. Milwaukee, WI.

Katzman, R., Brown, T., Fuld, P., Peck, A., Schecter, R., & Shimmel, H. (1983). Validation of a short orientation-memory-concentration test of cognitive impairment. *American Journal of Psychiatry, 140,* 734–739.

Miller, M. B. (1975). Iatrogenic and Nursigenic effects of prolonged immobilization of the ill aged. *Journal of the American Geriatrics Society, 23*(8), 360–369.

Monsour, N., & Robb, S. S. (1982). Wandering behavior in old age: A psychosocial study. *Social Work, 27*(5), 411–416.

National Center for Health Statistics (1979). *The National Nursing Home Survey: 1977 summary for the United States vital and health statistics.* Series 13, No. 43. Hyattsville, MD: Author.

Rader, J., Doan, J., & Schwab, M. (1985). How to decrease wandering: A form of agenda behavior. *Geriatric Nursing, 6*(4), 196–199.

Robb, S. S. (1987). Exercise treatment for wandering behavior. In H. J. Altman (Ed.), *Alzheimer's disease problems, prospects, and perspective* (pp. 213–218). New York: Plenum Press.

Roberts, B. L., & Algase, D. L. (1988). Victims of Alzheimer's disease and the environment. *Nursing Clinics of North America, 23*(1), 83–93.

Robinson, A., Spencer, B., & White, L. (1989). *Understanding difficult behaviors.* Ypsilanti, Michigan: Eastern Michigan University.

Synder, L. H., Rupprecht, P., Pyrek, J., Brekhus, S., & Moss, T. (1978). Wandering. *The Gerontologist, 18*(3), 272–280.

Weller, M. (1987). A biochemical hypothesis of wandering. *Medical Science Law, 27*(1), 40–41.

Wolanin, M. O., & Phillips, L. R. (1981). *Confusion: Prevention and care.* St.Louis: C. V. Mosby.

Young, S. H., Muir-Nash, J., & Ninos, M. (1988). Managing nocturnal wandering behavior. *Journal of Gerontological Nursing, 14*(5), 7–11.

14

Use of Physical Restraints and Options

Helen W. Lach

INTRODUCTION

The use of physical restraints in long-term-care facilities is the subject of a growing debate among nurses, physicians, nursing home administrators, and others with an interest in the care and quality of life of the elderly. Awareness of physical, psychological, and ethical problems associated with physical restraint has created a grass-roots movement and legislative action to decrease this common practice. However, several myths about providing safe care for frail elders lie behind the use of physical restraint, and change in practice is a slow and difficult process. This chapter will review factors in the use of physical restraints and explore alternative options for safely caring for frail elderly.

CHANGING PRACTICE

The largest force for change comes from new Federal regulations implemented in 1990 which take a strict view of the use of physical restraints. The Nursing Home Reform Act requires that "the resident has the right to be free from any physical restraints imposed . . . for purposes of discipline or convenience and not required to treat the resident's medical symptoms." Before this regulation went into effect in late 1990, the Health Care Financing Administration reported that 41.3% of nursing home residents were restrained daily (1988).

Even before the regulations, a grass-roots movement explored the use of physical restraints. Schwartz (1985), in "A Call for Help," sought out nurses who worked in facilities with programs or ideas for decreasing the overuse of physical restraints. At that time she received over fifty responses with suggestions or references. The Kendal Corporation, a non-profit organization with several nursing facilities, inititated a project called "Untie the Elderly." Kendal had been successfully operating restraint-free facilities for many years and wanted to increase awareness about the side effects of restraints and educate others on the alternatives available. To date, they have presented workshops around the country and published a newsletter to help disseminate information on restraint-free care (Kendal, 1991). Besides these professional initiatives, a series of newspaper articles across the nation has addressed the issue of restraints, generating support among the public for decreased use of restraints.

Because of these factors, most facilities are taking steps to decrease the use of physical restraints. It is helpful to explore the problems which physical restraints cause and the myths related to their use in order to understand the strong reactions this topic seems to generate.

THE PROBLEM OF PHYSICAL RESTRAINT

Few nursing home staff are aware of the adverse effects of physical restraint. Foremost are the physiological results of simple immobility, which have been well characterized by Miller (1975) and Harper and Lyles (1988). Immobility causes decreased muscle mass with resulting weakness, loss of balance and, along with bone demineralization, increased risk for falls and fractures. In addition, the metabolic rate slows, and changes in the circulatory system can include decreased cardiac output, venous stasis with increased risk of blood clots, and orthostatic hypotension. Constipation is a common gastrointestinal side effect and decreased volume of respirations can lead to increased risk of pneumonia. Increased incidence of skin breakdown and infections also have been associated with use in acute care settings (Lofgren, MacPherson, Granieri, & Sprafka, 1989).

Restraints can provide a barrier to meeting functional needs, resulting in urinary and fecal incontinence. Ability to eat or take fluids is often diminished, with the resultant risk of malnutrition and dehydration. Some incidents of contracture of the hands resulting from restraint have been reported (McLardy-Smith, Burge, & Watson, 1986), as well as brachial plexus injuries affecting the arms (Scott & Gross, 1989). But the most serious problems reported with restraints are incidents of strangulation or asphyxiation as a result of sliding down in a bed or chair or attempting to get out of restraints (Dube & Mitchell, 1986). Kendal (1990) has documented more than 60 cases of deaths related to restraints.

A different set of problems revolves around the psychological effects of restraint. Responses to restraints can include frustration, humiliation, confusion, and anger, which may be expressed in the mentally impaired as increased fear, agitation, or combative behaviors (Brower, 1991). These responses often prompt the use of medications which in turn exaggerate the behavior and cognitive problems. Long-term use of restraints can lead to regressive behavior, withdrawal, and finally, total apathy as the resident gives up trying. In a newspaper article, one 84-year-old woman reported her feelings after being restrained: "I felt tied up like a dog and I was so angry and ashamed. First I fought, then I cried and then I just went into myself" (Lewin, 1989). Loss of autonomy can result in loss of self-esteem and dignity (Folmar & Wilson, 1989). Staff themselves are uncomfortable when residents are upset about being restrained (Scherer, Janelli, Kanski, Neary, & North, 1991), but feel helpless to do anything else.

Ethical issues surrounding autonomy and the right to self-determination are often raised about the use of physical restraints. Historically, the rationale for restraint has always been safety, as seen in the case with the mentally impaired (Brower, 1991). But the humanistic movement dating back to the 1800s considered these devices inhumane, and the efforts to control their use have been effective in mental health settings. The issue has only recently been raised in regard to the elderly in long-term-care facilities. Another ethical dilemma lies in the incompatibility of restraint use with the goals of rehabilitation and maintenance of functional abilities (Johnson, 1990). Others have questioned the need for informed consent to control behavior with restraints which also has precedent in mental health practice (Evans & Strumpf, 1989).

WHY RESIDENTS ARE RESTRAINED

Given the above information, it is hard to understand why people are ever restrained. However, the average nursing home resident has a profile which makes her likely to be restrained. She is female, 85 years old and probably has osteoporosis. She is likely to have experienced a fall in the last year, causing staff to fear injury, particularly a hip fracture, a common injury in older women (Melton, Wahner, Richelson, O'Fallon, & Riggs, 1986). This resident needs assistance with bathing and dressing and a walker to ambulate steadily. She has to get to the bathroom right away or

TABLE 14.1 Misconceptions about Restraint Use

The old should be restrained because they are more likely to fall and injure
themselves.
It is a moral duty to protect residents from harm.
Failure to restrain puts individuals and facilities at risk for legal liability.
It doesn't really bother old people to be restrained.
We have to restrain because of inadequate staffing.

Adapted from Evans, L. K. and Stumpf, N. E., 1990.

she is incontinent. She also has a memory problem so she forgets to use
her walker. The staff would like to keep an eye on her at all times, but short
staffing and the many needs of residents prevent them from providing the
supervision they feel she needs. As a result, she is restrained in her bed
and wheelchair and is gradually becoming more confused, debilitated, and
incontinent, requiring even greater assistance and care.

This common scenario suggests several reasons why long-term-care
residents are restrained. These reasons are based on strongly held beliefs
of staff as well as others about the safety of frail elderly, the risk of injury,
and their liability. Evans and Strumpf (1990) present a framework for
understanding the assumptions of caregivers by outlining myths of elder
restraint (see Table 14.1). That these beliefs are still widely held is evidenced by the negative response to the new Federal regulations, with some
states even requesting waivers (Strumpf & Evans, 1991).

DEBUNKING THE MYTHS—GET THE FACTS

The best way to fight the myths of elder restraint is with the facts. First, the
prevention of falls in the elderly is probably not a realistic goal; 30% of
older adults living at home fall each year (Lach et al., 1991). It is a common
accident, and there is no scientific support to suggest that restraints
prevent falls (Evans & Strumpf, 1989). In nursing homes where restraint
use has been decreased or eliminated, the incidence of injuries from falls
has decreased (Blakeslee, Goldman, Papougenis, & Torell, 1991), though
some facilities report a modest increase in the number of falls.

Second, research has yet to show any benefits from customary use of
restraints (Johnson, 1990). Given the problems of physical restraints discussed, there are few instances where the benefits of restraint outweigh the
risks.

Concerns about liability represent another myth, commonly reinforced
by administrators. There are no reported successful legal claims against

long-term-care facilities based solely on the failure to restrain a resident (Montgomery, McCracken, Walker, & Rhoads, 1990). The responsibility of the facility for safeguarding residents requires that potential problems be assessed and reasonable action taken. Even when restraints are in place, this responsibility is not necessarily fulfilled. However, lawsuits over injuries to residents in long-term-care facilities are not common (Johnson, 1990). The damages that can be collected are low, and it can be difficult to prove the cause of the injury. In addition, the movement in regulations toward the least restrictive environment may play a role in future litigation.

Finally, many staff believe that it takes less time to care for restrained than nonrestrained residents. Given the amount of supervision and protection needed to comply with standards of care for the resident in restraints, this seems unrealistic. Studies by Blakeslee et al. (1991) have reviewed standards in Pennsylvania and have determined that residents in restraints take an estimated 4.58 hours per day of care compared with the 2.7 hours typically provided in that state. In addition, the functional declines associated with restraints can increase time needed to assist with all activities of daily living.

Given the facts, most people are willing to reconsider their positions on restraints. But the most important step involves providing options to dealing with the problems that cause restraints to be used in the first place. The rest of this chapter will focus on ideas and alternatives for restraints.

OPTIONS: THE KEY TO THE CHANGE PROCESS

The first step to changing practice regarding restraints involves support from all levels of the institution including administrators, physicians, and non-nursing staff (Blakeslee et al., 1991). Everyone must be involved in the change process to ensure success. Written policies should include clear guidelines on the use of restraints (Morrison, Crinklow-Wianko, King, Thibealt, & Well, 1987) to let staff know where the institution stands on their use.

A second step to change involves educating staff to explore myths about the use of restraints and replace their misconceptions with accurate information. In addition, staff need to know how to make good decisions about restraints. They should learn to explore the reason for the restraints, identify potential underlying causes, and explore the alternatives before initiating restraints (Masters & Favro, 1990). A useful aid to education involves assessing staff attitudes and knowledge. Table 14.2 provides a survey which can be used (Houston & Lach, 1990), and inservices can be focused on the most common concerns or misconceptions identified. Residents and families also may need information on changes in policies regarding restraints.

The final step is the identification of alternative options for managing resident's problems. The most common reason staff give for their reluctance to give up restraints is the lack of alternative measures. There is no magic remedy for reducing the use of restraints, but innovative ideas are being developed as staff look for new ways of coping with residents' problems. Alternatives tend to fit into one of four categories listed in Table 14.3: medical interventions, environmental changes, behavioral approaches, and rehabilitative measures.

Medical conditions often contribute to the need for restraints. Untreated illnesses such as infections can present with different symptomatology in the elderly: dizziness, falls, confusion, agitation, and postural hypotension. These reactions also can indicate adverse effects of medications. Any change in the behavior or functional capacity of an elderly resident should trigger a medical checkup and medication review. Medications for the treatment of behavior problems must be used judiciously; but appropriate medical treatment may alleviate symptoms and the need for restraint.

The environment of the facility should prevent problems that lead to restraints. First, overall safety measures must be in place. Nonslippery floors, adequate lighting, accessible grab rails, and furniture with adequate support should be standard for the prevention of falls. Additional precautions include rooms near the nurses' station, call lights within easy reach, and lower beds or mattresses on the floor (Evans & Strumpf, 1989). Avoid uncomfortable situations which might create agitated behaviors in residents with cognitive impairment: reduce glare from windows, and noise from bare walls and floors, and provide quiet opportunities during the day.

The use of color or objects can cue residents about areas that are appropriate for use or to be avoided. Doors where residents are not welcome can be painted to match the wall, doorknobs mounted in unusual spots, or a picture placed on the door. Alarm mechanisms can alert staff when residents enter areas that are off-limits. Rooms that residents might need, such as bathrooms, should be easy to find, preventing exploring and anxiety.

Behavioral techniques may be successful in dealing with other resident problems. One example is routine toileting. Some residents may get up unassisted or become agitated because of a need to go to the bathroom. Sometimes hunger or thirst can trigger agitation, which can be alleviated with snacks and offering of fluids. By anticipating the need, the problem is avoided.

TABLE 14.2 Restraint Questionnaire

1. Which of the following is considered a restraint?
   I.   Mittens
   II. Geri-chair
   III. Wheelchair safety bar
   IV. Tied bed sheet
       a. I and III
       b. I, III, and IV
       c. I, II, and III
       d. all of the above
2. When do restraints help residents?
   I.   To prevent falls or other accidental injuries
   II. To allow treatments to proceed without patient interference
   III. To improve functional abilities
       a. I and II
       b. II and III
       c. II only
       d. I, II, and III
3. Prolonged restraint use can cause:
   I.   Incontinence
   II. Skin breakdown
   III. Confusion
            Loss of calcium from bone
       a. I and II
       b. II and III
       c. III and IV
       d. all of the above
4. The patient in restraints should be checked every:
       a. 30 minutes
       b. 2 hours
       c. 1 hour
       d. 8 hours
5. What is the correct way to apply a vest restraint?
       a. With the opening in the front
       b. With the opening in the back
       c. Either way is acceptable
6. Restraint is an unusual and temporary measure.
       a. True
       b. False
7. Being restrained causes residents to get more confused.
       a. True
       b. False
Key: 1=d, 2=c, 3=d, 4=a, 5=a, 6=a, 7=a.

(Adapted from Houston, K. A., & Lach, H. W., 1990.)

TABLE 14.3 Categories for Interventions to Prevent Restraints

Medical: Appropriate diagnosis, medication, and treatment
Environmental: Safe, with modifications to meet resident needs
Behavioral: Provide for appropriate activities
Rehabilitative: Maintain strength and teach self-care skills

Structured activities and opportunities for socialization help meet needs for human contact and purposeful activity, use up excess energy, and aid rest as well. Activity therapists can provide varied programs for residents with different levels of cognitive and physical functioning. A good activity program will include opportunities for rest and quiet time.

Rehabilitation is indicated when resident problems relate to functional deficits or weakness. Physical therapists assess gait and evaluate residents for appropriate assistive devices. Exercises are done to improve strength and balance. In addition, problems with sitting posture can be addressed and recommendations for improving posture identified.

Occupational therapists provide adaptive equipment to help with activities of daily living. For example, stretch shoelaces could improve a resident's compliance with wearing shoes to walk, because they can easily slip shoes on and off without having to tie laces. A reacher bar could be used to pick up items that fall on the floor to avoid bending over or squatting, a difficult maneuver for those with poor balance.

Given these categories, clearly all members of the health team need to be involved in reducing restraint use. Each has expertise in areas where they can help solve resident problems and support this movement. Table 14.4 provides a list of alternatives for common challenges, and the following case studies provide examples of how these elements can work together to solve even some difficult resident problems.

CASE STUDIES

The strongest case for decreasing restraint use grows out of the many success stories which are being reported from almost every facility which is making an effort to move in this direction. The following are just a few of these stories from local facilities.

The Veterans Administration Nursing Home Care Unit in St. Louis has decreased the use of restraints to under 5% in less than a year. The unit attributes its success to a team approach. All new residents are evaluated by nursing, physical, and occupational therapy and are placed as needed in

TABLE 14.4 Restraint Alternatives for Common Challenges

Promote Residents' Function

Identify reason(s) for the resident's unsteadiness: need to get up, poor trunk control, medication, lack of exercise, hungry or thirsty, sitting too long, or needs to go to the bathroom.)

Eliminate medications or combinations of medications whose side effects distort resident's balance, perceptions, and/or cognitive function.

Increase ambulation skills by giving resident opportunities to exercise, for example: walking to and from meals or activities, developing formal exercise groups, etc.

Be sure residents wear comfortable, well-fitting shoes or sneakers and have appropriate foot and nail care.

Provide supportive devices to maximize function, for example: transfer disc, modified walkers, grab/safety bars in bathroom, elevated toilet seat, etc.

Address resident's vision and hearing impairments.

Minimize Likelihood of Resident's Needing to Get Up Unaided

Be familiar with the residents' lifelong roles and habits to anticipate personal needs and interests, such as bathroom routine, preferred snack times, or leisure activities.

Provide the resident with meaningful activity such as listening to music, assisting staff with simple tasks, or executing a repetitive task that satisfies a personal need.

Offer resident adequate stimulation such as reading materials, talking books, or an activities cart placed strategically on each unit.

Vary the locations where an individual sits. Sometimes quiet areas are appreciated, but often residents want to be "where the action is."

Explore possible alerting strategies/devices, i.e., attach call bell to resident garment or use of portable battery-operated alarms that monitor the individual's movements.

Customize Seating for Individual Postural Needs

Provide flexion at hips and knees and lateral support with wedge cushions, positioning pillows, and/or deep inclined seats to minimize slumping, falling to the side, or sliding out of chair.

Ensure that the most comfortable seating is available. Offer a variety of sitting arrangements, such as comfortable recliners, rockers, deep-seated high-backed chairs, or soft comfortable wing chairs.

Prevent tipping of wheelchairs with antitipping devices which are commercially available.

Ensure A Safe Facility

Monitor environment for safety hazards.

Modify environment with optimal lighting in residents' rooms and bathroom, appropriately placed safety bars, removal of wheels from overbed table, and other furniture, etc.

Note. From "Untie the Elderly: Newsletter" by Kendal Corporation, 1991. Copyright 1991 by Kendal Corp. Reprinted by permission (not for profit newsletter).

an Activities of Daily Living (ADL) program. Staff work with them to increase self-care skills and improve mobility. A daily walking program has been successful in improving strength. They describe particular success with an older resident with Huntington's chorea. The combination of appropriate medication (baclofen) to decrease random movement along with the ADL and walking programs improved his abilities, so that he no longer needs to be restrained.

The problem of falls has been addressed at the Jewish Center for the Aged. A "falls consultation service" has been developed to evaluate residents who fall and identify interventions to prevent future falls. The team consists of the physician, nursing clinical specialist, and physical therapist. An individualized plan is developed. For example, a 97-year-old man was admitted to the nursing home ambulating independently, but after two falls he was restrained. The consultation noted that his medications includede a benzodiazepine, a class of medications commonly implicated in falls. This was discontinued, and his gait improved, allowing the restraint to be discontinued.

Mrs. M., an intact resident with multiple sclerosis was interviewed about the problem of people with cognitive impairment wandering in and out of her room when they are not restrained. Before environmental changes were tried, she was constantly being interrupted by other residents. The staff put a yellow 36-inch-by-36-inch strip of fabric across her doorway which attaches by velcro strips for easy access in and out of the room. Mrs. M. reports that she can now have privacy when she wants. This facility also has had success with electronic monitoring devices which can detect if residents go through doorways to inappropriate areas.

SUMMARY

There is little to support the continued use of physical restraints in long-term-care facilities and the practice of using restraints is gradually changing. The side effects far outweigh the benefits and facilities find they are able to manage a number of resident problems by alternative measures. It is important for these facilities to share their innovative ideas and support each other's efforts, as care of the frail elderly moves into a new and hopefully more humane era.

RESOURCES

"Untie the Elderly Newsletter" and Resource Manual
The Kendal Corporation
PO Box 100
Kennett Square, PA 19348

"A Practical Guide to Reducing the Use of Restraints in Nursing Homes"
Contact: Laura Rice, Long-Term Care Specialist
Executive Office of Elder Affairs
38 Chancy Street, Boston, MA

REFERENCES

Blakeslee, J. A., Goldman, B. D., Papougenis, D., & Torell, C. A. (1991). Making the transition to restraint-free care. *Journal of Gerontological Nursing, 17*(2), 4–8.

Brower, H. T. (1991). The alternatives to restraints. *Journal of Gerontological Nursing, 17*(2), 18–22.

Dube, A. H., & Mitchell, E. (1986). Accidental strangulation from vest restraints. *Journal of the American Medical Association, 256*(19), 2725–2726.

Evans, L. K., & Strumpf, N. E. (1989). Tying down the elderly: A review of the literature on physical restraint. *Journal of the American Geriatrics Society, 37*, 65–74.

Evans, L. K., & Strumpf, N. E. (1990). Myths about elder restraint. *Image, 22*(4), 124–128.

Folmar, S., & Wilson, H. (1989). Social behavior and physical restraints. *The Gerontologist, 29*,(5), 650–653.

Harper, C. M., & Lyles, Y. M. (1988). Physiology and complications of bed rest. *Journal of the American Geriatrics Society, 36*(11), 1047–1054.

Health Care Financing Administration. (1988). *Medicare/Medicaid nursing home information 1987–1988*. Washington, DC: U.S. Government Printing Office. HE22.35

Houston, K. A., & Lach, H. W. (1990). Restraints: How do you score? *Geriatric Nursing, 12*(5), 231–232.

Johnson, S. H. (1990). The fear of liability and the use of restraints in nursing homes. *Law, Medicine & Health Care, 18*(3), 263–273.

Kendal Corporation (1990 & 1991). *Untie the elderly*. Kennet Square, PA: Newsletter.

Lach, H. W., Reed, A. T., Arfken, C. L., Miller, J. P., Paige, G. D., Birge, S. B., & Peck, W. A. (1991). Falls in the elderly: Reliability of a classification system. *Journal of the American Geriatrics Society, 39*, 197–202.

Legal consequences of the use or non-use of physical restraints in health care institutions. 1990, *3*(1). *New Horizons*, 2–4.

Lewin, T. (1989). Nursing homes rethink merits of tying the aged. *The New York Times*, pp. A1, B8.

Lofgren, R. P., MacPherson, D. S., Granieri, R., & Sprafka, J. M. (1989). Mechanical restraints on the medical wards: Are protective devices safe? *American Journal of Public Health, 79*(6), 735–838.

Masters, R., & Favro, M. (1990). The use of restraints. *Rehabilitation Nursing, 15*(1), 22–25.

McLardy-Smith, P., Burge, P. D., & Watson, N. A. (1986). Ischemic contracture of the intrinsic muscles of the hands: A hazard of physical restraint. *Journal of Hand Surgery, 11*(1), 65–67.

Melton, L. J. III, Wahner, H. W., Richelson, L. S., O'Fallon, W. M., & Riggs, B. L. (1986). Osteoporosis and the risk of hip fracture. *American Journal of Epidemiology*, *124*, 254–261.

Miller, M. B. (1975). Iatrogenic and nursigenic effects of prolonged immobilization of the ill aged. *Journal of the American Geriatrics Society*, *23*(8), 360–369.

Morrison, J., Crinklaw-Wiancko, D., King, E., Thibealt, S., & Well, D. L. Formulating a restraint use policy (1987). *Journal of Nursing Administration*, *17*(3), 39–42.

Scherer, Y. K., Janelli, L. M., Kanski, G. W., Neary, M. A., & Morth, N. E. (1991). The nursing dilemma of restraints. *Journal of Gerontological Nursing*, *17*(2), 14–17.

Schwartz, D. (1985). Replies to a call for help. *Geriatric Nursing*, *6*, 250.

Scott, T. F., & Gross, J. A. (1989). Brachial plexus injury due to vest restraints. *JAMA*, *259*, 598.

Strumpf, N. E., & Evans, L. K. (1991). The ethical problems of prolonged physical restraint. *Journal of Gerontological Nursing*, *17*(2), 27–30.

15

Aggressive Behaviors and Chemical Restraints

Adam J. Sky
George T. Grossberg

The aging of the North American population in the coming decades will mean a rise in both the incidence and prevalence of progressive dementias. Recent literature has suggested nearly 50% of the population over age 85 will be affected (Larsen, 1989), highlighting the importance of effective treatment strategies for behavioral problems associated with dementia. The recent enactment of the Omnibus Budget Reconciliation Act (OBRA) of 1987 regulations has further brought this issue to the forefront. In this chapter we will review the common types of behaviors seen in the dementing disorders and summarize the pharmacologic agents available for their treatment; we will conclude with several actual case reports.

Agitation has been defined as the clinical term for inappropriate verbal or physical activity that is not an overt expression of needs or confusion (Cohen-Mansfield, 1989). Agitation is not a diagnostic term per se; rather, it represents a constellation of symptoms. Agitation may reflect functional or psychotic disorders, medical illnesses, iatrogenic effects of medications, sensory or communication difficulties, or combinations of all of the above. Common behaviors found in dementia include striking out and hitting, verbal agitation and screaming, accusatory or paranoid ideations, catastrophic reactions, and wandering. Oftentimes, varying combinations of these symptoms present.

The prevalence of behavioral problems in nursing home residents has been estimated to be 50% to 70%, according to some studies (Knopman, Deinard, & Kitto, 1985). The advantage of treating these behaviors effectively is that it can lead to an enhanced quality of life for the resident and decreased burden for the caregivers.

The necessity of specifically identifying the problem behaviors cannot be understated, because they will be prime determinants of treatment and medication choice. However, when treating behavioral manifestations of the dementing disorders, the clinician should not automatically consider the exclusive use of medications. The management of these behaviors should be done in the context of an integrated approach, one that incorporates environmental, medical, and psychological issues. Frequently, alternative modes of treatment are available which can be utilized prior to initiating pharmacologic management of these problems. It is obviously essential that clinicians who treat these residents be familiar with the evolving number of medications and innovative treatments used in the management of problem behaviors.

MEDICATIONS USED IN THE TREATMENT OF BEHAVIORAL PROBLEMS

Neuroleptics

Neuroleptics (major tranquilizers) have been used for treating problem behaviors since shortly after their introduction in the early 1950s. While there have been numerous citations in the literature attesting to their efficacy, a recent meta-analysis of these studies showed neuroleptics to be only marginally effective in treating problem behaviors associated with dementia. In fact, their effectiveness may have stemmed primarily from their sedative rather than antipsychotic effects (Schneider, Pollock, & Lyness, 1990; Grossberg, 1990).

Neuroleptics were designed for and are effective in treating psychotic symptoms (i.e., hallucinations, paranoid ideations, and delusions). These common manifestations of cognitive impairment are effectively managed with neuroleptics in much the same manner as with younger, cognitively intact, psychotic patients. Neuroleptics can also be used on a short-term basis to manage acute agitation, though for these purposes their use would be almost exclusively a function of their sedative potential.

There are a number of general principles to consider in order to safely and effectively prescribe neuroleptics in demented, elderly patients. The first is that older patients and especially those with cognitive dysfunction are exquisitely sensitive to psychotropic medications (Shamoian, 1988). Therefore, the axiom of "start low and go slow" is fundamental in this regard. The second concept to keep in mind when choosing neuroleptics is to consider their side effects. The low-potency neuroleptics, such as thioridazine and chlorpromazine, have lower incidences of tardive dyskinesia and extrapyramidal symptoms; however, they have a rather high incidence of anticholinergic and cardiovascular side effects. Furthermore, they can be quite sedating. Conversely, the high-potency neuroleptics have little effect relative to anticholinergic and cardiovascular side effects; however, they expose the patient to a significant risk of movement disorders, such as tardive dyskinesia and extrapyramidal symptoms.

Generally speaking, when the problem behavior is in the psychotic arena, starting the patient on a small dose of a high-potency neuroleptic will usually be safe and effective. An appropriate initial dosage would be 0.25 mg of haloperidol, once or twice daily. This low, initial dosage can be gradually increased or decreased, depending on tolerability and clinical response. If a poor patient response or side effect develops when using a high-potency neuroleptic, substituting a more intermediate-potency medication (such as loxapine or mesoridazine) may be effective.

In cases of acute agitation or severely violent behavior, the clinician can be more liberal in dosing neuroleptics. Some rough guidelines for this scenario would range from 1 to 15 mg or more of haloperidol equivalent daily. However, in the acute situation, neuroleptic use should be considered short-term treatment, and a safer alternative should be sought as soon as the crisis has receded.

Relative to the OBRA 1987 regulations, neuroleptics may be prescribed. However, use is limited by specific guidelines and criticism as noted in Table 15.1.

Benzodiazepines

Benzodiazepines, like neuroleptics, have been studied extensively for use in elderly patients since shortly after their introduction in the 1960s. Agitation, restlessness and wandering behaviors, commonly seen in demented patients, may be regarded as manifestations of anxiety, especially in the earlier disease stages (Risse & Barnes, 1986; Petrie, 1983; Post, 1975). Therefore, a logical postulate is that anxiolytics, such as benzodiazepines, would be useful in the treatment of such symptomatology.

Interestingly, the studies comparing benzodiazepines to neuroleptics have shown benzodiazepines to be inferior in the management of physical and verbal agitation (Cerevra, 1974; Chesrow, Kaplitz, & Vetra, 1965; Kirven & Mantero, 1973; Stotsky, 1984; Twefik, Jain, Harcup, & Magowan, 1970).

Table 15.1 Omnibus Budget Reconciliation Act (OBRA)

Neuroleptics may be used if the clinical record documents that the patient has one
  or more of the following "specific conditions":

Schizophrenia

Schizo-affective disorder

Delusional disorder

Psychotic mood disorders (including mania and depression with psychotic
  features)

Acute psychotic episodes

Brief reactive psychosis

Schizophreniform disorder

Atypical psychosis

Tourette's disorder

Huntington's disease

Organic mental syndromes (including dementia) with associated psychotic
  and/or agitated features as defined by:

  Specific behaviors as quantitatively (number of episodes) and objectively
  (e.g., biting, kicking, and scratching) documented by the facility, that
  cause residents to:

    Present a danger to themselves,

    Present a danger to others (including staff), or

    Actually interfere with the staff's ability to provide care

    Psychotic symptoms (hallucinations, paranoia, delusions) not exhibited
    as specific behaviors listed above but which cause the resident frightful
    distress

Short-term (seven days) symptomatic treatment of hiccups, nausea, vomiting, or
  pruritus

In more severely impaired patients, the benzodiazepines have even been
associated with a worsening of symptoms via a paradoxical disinhibition-
type mechanism. In the above studies, benzodiazepines were demonstrated to be effective in treating anxiety manifestations of dementia,
especially in those with mild, cognitive impairment.

When considering the use of benzodiazepines, one with a short to
intermediate half-life (which is metabolized through conjugation, and has
no active metabolites) should be chosen (Salzman, Shader, & Greenblatt
1983). Such medications include alprazolam, lorazepam, and oxazepam.

In order to minimize side effects, caution should be taken when dosing
benzodiazepines in the elderly. Prominent among these side effects are:
sedation, confusion, dysarthria, unsteady gate, uncoordination, and disinhibition with paradoxical agitation. Benzodiazepines should be discontinued slowly in order to minimize the risk of uncomfortable and potentially dangerous withdrawal symptoms.

Serotonergic Agents (Trazodone)

One of the more innovative medications which has been used in the treatment of agitation is the antidepressant trazodone. In 1973, the Nair, Ban, Hontela, & Clarke studies reported the use of trazodone to improve behavioral manifestations of dementia and organic brain syndromes. The mechanism of action of trazodone in this context is somewhat unclear. As an antidepressant, trazodone may lead to clinical improvement by relieving a concurrent underlying depression. Some studies have further suggested that trazodone's calming effects are a result of its serotonergic-reuptake-blocking properties. Reduced serotonin has been hypothesized to be a factor in aggression (Salzman, 1987).

At least six case reports or studies attest to trazodone's efficacy in treating behavioral problems associated with dementia. Some of those studies noted improvement in patients who had failed prior treatments with various neuroleptics (Greenwald, Marin, & Silverman, 1986; Nair et al., 1973; O'Neal, Page, Adkins, & Eichelman, 1986; Simpson & Foster, 1986; Tingle, 1986; Wilcock, Stevens, & Perkins, 1987). Among symptoms noted to improve with trazodone were hostility, appetite, verbal agitation, physical agitation, and dysphoria. For use as an antiagitant, trazodone doses have been reported as ranging from 25 to 600 mg per day (given in divided doses). Trazodone's purported clinical efficacy is enhanced by its relatively benign side effect profile. Among its more common side effects are sedation, hypotension, and gastrointestinal (GI) upset. However, these tend to be well tolerated and relatively minimal in comparison to other psychotropics.

Unfortunately, double-blind controlled studies relative to the treatment of hostility and aggression with trazodone have been lacking. However, given the existing literature, trazodone would appear a very promising alternative to the neuroleptics in the management of patients with these symptoms.

Azapirones (Buspirone)

Buspirone is an anxiolytic which has been noted to have a high affinity for the 5HT1 receptor site. This agonist potential has led to the postulation that buspirone may be a useful tool in managing aggressive behaviors.

Buspirone's precise effect in serotonin metabolism is somewhat controversial, but its general effect has been confirmed in animal studies (Smith & Peroutka, 1986). The few case studies of buspirone treatment in elderly, demented patients have certainly been promising (Colenda, 1988; Tiller, Dakis & Shaw, 1988), and other studies of its efficacy in demented patients are currently under way. Symptoms reported to improve with buspirone are: angry outbursts, wandering, sexual disinhibition, physical agitation, and oppositional-type behavior.

Buspirone's promising utility is (similar to trazodone's) enhanced by its mild side effect profile. The most common side effects include dizziness, drowsiness and headache; however, these only occur in a low percentage of patients and tend to decrease in frequency with time. Buspirone dosages reported in the literature have ranged from 5 mg thrice daily to 15 mg thrice daily with an observed five-day to two-month onset of action.

Beta Blockers

Beta adrenergic blocking agents such as propranolol and pindolol have been long advocated for treatment of agitation and hostility in organically impaired patients (Cole, Altesman, & Weingarten, 1979; Elliot, 1977). However, the literature on the use of beta blockers tends to focus on younger organically impaired patients.

Though the efficacy of beta blockers in reducing agitation in demented elderly patients has been documented in a number of case reports (Jensen, 1989; Weiler, Mungas, & Bernick, 1988) and studies (Greendyke & Kanter, 1986; Greendyke, Schuster, & Wooten, 1984; Petrie & Ban, 1981;), the precise mechanism of action remains vague. It has been hypothesized that beta blockers increase presynaptic norepinephrine output in response to postsynaptic antagonism, leading to an overall increase in noradrenergic activity with a concomitant decrease in rage response (Weiller, Mungas, & Bernick, 1988). There has been evidence that central adrenergic deficiencies (Davis, 1983) (demonstrated in Alzheimer's disease) have been implicated in hostile and agitated behavior (Stevens & Jermann, 1981). Symptoms reportedly helped by beta blockers include physical outbursts (particularly those that have been more chronic), pacing, and verbal outbursts.

The existing literature has shown beta blockers to be well tolerated even at higher doses. As with all medications, they must be used with caution. Among the beta blockers' more common side effects are confusion, depression, hypotension, and bradycardia. The effective beta blocker dosage cited in the literature has been suggested as ranging from 40 mg to 520 mg per day of propanolol and from 60 mg to 100 mg per day of pindolol. The response time of beta blockers has been reported as varying from several days to several months. Beta blockers should be prescribed judiciously in patients with a history of cardiac failure, chronic obstructive pulmonary disease, diabetes, asthma, or hyperthyroidism. Propanolol can also increase the plasma levels of other drugs, such as anticonvulsive medications and antipsychotics.

Seemingly beta blockers are a useful alternative in the management of behavioral difficulties associated with dementias. However, as with other innovative treatments, a sizable double-blind study in the older population has yet to be done.

Carbamazepine (Tegretol)

The iminostilbene anticonvulsant carbamazepine has been shown to be effective in decreasing impulsivity and aggression in a wide variety of organically impaired psychiatric patients (Essa, 1986; Patterson, 1987). It has been noted to be particularly useful when the problem behaviors occur in a more episodic or unpredictable fashion.

Carbamazepine is thought to work via a limbic antikindling mechanism combined with increased locus ceruleus firing rates, increased tryptophane levels, and possible enhancement of dopaminergic release (Post, 1987). Dysfunctions in all of the above areas have been associated with the dementing disorders, thus providing a theoretical framework for carbamazepine's mechanism of action (Gleason & Schneider, 1990; Leibovici & Tariot, 1988).

Several studies to date relative to carbamazepine's effect on problem behaviors in elderly patients have been encouraging. Carbamazepine has been specifically reported to be effective in helping manage tension, hostility, and intermittent agitation, especially during nursing care (Gleason & Schneider, 1990; Leibovici & Tariot, 1988; Patterson, 1988; Marin & Greenwald, 1989). The current literature has also suggested that carbamazepine may be effective in patients who had been previously treated unsuccessfully with neuroleptics. Electroencephalograms of a number of the patients who were treated with carbamazepine showed increased slow waves and decreased alpha waves; however, no seizure activity was noted (Gleason & Schneider, 1990).

Carbamazepine dosages quoted in the literature range from initial doses of 50 mg per day to maintenance doses of up to 1,000 mg per day. The serum carbamazepine levels were quoted as ranging from 1.5 ug/ml to 9.6 ug/ml. Ten days to seven weeks was the range of time lapse before improvement was seen. Carbamazepine is not a totally benign medication. Carbamazepine's more common and potentially toxic side effects include leukopenia, hepatotoxicity, thyroid abnormalities, ataxia, cardiac problems, and rashes.

Valproic Acid

The anticonvulsant valproic acid deserves mention, as it has been shown effective and safe in managing agitated behaviors in younger organically impaired patients. Valproic acid may have fewer side effects than carbamazepine. However, no studies to date have been done on valproic acid's use in elderly demented patients.

Lithium Carbonate

Lithium carbonate has been long used for the management of bipolar affective disorder and has also been used successfully in younger agitated patients. Patients reported to have been helped by lithium have had various diagnoses such as closed head injuries, mental retardation, and stroke (Goetzel, Grunberg, & Berkowitz, 1977; Herlihy & Herlihy, 1979; Sargent, 1979; Souver & Hurley, 1981). However, the only sizable study of lithium's use in elderly demented, agitated patients showed it to be ineffective (Holton & George, 1985). The few patients in the literature who have responded to lithium were generally exhibiting manic-like symptoms of hyperactivity, hypertalkativeness, pressured speech, sleeplessness and intrusiveness. Therefore, its use in demented patients would probably be best reserved for that subtype of patient.

CASE EXAMPLES

Case 1.

Mr. R. was a 77-year-old white male with an approximately four-year history of probable dementia of the Alzheimer's type. For the four to five months prior to evaluation, he had been hitting himself and others, leading to his ejection from two nursing homes. This violent behavior was noted to occur on an almost constant basis without any precipitating factors. At the time the resident was initially evaluated, he was nonverbal and could not express himself. He had a medical history of a myocardial infarction two years prior and of chronic renal insufficiency. The resident had been started on a relatively small dose of haloperidol several months prior to evaluation, and by the time he was seen, a rather pronounced movement disorder had developed. Aside from the haloperidol, this resident's only other medication was diltiazem.

As no physical or environmental trigger to his behaviors could be found, a decision was made to treat his agitation pharmacologically. The resident's neuroleptic regime was discontinued, and after no improvement in behavior, he was started on trazodone. The initial dosage of 50 mg thrice daily was gradually increased to 150 mg four times a day before any improvement in his symptoms were noted. Behavioral symptoms were noted to improve by both the family and the nursing staff.

After several months of Mr. R.'s doing well, an attempt was made to decrease the resident's trazodone. The resident's behavioral symptoms markedly worsened when the dose was decreased to 100 mg t.i.d. and remitted when his medication was again increased.

Case 2

Mr. S. is an 83-year-old black male with an approximately two-year history of probable dementia of the Alzheimer's type who was brought for evaluation because he had recently become very frightened of the staff at his nursing home. He additionally felt people were stealing his possessions and was convinced his roommate was having sex with the nurses. The resident's past medical history was remarkable for congestive heart failure and arthritis. His medication regime at the time of evaluation consisted of a diuretic and a nonsteroidal anti-inflammatory drug. Given this resident's suspicion and paranoia, it was felt he would be an appropriate candidate for neuroleptics. It was also felt that there were issues that could be addressed environmentally and socially.

In terms of a treatment approach, the resident was first placed in a private room and then started on haloperidol, 0.25 mg p.o., twice daily. After approximately 10 days, his symptoms improved markedly, and his mood seemed to be much more relaxed and calm. He did not express further paranoid ideations and did so well that the medications were tapered and discontinued. Placing him in a private room helped minimize the symptoms caused by his misinterpreting environmental cues and by his being overstimulated. Short-term neuroleptics effectively treated his psychotic symptoms.

Case 3

Mrs. B. is a 79-year-old white female with an approximately 2½ year history of probable multi-infarct dementia. Throughout that time she had been displaying symptoms of screaming, wandering, and restlessness. She had been tried on numerous neuroleptics without any success. She had a past medical history remarkable for cardiac arrhythmia as well as mild congestive heart failure. After she was admitted to the geriatric psychiatry inpatient ward, her cardiac problems were addressed. Stabilization of her cardiac problems did not, however, decrease her behavioral symptoms. Because her primary symptom seemed to be in the anxiety spectrum, she was begun on a regimen of alprazolam 0.5 mg twice daily. This was gradually increased to 1 mg twice daily, and in approximately two weeks the resident's symptoms improved markedly. She was discharged back to the nursing home, where she continued to do well even when the benzodiazepine was reduced. She was noted to be able to converse more appropriately, she longer tried to run away, and she seemed to be generally more comfortable.

Case 4

Mr. K. is a 76-year-old white male who presented with an approximately five-year history of hyperactivity, hypertalkativeness, inappropriate joking, wandering, and intrusiveness. He had an essentially negative medical history at the time of evaluation. An MRI of his brain and neuropsychiatric tests obtained suggested he had probable multi-infarct dementia, and his psychiatric symptoms were described as being consistent with an organic affective disorder. The resident was begun on lithium carbonate, and therapeutic levels were obtained. After approximately three weeks the resident's family noted that he became more controllable and manageable, and he began sleeping better and listening to directions. They did note that he had developed a slight tremor but was not bothered by it.

CONCLUSION

An increasing number of alternatives are available in the treatment of problem behaviors in the dementias. However, large, well-controlled studies relative to the usage of these medications are needed. It would also behoove the clinician to thoroughly investigate any underlying instigators of behavioral change in dementia rtesidents and target the treatment to such disorders.

REFERENCES

Cervera, A. A. (1974). Psychoactive drug therapy in the senile patient: Controlled comparison of thioridazine and diazepam. *Psychiatric Digest, 35,* 16.

Chesrow, E. J., Kaplitz, S. E., Vetra, H. (1965). Double-blind study of oxazepam in the management of geriatric patients with behavioral problems. *Clinical Medicine, 72,* 1001–1005.

Cohen-Mansfield, J. (1989). Agitation in the elderly. *Issues in Psychiatry, 19,* 101–103.

Cole, J. O., Altesman, R., & Weingarten, C. (1979). Beta blocking drugs in psychiatry. *McLean Hospital Journal, 8,* 40–68.

Colenda, C. C. (1988). Buspirone in treatment of the agitated demented patient [Letter to the editor] *Lancet, 1*(8595), 1169.

Davis, P. (1983). The neurochemistry of Alzheimer's disease in senile dementia. *Medical Research Review, 3,* 221–236.

Elliot, F. A. (1977). Propranolol for control of belligerent behavior following acute brain damage. *Annals of Neurology, 1,* 489–491.

Essa, M. (1986). Carbamazepine in dementia. *Journal of Clinical Psychopharmacology, 6,* 234–236.

Gleason, R. P., & Schneider, L. S. (1990). Carbamazepine treatment of agitation in Alzheimer's outpatients refractory to neuroleptics. *Journal of Clinical Psychiatry, 51*(3), 115–118.

Goetzel, U., Grunberg, F., & Berkowitz, B. (1977). Lithium carbonate in the management of hyperactive aggression behavior of the mentally retarded. *Comprehensive Psychiatry, 18,* 599–606.

Greendyke, R. M., & Kanter, D. R. (1986). Therapeutic effects of pindolol on behavioral disturbances associated with organic brain disease: A double-blind study. *Journal of Clinical Psychiatry, 47,* 423–426.

Greendyke, R. M., Schuster, D. B., & Wooten, J. A. (1984). Propranolol in the treatment of assaultive patients with organic brain disease. *Journal of Clinical Psychopharmacology, 4,* 5.

Greenwald, B. S., Marin, D. B., & Silverman, S. M. (1986). Serotoninergic treatment of screaming and banging in dementia. *Lancet, 2*(8521-22), 1464–1465.

Grossberg, G. T. (1990). The pitfalls of meta-analysis. *Journal of the American Geriatrics Society, 38,* 607.

Herlihy, C. E., & Herlihy, C. E. Jr. (1979). Lithium in organic brain syndrome [Letter to the editor]. *Journal of Clinical Psychiatry, 40,* 455.

Holton, A., & George, K. (1985). The use of lithium carbonate in severely demented patients with behavioral disturbance [Letter to the editor]. *British Journal of Psychiatry, 146,* 99–100.

Jensen, C. F. (1989). Hypersexual agitation in Alzheimer's disease [Letter to the editor]. *Journal of the American Geriatrics Society, 27*(9), 917.

Kirven, L. E., & Mantero, E. F. (1973). Comparison of thioridazine and diazepam in the control of nonpsychotic symptoms associated with senility: A double-blind study. *Journal of the American Geriatrics Society, 21,* 546.

Knopman, D., Deinard, S., Kitto, J., Hartman, M., & Mackenzie, T. (May 1985). A clinic for dementia: Two years' experience. *Minnesota Medicine, 68,* 687–692.

Larson, E. B. (1989). Alzheimer's disease in the community. *Journal of the American Medical Association, 18,* 2591–2592.

Leibovici, A., & Tariot, P. N. (1988). Agitation associated with dementia: A systematic approach to treatment. *Psychopharmacology Bulletin, 24*(1), 39–42.

Marin, D. B., & Greenwald, B. S. (1989). Carbamazepine for aggressive agitation in demented patients during nursing care [Letter to the editor]. *American Journal of Psychiatry, 146*(6), 805.

Nair, N. P. V., Ban, T. A., Hontela, S., & Clark, R. (1973). Trazodone in the treatment of organic brain syndrome, with special reference to psychogeriatrics. *Current Theory and Research, 15*(10), 769–775.

O'Neal, M., Page, N., Adkins, W. N., & Eichelman, B. (1986). Tryptophane-trazodone treatment of aggressive behavior. *Lancet, 2*(8511), 859–860.

Patterson, J. F. (1987). Carbamazepine for assaultive patients with organic brain disease: An open pilot study. *Psychosomatics, 28,* 579–581.

Patterson, J. F. (1988). A preliminary study of carbamazepine in the treatment of assaultive patients with dementia. *Journal of Geriatric Psychiatry and Neurology, 1,* 21–23.

Petrie, W. M. (1983). Drug treatment of anxiety and agitation in the aged. *Psychopharmacological Bulletin, 19,* 238–246.

Petrie, W. M., & Ban, T. A. (1981). Propranolol in organic agitation [Letter to the editor]. *Lancet, 1*(8215), 324.

Post, R. M. (1987). Mechanisms of action of carbamazepine and related anticonvulsives in affective illness. In H. Y. Meltzer (Ed.), *Psychopharmacology: A generation of progress* (p. 567). New York: Raven Press.

Post, F. (1975). Dementia, depression, and pseudodementia. *In* P. F. Benson & D. Bloomer (Eds.), *Psychological aspects of neurological disease* (pp. 99–101). New York: Grune and Stratton.

Risse, S. C., & Barnes, R. (1986). Pharmacologic treatment of agitation associated with dementia. *Journal of the American Geriatrics Society, 34*(5), 368–376.

Salzman, C. (1987). Treatment of the elderly agitated patient. *Journal of Clinical Psychiatry, 48*(Suppl.), 19–22.

Salzman, C., Shader, R. I., Greenblatt, D. J., & Harmatz, J. S. (1983). Long vs. short half-life benzodiazepines in the elderly. *Archives of General Psychiatry, 40,* 293.

Sargent, M. (1979). Treating non-affective disorders with lithium. National Institute of Mental Health Report. *Hospital and Community Psychiatry, 40,* 579–581.

Schneider, L. S., Pollock, V. E., & Lyness, S. A. (1990). A meta-analysis of controlled trials of neuroleptic treatment in dementia. *Journal of the American Geriatrics Society, 38*(5): 553–563.

Shamoian, C. (1988). Somatic therapies in geriatric psychiatry. In L. Lazarus (Ed.), *Essentials of geriatric psychiatry.* New York: Springer. pp. 173–188.

Simpson, D. M., & Foster, D. (1986). Improvement in organically disturbed behavior with trazodone treatment. *Journal of Clinical Psychiatry, 47*(4): 191–193.

Smith, L. M., & Peroutka, S. J. (1986). Differential effects of 5 hydroxytryptamine 1a. selective drugs on the 5-HT behavioral syndrome. *Pharmacology, Biochemistry and Behavior, 24,* 1513–1519.

Stevens, J. R., & Jermann, B. P. (1981). Temporal lobe epilepsy, psychopathology and violence: The state of evidence. *Neurology, 31,* 1127–1132.

Souver, R., & Hurley, A. (1981). The management of chronic behavior disorders in mentally retarded adults with lithium carbonate. *The Journal of Nervous and Mental Diseases, 169,* 191–195.

Stotsky, B. (1984). Multicenter study comparing thioridazine with diazepam and placebo in elderly, nonpsychotic patients with emotional and behavioral disorders. *Clinical Therapies, 6*(4), 546–559.

Tiller, J. W. G., Dakis, J. A., & Shaw, J. M. (1988). Short-term buspirone treatment in disinhibition with dementia [Letter to the editor]. *Lancet, 2* (8609), 510.

Tingle, D. (1986). Trazodone in dementia [Letter to the editor]. *Journal of Clinical Psychiatry, 47*(9): 482.

Twefik, G. I., Jain, V. K., Harcup, M., & Magowan, S. (1970). Effectiveness of various tranquilizers in the management of senile restlessness. *Gerontologic Clinics, 12,* 351–359.

Weiler, P. G., Mungas, D., & Bernick, C. (1988). Propranolol for control of disruptive behavior in senile dementia. *Journal of Geriatric Psychiatry and Neurology, 1*(4), 226–230.

Wilcock, G. K., Stevens, J., & Perkins, A. (1987). Trazodone/tryptophane for aggressive behavior. *Lancet, 1*(8538), 929–930.

16

Special Care Units

Susan Bass
Gloria Crumpton
Linda K. Griffin
Rakhshanda Hassan
Raymond F. Rustige

Due to an ever increasing awareness, larger numbers of nursing home residents are diagnosed with serious cognitive impairments. It is currently estimated that 50% to 80% of nursing home residents are cognitively impaired (Weiner & Reingold, 1989). The number of persons with senile dementia of the Alzheimer's type increases significantly for those 85 years and over.

In spite of efforts to improve overall quality of nursing home care, the adequacy of care of residents with dementia remains a significant problem. In order to improve care of these residents, the Philadelphia Geriatric Center (1974) opened a treatment unit especially designed for this population. Since then, special care units (SCUs) have become a growth industry (Leon, Potter, & Cunningham, 1990). In 1987, 8% of all nursing homes had special care units, and this proliferation continues rapidly.

In this chapter, the authors will address the issues in developing special care units, specifically discussing administrative concerns, staffing issues, and design considerations for the special care unit resident. As important, programming activities and intervention in the behavioral sequelae of the disease will be elaborated.

DEFINITION OF SPECIAL CARE UNITS

To begin with, the basic definition of a special care unit is a specially designed environment with a skilled staff to provide ongoing care and programs addressing the special needs of the resident with dementia.

The basic rationale for SCUs is to provide better care. Physical design, programs, and staffing in the traditional nursing home often fail to meet the needs of the increasing cognitively impaired. Further planning for the deteriorating course of these illnesses is an integral part of the SCU. This will require different services over time with increasing amounts of nursing care. Increasing physical dependence should be considered in developing long-term services for SCU residents. There is a need to provide for appropriate physical and mental stimulation. As important is the safety of this resident, as well as protection from exploitation and abuse. For example, a resident who has physical problems but who is cognitively intact places great value on privacy and choice. These residents have the right to an environment that is not disrupted by inappropriate behaviors exhibited by residents with dementia, such as rummaging through others' possessions and problem wandering.

In the process of developing an SCU, the administrator's role requires thorough investigation of the feasibility of need and potential for such a unit. Several fundamental issues should be addressed:

- Will this venture be consistent with the mission of the organization? Given the ongoing mission of all long-term-care facilities for providing quality of life, the SCU should be viewed as an enhancement.
- Presuming that the nursing home already has residents who would benefit from the SCU, the next step would be the evaluation of an ongoing market share. How many other facilities in the area provide the specialized care that is envisioned?
- Will the anticipated SCU provide an avenue for continued occupancy levels needed for stability and financial viability?

In evaluating the organization's resources, it is important to detail the project's objectives, which center upon the resident's care, family satisfaction, staff education, and organizational stability. Meeting these objectives will require initial expenditures for construction and renovation. Ongoing costs will include possibly increased staffing and certainly staff in-service education. Program planning will also require an appropriate allocation of staff time. (This will be further addressed later in this chapter.)

COST IMPLICATIONS

As indicated above, current occupancy of an existing facility and the percentage of cognitively impaired residents will signal whether the renovation of existing space, an addition, or new construction will be warranted. In some states, a Certificate of Need is necessary. An evaluation of the organization's current assets and abilities to meet incurred debts for construction and/or renovation is crucial. Where will the revenues be generated to offset these increased costs? In general, facilities tend to charge private pay residents 15% to 25% more for the SCU than the regular rate. It is too early to evaluate the benefits of private long-term-care insurance. State Medicaid reimbursement rates fall about 10% below actual costs for the SCU. The costs of special care units and concerns for residents who would benefit but cannot afford them must be addressed, not only in terms of direct cost but costs to residents, their caregivers, and overall public relations of the facility.

UNIT DESIGN

The organization's current facility utilization and the capital resources for expansion will determine whether an entirely new unit will be designed and built or if an existing unit could be renovated. In either instance, there are basic elements to consider for the most desirable environment.

Zarit, Zarit, and Rosenberg-Thompson (1990) suggest a homelike atmosphere, with areas both inside and out to allow for wandering. In renovation or new construction, physical design should include a secured unit. Enclosed courtyards, landscaped with comfortable sitting areas, allow for visual and tactile stimulation. The evaluation of adequate lighting, including night lights, is a necessity for safety and reassurance. Security measures surface as one of the most important considerations. Some units with fewer residents have been successful in keeping the exit doors closed without locking devices. Use of stop signs at exit doors and color coding have been mechanisms to cue residents or "prompt" memory. Various alarm systems are also available. Dialogue between designers and staff caregivers can elicit practical information about successful security and cognitive cuing techniques. (Further elaboration of design are discussed in another chapter.)

INCLUSION CRITERIA

One of the most important aspects in the development of the unit will be deciding on the inclusion/exclusion criteria. Idealism must co-exist with realism. The unit program must clearly offer what is not readily available in the rest of the facility. Otherwise, it will not serve as a specialized environment to its population.

Basic criteria for the resident should include: a current diagnosis of dementia with completed workup, stage of the disease, medication review, functional assessments, and mental status examination. Discussion should include the benefits to the resident as compared to his/her present environment. It is imperative to define preadmission screening criteria. Not all residents with dementia will benefit from, or be appropriate for the goals of the unit.

If the potential resident does not yet reside in the facility, a visit to their present environment for assessment and observation should be considered. Family members' or primary caregivers' input is essential in obtaining history, medication compliance, and behavioral style. Individuals with a lifelong history of violence or some chronic mental illnesses, and those whose family and/or physician are not agreeable may not be acceptable in many facilities. Administration and staff will need to decide on the stage or levels of abilities the unit will be most effective with. Further, policy needs to be addressed to anticipate the resident's deterioration of abilities and what happens when he no longer fits the goals of the unit. How is this to be handled, and where does he go? Ultimately, the final determination of who will be admitted to the unit should be made by the SCU's multidisciplinary treatment team.

STAFFING

Staffing requirements and development are important for successful implementation of the unit program. Much time and energy must be expended in this facet of development. Innovative staffing patterns should be considered in order to offer flexible schedules, rotations, and overlaps that can accommodate resident's needs such as, "sundowning" which is late afternoon confusion. Basic staff requirements include those experienced in long-term care and with enthusiastic desire to work in an SCU. The interview process should elaborate clear understanding of the goals of the SCU and the expectation of staff responsibilities in implementing this program. Increased staffing appears to be a reality in the SCU. Surveys indicate that the staff-resident ratio increases when implementing programmatic changes (Sandel, Fisher, & Hollander, 1989). Some facilities surveyed preferred around-the-clock registered nurse (RN) coverage. In addition, evening and night shift staffing was not reduced as significantly as in other nursing home units. For adequate staffing, the rate of professional staffing should comprise one third of the total staff and the remaining two thirds paraprofessional. The optimum ratio of Certified Nurse Aide (CNA) to resident is one to three. A full-time activity therapist should be considered as well as a unit psychiatrist, preferably a geriatric psychiatrist. The facility's education and social service directors can normally serve the unit's needs, though the start-up phase may require their intensive involvement for several months. Allocation of monies for outside consultants and use of part-time personnel when needed should be included in the budget and programing.

It is essential that prior to the unit opening, the core staff has completed a training program specific to dementias and behavioral theories. Ronch (1987) suggests a minimum of a two-week staff preparation prior to the admission of residents. This training is often overlooked in its importance. New employees should have a thorough orientation program, including a review of normal aging, the dementias, behavioral approaches, program goals, and medications. This knowledge must be routinely confirmed through feedback, observation of approaches, and application, so that educational needs can be updated. Sufficient resources have to be allocated for staff education.

All institutions caring for the elderly have a responsibility to their residents and staff to provide progressive, ongoing in-service programs. Ancillary staff involved with the unit, i.e., housekeeping, dietary, and maintenance should also be included in the training. In-service programs should include: promotion of professional growth at every level, strengthening of skills, encouragement of staff creativity, and dialogues about new methods of dealing with old problems. Staff meetings help identify and develop team treatment approaches to work together on problems. Conference attendance and networking activities also foster and promote staff growth.

A forum for staff to ventilate frustrations and feelings needs to be established. The difficulty of being the target of residents' frustration and of continued loss must be acknowledged and discussed as a frustration shared by all. (Further discussion of caregivers' stress is addressed elsewhere in this text.) Group experiences can encourage support and offer creative ways to handle these situations. An outside consultant may be necessary to allow staff to be candid.

SCU PROGRAM

Specialty units need to be just that. Program development is the basic component of an SCU. What will the staff and residents do routinely? Program flexibility and adaptability to the abilities of the residents in an ongoing process, plus a daily routine of both group and individual activities, need to be planned. Suggested activities include: social skills activities to stimulate language, interaction and orientation; exercise or movement activities to encourage range of motion and diffuse excessive energy; reminiscence groups to stimulate use of old memories, language, and identification of one's sense of history; sensory stimulation activities to incorporate use of senses; and supportive talk therapy to foster trust and help with coping.

All activities have a purpose, to encourage function, and should ensure success. Activities will have to be tailored to meet the ability levels of residents. Ongoing assessment is an integral component of the program to identify and meet the needs of the residents as their disease progresses and functional abilities deteriorate. Routine cognitive, functional, and medical assessments need to be completed in order to plan for changes but also to document changes in levels of functioning. This documentation also supports need for increased staffing requirements and assists in evaluating the success of the SCU.

The most successful activity program allows for separate activities for residents of the SCU. Residents with a dementia may exhibit a shorter attention span, poor concentration, and the inability to follow multistep directions. Large group activities may be overstimulating. Short-term activities offered several times a day work well. Small-group discussions lasting approximately 30 minutes have proven successful. The activity therapists need to discuss previous activities and hobbies with the resident's family. These activities can be modified to fit the resident's functional level. Life review or reminiscence activities allow all group members to share their experiences. Simple discussion topics may include a first car, school, or first date; are all subjects to which most residents can contribute. Group facilitators should feel comfortable taking an active role and intervening in behaviors such as shyness or intrusiveness.

Daily exercise is another important aspect of the unit. A 15-30-minute exercise session can assist in relieving tension and anxiety, and decreasing wandering behaviors. Exercise programs help maintain balance, strength, and coordination.

Music and entertainment is an easily facilitated activity encouraging interaction and movement. Using a small room for these activities allows the resident to wander safely about during the session. Residents with short attention spans may show limited interest in television or movies, and in the authors' experience, these offer limited benefit as part of a therapeutic program.

Staffing will need to be adjusted to address different resident needs, for example, for moderately or severely impaired. When possible, higher-functioning residents may be able to participate in activities off the SCU.

The goal is to find the appropriate fit for the resident and to develop activities to ensure success.

It is important to emphasize those skills which residents can still perform successfully. This applies to all activities which help a resident to maintain dignity despite deficits. Adhering to a simple, predictable schedule can help staff and residents cope with activities throughout the day.

FUNCTIONAL ASSESSMENT AND ACTIVITIES OF DAILY LIVING

A thorough functional assessment can be a valuable tool when identifying abilities of the residents in the special care unit. Activities of Daily Living (ADLs) include toileting, bathing, dressing, and feeding. The activity therapist and nursing staff can perform the functional assessment. A bathing assessment may require one or more persons. The therapist should discover whether the resident's preference is for a bath or shower and at what time of the day she/he is accustomed to bathing. Preparation should include an uncluttered, simplified environment to prevent confusion. Many residents find dressing difficult. Body awareness and coordination can decrease during the course of a dementing illness. Simple, washable clothing with elastic waists and shirts with zippers or large buttons allow the resident to dress with minimal assistance. Some residents find the selection of clothing overwhelming. Clothing hung together as outfits can minimize the choices the resident must make. Choice of clothing should include ease, comfort, and safety.

Use of bowel and bladder routines may be necessary for many residents. This assessment includes the impact of fluid intake, degree of confusion, location of toilets, and complicated clothing. Innovative and creative approaches as well as individualized bowel and bladder routines create a challenge for staff.

NUTRITION

Eating and maintaining nutrition can be a problem. Discovering a resident's favorite foods may be helpful. Small, frequent meals instead of three larger meals may be indicated. Residents often have poor appetites, and seeing a meal tray with many dishes can cause confusion. As manual dexterity declines, the use of silverware can also be a problem. Finger foods work well, and many foods can be adapted to this method. A consultation with the occupational therapist is a good resource for adaptive eating. Meal times should be as pleasant as possible. Segregating residents according to their eating abilities may be necessary. Those who are more independent should be allowed to eat their meals with less impaired residents. And it may be appropriate for agitated residents to eat alone.

COMMON BEHAVIORAL PROBLEMS

Behavioral problems associated with dementia pose management concerns. The advantage of the SCU is that many of these behaviors are tolerated and redirected. This section will address common behaviors and suggest interventions. When interviewing a resident with behavioral problems, sensitivity to the resident's responses is essential. Frustration or negative feelings lead to problem behaviors such as aggression or screaming. Establishing and maintaining a warm therapeutic relationship with the cognitively impaired resident encourages support and trust, and helps set limits with their behaviors.

Agitation

Residents who are easily agitated and at risk for becoming physically aggressive can hinder the safety of others. Establishing a safe environment where the resident can be assessed and treated is necessary. It must be determined if there is a pattern to the acting-out behavior and, if so, what triggers it. Behavioral charting noting time, activity, staffing, and what is occurring during the outbursts can be extremely beneficial and easy to implement. Refer to Table 16.1 for a sample of questions to ask in assessing behaviors. This information will help in developing a treatment care plan. With this data, the staff can intervene early, possibly preventing major catastrophic reactions. Use of chemical or physical restraints is considered only as a last resort.

Wandering

The management of wandering and rummaging behaviors depends upon the cause of the behavior. Residents may wander because they feel lost in the environment, or they may be trying to relieve tension.Wandering may also be a search for home. Reinforcement of belonging by talking about what "home" means can be comforting and can divert residents' attention. Wandering and rummaging behavior often indicates feeling lost or out of place. Reassurance about where she/he is can alleviate a distressing moment. When providing a safe, enclosed area is provided, wandering can be tolerated. Rest periods can be facilitated by strategically placed seating.

TABLE 16.1 Behavioral Charting Questions

Does the resident feel threatened?
Is the environment too stimulating or not stimulating enough?
Are too many demands being made of the resident?
Can the task or expectation be simplified to ensure success?
Is there some physical reason for the agitation?

Directional signs can assist with orientation and mark ownership, for example, Mrs. Jane Jones' room. Even with the above approaches, the resident may insist that this is not home and continue attempts to leave. It is an ongoing challenge to find ways to help the resident feel at home.

Screaming and Repetitious Behavior

Screaming and repetitive behaviors may be the most disruptive to any unit. As previously noted, behavioral symptom charting can be useful. Further investigation of screaming behavior should include assessment of pain, boredom, hunger and thirst, isolation, and other basic needs. Repetitive questioning may respond to written cues as well as supportive strategies to minimize residents' fears and anxieties. Teri and Logsdon (1990) reported medication may be a necessary adjunct with behavioral approaches in these behaviors. Even the most creative and compassionate staff person may find they have tried everything without much success. After evaluation of the treatment plan, staff may have to realize they have done all they can. They may accept this behavior and alter the environment to accommodate the resident's behavior.

In developing the SCU, consideration and design of a sound-reduction room, where a disruptive resident could be comfortable and well cared for without disrupting the unit, may be indicated. It must be emphasized this is not an isolation room, but a room that has been designed to considerably reduce noise, and it should be used to allow a "noisy" resident freedom without restraint.

FAMILY

As an ongoing part of the assessment, family dynamics and assessment of their understanding of dementia need to be explored. The family assessment provides an opportunity for family members to express their fears and concerns. Initially, staff may provide information and emotional support. In subsequent contacts, evaluation of the families' understanding and discussion of involvement with their relative, as well as progress reports, are appropriate. Family conferences may be warranted. An informed staff member can assist families by clarification of concerns such as diagnosis, treatment approaches, and prognosis. Potential ethical and legal issues can also be explored. Periodically, the family may need assistance as the disease progresses and further decline is noted. Families should be referred to appropriate resources such as the Alzheimer's Association for assistance, information, and additional support.

DRAWBACKS OF THE SCU

There are many issues concerning the SCU that need to be addressed in their potential for negative use. First, there is the need for families to understand that quality care will be provided throughout the facility and not only in the special care unit. Conversely, SCUs do not warehouse the "difficult" and "troublesome" residents. Second, with the progressive nature of dementing illness resulting in increased care needs, monies to provide that care need to be allocated. Third, recruitment may be difficult if the intensity of care is not planned for and appropriate measures introduced. And last, there is the potential for misuse of the label "special care unit" as a marketing tool rather than as a developed program.

POSITIVE OUTCOMES

The outcomes of the special care units are presently difficult to assess because of the paucity of research. Several attempts at objective evaluation of special care units have been somewhat difficult, because the existing special care units vary tremendously in their underlying philosophy, physical design, staff training, ratio between staff and residents, activities, and so on. More systematic research is needed to develop licensing guidelines to standardize the quality of the special care units. These units have the potential to provide important research data about dementia and techniques of care, and can become much needed educational training sites for training health-care providers. As indicated initially, the SCU provides a way of meeting the mission of the long-term-care facility. It offers freedom and security to the cognitively impaired resident. Given this appropriate care, the resident will be able to experience a level of quality of life appropriate to his/her condition.

Reports consistently point to increased staff morale rather than increased burnout in the SCU. Employees do see their work as "special." Enthusiasm develops as personal relationships are formed. Staff committed to SCUs do not want to be rotated from their divisions.

Experiencing the SCU will enable family members to be satisfied that they are providing appropriate care for their loved ones. Families will have the opportunity for additional education and increase their understanding of the changes taking place as the disease progresses. Available staff will assist them throughout the illness.

SUMMARY

A model SCU presented in this chapter is derived from the survey efforts of the experienced professionals in field (Hepburn, Severance, Gates, & Christensen, 1989; Myer, 1990). A model SCU is designed for the resident as well as the family. Training staff is a key component of this model.

The goals of special care units include:

(a) Evaluation of potential residents' needs and the meeting of these needs through physical design, a stable and personalized environment, and care with dignity. This includes frequent reevaluation of residents for their needs, evidence of excessive disabilities, worsening of dementia, and causes of mental status changes, for example, medications, other illnesses, etc.

(b) Establishment of a stable and secure environment defined as "secured freedom" (Hall et al., 1986). This will not be with inappropriate barriers, but with redundant cues and signs, to assist residents with orientation and redirection.

(c) De-emphasis of the traditional medical model of a nursing home and the provision of specialized meaningful programs which are integrated with this environment. Efforts are aimed at maximizing levels of functioning, while encouraging appropriate autonomy and enhancing social interaction with others. Lastly, ongoing behavioral assessment and behavioral intervention over traditional medical treatment are emphasized.

Family

(a) Educating the family, assisting them with reasonable expectations, providing information regarding the diagnosis and prognosis of the resident's illness, and defining the program and goals of the special care unit.

(b) Providing support groups for counseling and referral to the Alzheimer's Association and other support groups.

(c) Maintaining family involvement both in care as well as in the decision-making process.

(d) Developing a confident, competent, multidisciplinary team who are comfortable in their skills and abilities to plan and act appropriately and compassionately. Further, the staff is committed not only to the program and their residents but to each other in developing continued professional growth and support.

REFERENCES

Hall, G., Kirschling, M., & Todd, S. (1986). Sheltered freedom: An Alzheimer's unit in an ICF. *Geriatric Nursing 7*(3), 132–136.

Hepburn, J., Severance, J., Gates, B., & Christensen, M. (1989). Institutional care of dementia patients: A statewide survey of long-term care facilities and special care units. *American Journal of Alzheimer's Care and Related Disorders and Research, 4*(2), 19–23.

Leon, J., Potter, D., & Cunningham, P. (1990). *Current and projected availability of special nursing home programs for Alzheimer's disease patients.* (DHHS Publication No. PHS 90-3463). Public Health Services, Rockville, MD: National Medical Expenditure Survey Data Summary 1, Agency for Health Care Policy and Research.

Meyer, D. (1990). A special care home for Alzheimer's disease and related disorders: An 18-month progress report. *The American Journal of Alzheimer's Care and Related Disorders and Research,* January/February, 1991, 18–23.

Ronch, J. L. (1987). Specialized Alzheimer's units in nursing homes: Pros and cons. *American Journal of Alzheimer's Care and Research, 2*(4), 10–19.

Sandel, S., Fisher, J., & Hollander, A. (1989). A program for patients with dementia: A management challenge. *The Journal of Long Term Care Administration, 17*(1), 20–23.

Teri, L., & Logsdon, R. (1990). Assessment and management of behavioral disturbances in Alzheimer's Disease. *Comprehensive Therapy, 16*(5), 36–42.

Weiner, A., & Reingold, M. (1989). Special care units for dementia. *The Journal of Long Term Care Administration, 17*(1) 1989, 14–19.

Zarit, S., Zarit, J., & Rosenberg-Thompson (1990). A Special Treatment Unit for Alzheimer's Disease: Medical, Behavioral, and Environmental Features. The Haworth Press: 47–63.

SUGGESTED READINGS

Ackerman, J. O. (1985). Separated, not isolated—as basic as administrative backing and commitment. *The Journal of Long-Term Care Administration, 13,* 90–94.

Benson, D. M., Cameron, D., Humbach, E., (1987). Establishment and impact of a dementia unit within the nursing home. *Journal of the American Geriatrics Society 35,* 319–323.

Calkins, M. P. (1987). Designing special care units: A systematic approach. *American Journal of Alzheimer's Care and Research and Related Disorders and Research 2*(3), 30–34.

Cameron, D. J., Gambert, S. R., Bashian, N. (1987). A specialized dementia unit: Cost and benefit analysis. *The New York Medical Quarterly, 7,* 103–107.

Coleman, E. A., Barbaccia, J. C., & Croughan-Minihane, M. S. Hospitalization rates in nursing home residents with dementia: A pilot study of the impact of a special care unit. *Journal of the American Geriatrics Society 38,* 108–112.

Coons, D. H. (Ed.) (1990). *Specialized dementia care units.* Baltimore: Johns Hopkins University Press.

Folstein, M. F., Folstein, S., & McHugh, P. R. (1975). Mini Mental State: A practical Method of Grading the Cognitive State of Patients for the Clinician. *Journal of Psychiatric Research, 12,* 189–198.

Hyde, J. (1989). The physical environment and the care of Alzheimer's patients: An experimental survey of Massachusetts' Alzheimer's units. *American Journal of Alzheimer's Care and Related Disorders and Research, 4*(3), 36–43.

Johnson, C. J. (1989). Sociological interventions through developing low stimulus Alzheimer's wings in nursing homes. *American Journal of Alzheimer's Care and Related Disorders and Research, 4*(2), 33–41.

Mayers, K., Block, C. (1990). Specialized services for demented residents in Washington state nursing homes: Report of a survey. *American Journal of Alzheimer's Care and Related Disorders and Research 5*(4), 17–21.

Meyer, D., Jacques, J., O'Rourke, J. (1990). A special care home for Alzheimer's disease and related disorders: An 18-month progress report. *American Journal of Alzheimer's Care and Related Disorders and Research, 5*(1), 18–23.

Ohta, R. J., & Ohta, B. (1988). Special units for Alzheimer's disease patients: A critical look. *The Gerontologist, 28,* 803–808.

Rabins, P. (1986). Establishing Alzheimer's disease units in nursing homes: Pros and cons. *Hospital Community Psychiatry, 37,* 120–121.

Robinson, A., Spencer, B., & White, L. (1989). *Understanding difficult behaviors: Some practical suggestions for coping with Alzheimer's disease and related illnesses.*

Rovner, B. W., German, P. S., Broadhead, J. (1990). The prevalence and management of dementia and other psychiatric disorders in nursing homes. *International Psychogeriatrics, 2,* 13–24.

Schiff, M. R. (1990). Designing environments for individuals with Alzheimer's disease: Some general principles. *American Journal of Alzheimer's Care and Related Disorders and Research, 5*(3), 4–8.

17

Design Issues in Nursing Homes and Special Care Units

David V. Kromm
Young-Hie Nahm Kromm
Laura Wehrenberg

INTRODUCTION

The intentions of this chapter are to create a starting point for making the design process accessible to administrators and staff of nursing homes, to set some guidelines for working with design professionals, and to outline some of the key design issues in housing and caring for the elderly and cognitively impaired.

DESIGN AND PLANNING TEAM

Because of the complexity of program and user needs in nursing homes and special care units, the development of appropriate design solutions involves a team. Key members of this team include the staff of a facility, members of the administration, resident representatives, and design professionals: planners, architects, interior designers, and engineers.

The planning and design team identifies problems, develops alternatives to resolve the problems, and ultimately, chooses alternatives to best meet the goals and needs of the facility. The role of the design professional is to ask questions and to work with staff, administration, and resident representatives in clarifying the goals and needs of the facility.

Staff, administration, and resident representatives examine the questions generated by design professionals. The administration addresses questions related to broad program concerns, such as:

1. What is the philosophy of care in the facility?
2. What are the programs/activities/levels of care offered within the facility?
3. What additional programs/services should be offered?
4. What spaces/relationships work well for current programs and activities?
5. What do you see for your facility/programs in the future?
6. What is the level of your staff's involvement with residents?

Staff input provides information about routines and schedules, required practices and activities, and the effectiveness of existing facilities. Some questions to examine with staff are:

1. What are daily routines? Weekly? What tasks are regular but unscheduled?
2. What tasks are required by Federal or state agencies? What activities are performed as a result of the facility's programs?
3. What spaces and space relationships are effective? Which ones are ineffective?
4. Under ideal circumstances, what spaces/relationships/equipment/furnishings would you have to accomplish your job?

Residents are also users of a facility and should be represented on the planning and design team. A representative for the residents may be a staff social worker or psychologist, an independent consultant, someone affiliated with an agency that serves the elderly, or an actual resident in the facility. This person's responsibility is to present information from the resident's point of view. The questions they deal with are similar to questions that the staff responds to regarding daily activities, what is effective and ineffective in the existing facility, and the physical limitations to be accommodated in designing a physical environment (Koncelik, 1976).

The questions listed here will ideally produce an interactive planning process in which goals and needs are clearly defined before design solutions are generated. The design professional creates a bridge between the verbal responses of planning team members and the visual and spatial organization of a nursing home or special care unit. Program goals and staff and resident needs can be expressed as diagrams showing key ideas, relationships, and important issues. These diagrams begin to suggest a comprehensive space and arrangements within the space to meet identified goals and needs. This process is by nature interactive, as team members respond to the efforts of the design professional and provide additional information to be incorporated into the planning process.

Using a team for planning and design has several benefits. Including the end users gives them an opportunity to express their needs and concerns and to incorporate their input into program development. Including philosophy of care and long-range needs provides a flexible program to accommodate both immediate and future needs. Patterns of usage and philosophy of care vary from facility to facility; it is a critical step to uncover these elements because a single design solution does not work for all facilities.

An examination of the level of staff involvement with residents quickly reveals implications in planning and design. If a facility's philosophy of care encourages a high level of interaction between staff and residents, both the size of a facility and the number of residents are limited by the amount of staffing required and the demands placed upon them. Private staff space becomes important for completing paperwork and for breaks. The nursing station will be small, because it is not a focal point for interaction.

Conversely, if a facility's emphasis is on supervision of residents, the facility can be larger and more residents can be taken care of. The nurse station will be larger and will provide space for staff to complete paperwork. It will be located where the largest number of rooms and activities can be supervised. Residents will tend to congregate in the area because it is the focus of activity on a wing. Private space for staff is not as critical.

KEY DESIGN ISSUES

Regardless of program goals and philosophy of care, there are issues that must be considered in the design of nursing homes and special care units. These issues are shown in Table 17.1 as the end points of a continuum. Individual facilities, through clarification of their own needs and goals, will find themselves at different points on this continuum.

Within an individual facility or program, there will be variations based upon activities, spaces, and different needs. In developing a plan for environmental intervention, it is useful to rank specific spaces and programs as well as the total facility. This process provides a framework in which

TABLE 17.1   Continua

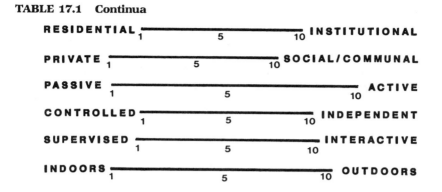

specific design alternatives can be examined, resulting in a constant reference point for design choices.

A final design issue stands by itself: safety and security of the residents. Local, state, and Federal regulations exist to provide parameters for life safety and handicapped accessibility. A knowledgeable and experienced design professional will thoroughly review these regulations in the planning and design process. The professional should establish good working relationships with design review officials in order to accurately interpret and meet regulations and to incorporate them into an overall plan for the facility.

For each key design issue, there are specific elements to consider. The following checklists are intended as a starting point, as the interactive planning and design process will generate more questions.

RESIDENTIAL/INSTITUTIONAL

Current opinion indicates that a residential "feel" to a facility eases the transitions that residents make and gives them a sense of being in a familiar place (Calkins, 1988; Koncelik, 1976). Some of the elements that affect the residential or institutional appearance of a facility are included in the following list.

1. Colors: Which colors say "institution?" Residence? Physical limitations in distinguishing colors will influence color selections; residents tend to respond to warm colors (reds, yellows, oranges) and may have trouble distinguishing between blues and greens. The yellowing of the lens that occurs with age can cause problems in differentiating between the same values of several colors; for example, deep or pastel tones will be read as the same color (Hiatt, 1981a). As a consequence, contrast between colors

is probably more important than actual colors chosen. Walls should stand out clearly from floors; changes in color on floors may be perceived as changes in level.

2. Finishes/furniture: Which finishes/furnishings are institutional? Residential? Where is a hard surface appropriate? Carpet? Does carpet surface allow for easy movement of walkers and wheelchairs? What new products have been designed specifically to meet the needs of elderly residents? Product representatives are a valuable resource in this area.

3. Sizes of rooms: What are the optimal locations of large rooms? Small rooms? Most people have spent their lives within environments that are immediately understandable. What happens to cognitively impaired residents when they are confronted with spaces without windows or where they can't see walls?

4. Lighting/light fixtures: What is associated with institutions? Residences? Hiatt has documented the effect of inadequate levels of lighting on further deterioration of vision (Hiatt, 1980a). What levels of lighting are needed in different areas? In general, older residents require higher levels of illumination than the general population.

5. Corridors: These are perhaps the most important element in determining a residential or institutional atmosphere. Long corridors at the minimum width of eight feet, with doors to resident rooms opening on each side, are institutional. Clustered arrangements of rooms can reduce corridor length and provide alcoves to mark individual room entrances. Changes in corridor width allow for seating areas to shorten the distance that residents have to travel. These seating areas can be places for social interaction or gathering with family members. Seating arrangements should be for groups of two to six (Calkins, 1988), can also be used for residents to observe activity, and for additional gathering places. Where are there opportunities to make a corridor more than a place to walk? Deep windowsills can be used for potted plants, creating an indoor "garden." Corridors are indoor streets. What can be done to provide as much interest along them as along exterior streets?

PRIVATE/SOCIAL

1. Resident rooms: Two basic arrangements of resident rooms are most often used. One is to locate rooms along both sides of a corridor; the other is to cluster rooms around a central space. The choice of room arrangement will depend upon facility and program goals. Rooms along a corridor provide residents with a "path" for walking but may present problems in identifying the resident's individual room. Rooms clustered around a cen-

tral space provide clear definition of private and group space but may be difficult to supervise. Size of rooms, furniture arrangements within rooms, provision of bathrooms, and storage space are also issues to consider in relation to residents' capabilities and program goals.

2. Activity rooms: One large room or several smaller rooms for activities? Will a dining area be used as an activity space or have its own separate location? Clear definition of separate spaces within a special care unit may help to decrease confusion. How can separate spaces be defined without walls?

3. Private spaces: Where will family members meet privately with residents? With staff? In the event of catastrophic reactions from residents, will space for a resident to regain control be provided? Around areas of activity (nurse station, entrance, lobby), will the gathering of residents be encouraged or discouraged? Will space or seating arrangements be provided for those who want to observe without participating?

4. Staff rooms and work stations: What level of staff interaction is expected? Where a high level of interaction between staff and residents is desired, the staff needs private space for relief from the demands of residents as well as an area for charting. Where supervision of residents is emphasized, paperwork and supervision can take place at a nurse station located for optimal supervision.

5. Offices: Where will offices for administration, doctors, social workers, counselors, physical and occupational therapists and other staff members be located? Is it better to concentrate these offices in a central location or to spread them throughout the facility? Should administration be separate from services?

6. Spaces, relationships, connections: Which services should be or already are centrally located? Are there changes to be made to improve operations or to make it easier for residents to move throughout the facility or wing on their own? What is the best location for support services such as laundry, kitchen, maintenance? Responses to some of these questions will depend upon existing spaces and relationships and budgets.

7. Dining areas: Eating is one of the most basic human activities, and meals are often the focal point of a resident's day. Questions range from operational concerns about the size and location of the kitchen and delivery of food to color choices for tabletops and place settings. In general, a separate dining area should be provided for each level of care in a facility. Choices for furnishings and finishes will be related to residents' physical and cognitive limitations. A dining area for congregate apartments might be carpeted, with fabric-covered chairs. For a skilled nursing unit, a tile floor may be more appropriate, and tabletops must be high enough for wheelchairs.

Will the dining area be used for other activities? Should a private dining room for special occasions be provided? How many people will be seated together at a table? Groups of more than six or large circular tables may make it difficult for people to carry on conversations. Contrast between tabletop and place settings makes it easier for residents to distinguish and manipulate silverware and china. Will meals be served to residents or will they go through a cafeteria line? Trays, plastic, and paper for food service will give a more of an institutional feel to the dining area than china, silver and individual service.

Food service and operations should be closely examined with the staff dietitian and food service staff. A careful evaluation of program goals and current or desired operations is critical in planning and designing dining and food service areas.

PASSIVE/ACTIVE

In general, knowledge of the physical limitations of aging residents can bring about awareness of how the physical environment supports or hinders activity. If residents feel in control of their surroundings, they will often become more active.

1. Multiple cuing: Color is one element that can provide multiple cues for residents. Specific corridors can be identified by signage, color changes, individual color schemes, or texture changes (e.g., floor surface changes from carpet to tile or wall surface changes from smooth to bumpy). A dining area may be identified by a color change on the floor, by a railing, or by a dropped or raised ceiling. How many cues involving different senses can be provided in identifying important spaces and pathways?

2. Patterns: Patterns should be selected with care; too much information may be confusing to residents. Expanses of solid color on walls can be broken up with wall hangings or special displays.

3. Edges: Because of the loss of depth perception, changes in level and the difference between walls and floors should be clearly marked. Different edges can be marked by color and texture changes. This applies in individual rooms as well as in corridors and common spaces. An example is the use of an edge of a different color or material for dining room tables.

4. Tactile surfaces: Surfaces that can be distinguished by touch allow residents to interact with the environment as well as reinforcing visual cues. A surround for doorways to resident rooms that can be touched may

help residents to identify their own rooms. Several facilities have used interactive wall hangings or art work to provide tactile experiences for residents (Calkins, 1988).

5. Ventilation systems: The sense of smell is extremely powerful in providing orientation/familiarity. Some facilities have experimented with exhausting cooking and baking smells into resident wings to stimulate appetites and to cue residents before meals (Hiatt, 1990).

6. Doors: Doors are a signal to enter. What steps can be taken to avoid creating an attractive nuisance? How can residents be encouraged in finding their own rooms and discouraged from entering other areas? Individualization of doorways with photographs and personal memorabilia has become almost a standard practice. Room signs should be easy to read, with either light lettering on a dark ground or dark lettering on a light ground (Calkins, 1988).

Exit doors can be minimized by painting them the same color as surrounding walls or minimizing hardware and locks. Conversely, the message not to use an exit door can be reinforced by a stop sign or a fence painted on the door. Storage closets, mediprep areas, and other areas that pose a danger to residents should be locked. Doors that provide access to secured outdoor space can be clearly marked. At both interior and exterior doors, be careful of level changes immediately before or after the door.

CONTROLLED/INDEPENDENT

The issue of controlled/independent is closely related to passive/active. The goal is to provide freedom for residents in orienting themselves within an environment and in negotiating that environment.

1. Communication systems: From a resident's standpoint, where are nurse call buttons located? Can residents reach them easily? What sound does the call system make at the nurse station? Do residents wear some kind of monitoring device? What sound does the monitoring device make if a resident leaves a special care unit?

From a staff point of view, what are the least disruptive ways of monitoring residents? Where should the control panel for call systems and alarm systems be located? How should staff be alerted to a resident's call or to an alarm being triggered? Silent alarms can warn the staff without upsetting other residents. It may be useful to have someone on the planning team to research new products and technology in this area.

2. Barrier-free access: What aids to mobility are used by residents? Are all areas of the facility accessible to residents using wheelchairs, canes,

walkers? Areas to pay special attention to are individual bathrooms, kitchens, and bathing rooms. Kitchen counter tops without storage below
provide more mobility and room for a resident in a wheelchair to face a
task directly. Lowered counter tops and wall cabinets make it easier for
those in wheelchairs to reach and to work.

3. Lighting: Older eyes are sensitive to glare. Are there reflective surfaces that create glare? Are windows located so they are not a single
opening against a dark wall? Is the entire building oriented to make use of
indirect sunlight? Where can clerestory windows or skylights be used?
Roof overhangs to shade windows? Trees or plantings to filter light?
Window coverings that allow diffused light? Can a combination of both
fluorescent and incandescent lighting be used? The levels of light required
for residents will often make it easier for staff to do their work. An electrical
engineer or lighting consultant can provide additional information.

4. Hardware/switches/controls: Adaptations for use by the elderly can
be effective for the general population as well. Examples are the use of
levers rather than knobs, the placement of locks and electrical switches at
a lower than usual height to offset decreased mobility, and the use of
handles large enough to grasp easily. Timers can help to prevent injury if
appliances are turned on and forgotten (Calkins, 1988). Electrical outlets
can be placed high on walls for easier access; unused outlets may be
plugged to prevent accidental shock. Open shelving in kitchens allows
access to contents without having to pull cabinet doors open. A question to
ask is whether someone with decreased mobility will find this location or
piece of hardware easy to use.

5. Acoustics: What distracting background noises can be filtered out?
How can they be muffled without absorbing too much sound? Soft surfaces
absorb sound; hard surfaces reflect it. A large open space should have
some soft surfaces to absorb sound; carpeting and fabric will help deaden
noise in these spaces. Applying wall carpet up to the height of handrails in
corridors will absorb sound, protect both residents and walls from bumps,
and provide a tactile cue to identify a corridor. In new construction, sound
baffles can be provided in walls and ceilings that separate noisy areas from
quieter areas.

6. Bathrooms: Are mirrors set at a height and angled so that they can be
used by people in a wheelchair? Commodes should be set higher; wall-
mounted units allow for easy maintenance. In individual apartments, show-
ers are easier to use than tubs; can shower units be equipped with a seat?
In shared toilet rooms, can personal storage space be provided for each
resident? If there are shared toilets, can a sink and mirror be provided in
each room, separate from the toilet? In bathing rooms, consider the use of
a tub which allows for direct transfer of residents without placing them in a
hoist. Bathing room finishes are often white, shiny ceramic tile; matte-

finish tile, soft colors, and noise reduction can provide a less institutional appearance (Hiatt, 1990).

7. Individualization of resident rooms: What choices can be allowed for residents? In a new facility, can they choose their own wall or carpet colors? What personal furnishings can be used? Can family members or staff create a memory wall within a room? Can built-in storage units create some privacy in shared rooms? In special care units, the use of personal mementos and furnishings can help to identify a room clearly for the resident.

8. Pathways through a facility: In planning and designing a new facility or wing, ease of movement through the facility should be considered carefully. In renovating an existing facility, are pathways easy to identify? Will the addition of signage make the pathways clearer? Do pathways have a clear goal? In special care units, can a closed circulation loop provide a path for walkers?

9. Handrails: Can they be reached by those in wheelchairs as well as those who are walking? Are they easy to grasp and sturdy? A rounded shape is easier to grab than one which is squared off. Is the handrail differentiated from the wall? A contrasting color is more visible than one which matches the wall.

SUPERVISED/INTERACTIVE

Design responses to this issue will vary based upon the level of care provided, the program goals of a facility, and even the time of day. The maximum number of beds that can be supervised from a single nursing station is 60; nursing sub-stations can be used to reduce this number for a more residential atmosphere and individual attention. Elements to consider are:

1. Size of facility/number of residents: As these increase, the potential for confusion increases. In large facilities, are individual wings or units clearly identified? Nursing substations, separate dining areas, activity spaces, and common spaces can give residents a sense of belonging in a specific wing. In general, it is easier to move staff for activities than it is to move residents. In a smaller facility, a single activity area may serve for all residents and encourage them to move beyond their own rooms.

2. Location and size of nurse stations: What activities are encouraged by a single nurse station? By substations? What size and location fit with facility goals and needs? Residents tend to congregate around the nurse station as a place of "normal" activity; smaller substations can alleviate this occurrence. Decisions about the size and location of nurse stations

will have other consequences: the location of chart areas, mediprep room, soiled and clean utility rooms, communication systems, staff work spaces and lounges.

3. Entrance: The entrance is a place where residents gather. Depending on program needs or goals, this may or may not be desirable. Residents may be provided with a commons near the entrance where they can observe or participate in the activity that goes on. Conversely, the entrance may be small with limited seating to discourage gathering. In a facility that provides multiple levels of care, separate entrances for nursing and residential levels of care should be considered. Site planning should include elements such as parking, circulation of vehicles, service and delivery entrances, and weather protection in going from indoors to outdoors.

4. Pathways: How do corridors function? Are they for movement from one point to another or are there places to stop along the way? If there are places to stop, how are they supervised? Does everyone travel along the same pathways, or are there separate service corridors? What specific functions do service corridors provide? In a smaller facility, a single corridor can bring staff and residents together. In a larger facility, a staff corridor can keep cart traffic from "institutionalizing" resident spaces.

5. Mailboxes/bulletin board/kiosks: Separating these functions from a central administrative area provides residents with alternate gathering places and give them some independence in picking up their own mail. Bulletin boards can be used for cuing and information. Kiosks provide a three-dimensional cue for orientation, gathering, privacy, or special activities.

INDOORS/OUTDOORS

1. Windows: Residents who cannot go out can have access to the outdoors through windows. What are the best views on the site? How can windows be located to provide those views? Views for dining areas, resident rooms, and staff lounges should all be considered in locating a building. Orienting a building so that it does not receive direct eastern or western light can reduce glare as well as heat gain in the summer. Preferably, windows in resident rooms should be operable but should not be large enough for residents to crawl out of. One possibility is to provide fixed windows with an awning opening. Residents can operate these windows but cannot crawl through (Calkins, 1988).

2. Ease of access to outdoor spaces: Are thresholds level so that residents won't trip? What grade changes are there in outdoor spaces? How

will these be handled for accessibility? Are steps shallow and clearly marked? Are treads deep enough for firm placement of feet? Are ramps sloped gently for wheelchairs?

3. Circulation loop: Can outdoor spaces be part of a loop for walking? Can a loop and its enclosure provide a courtyard?

4. Enclosure: How are residents supervised when they are outdoors? What measures need to be taken for their protection? Are covered or shaded spaces provided? Porches, verandas, and shady places to sit are often part of familiar past patterns and can give residents a protected place to observe activities. Enclosure of outdoor spaces should not be readily visible to residents; they may perceive it as a barrier and try to escape. One technique for screening an enclosure is to plant shrubbery in front of it.

5. Activities: What activities can be incorporated into outdoor spaces? Raised beds can be built so that residents do not have to bend over as they tend their gardens. Special products are available to make raised beds for wheelchair gardening. Local university extensions and gardening clubs can provide a wealth of information about gardens for touch and smell.

PROGRAM GOALS AND NEEDS IN THE DESIGN OF THE NURSE STATION

Nurse stations are a work center for staff; they are a center for social interaction with residents; they may function on several levels within this range. Nurses themselves are the agents through which these functions are performed, and the design of the nurse station should support their activities. The diagrams below (Figures 17.1–17.4) show four different ways of accommodating the activities around a nurse station. These concepts have been developed to meet specific program goals.

CONCLUSIONS

1. Effective planning and design are the result of an interactive process involving a team.

2. Clear identification of program goals and needs provides a framework for evaluating the advantages and disadvantages of specific design choices.

3. Interventions in the environment to encourage or discourage specific behaviors can be made without major programs of renovation or new construction.

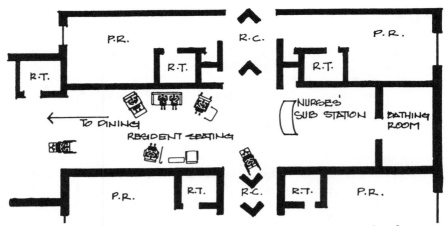

FIGURE 17.1. Program goal is to provide maximum interaction between nurses and residents. This is accomplished by providing a nurse sub-station at the intersection of two corridors.

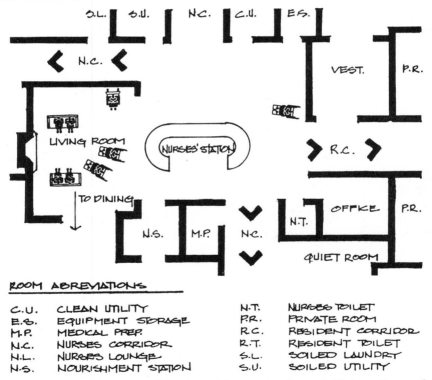

ROOM ABREVIATIONS

C.U.	CLEAN UTILITY	N.T.	NURSES TOILET
E.S.	EQUIPMENT STORAGE	P.R.	PRIVATE ROOM
M.P.	MEDICAL PREP	R.C.	RESIDENT CORRIDOR
N.C.	NURSES CORRIDOR	R.T.	RESIDENT TOILET
N.L.	NURSES LOUNGE	S.L.	SOILED LAUNDRY
N.S.	NOURISHMENT STATION	S.U.	SOILED UTILITY

FIGURE 17.2. Program goal is to provide a center for social interaction and a work center, with emphasis on the work center. This is accomplished by locating a living room next to the nurse station and providing work surfaces as part of the nurse station.

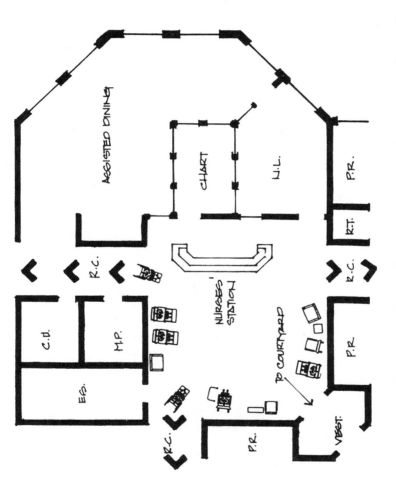

FIGURE 17.3. Program goal is to provide a work center for nurses and to encourage interaction with residents, with emphasis on social interaction. This is accomplished by providing a commons adjacent to the nurse station and a separate chart area and nurses' lounge.

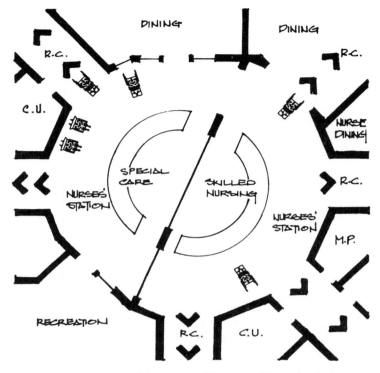

FIGURE 17.4. Program goal is to provide a work center for nurses, with emphasis on supervision of residents. Two large back-to-back nurse stations are provided to supervise five corridors. The back-to-back location allows the door to the special care unit to be left unlocked.

REFERENCES

Calkins, M. P. (1988). *Design for dementia: Planning environments for the elderly and the confused.* Owings Mills, MD: National Health Publishing.

Hiatt, L. G. (1980). Is poor lighting dimming the sight of nursing home patients? *Nursing Homes*, September/October 1980, 32–41.

Hiatt, L. G. (1982). The importance of the physical environment. *Nursing Homes*, September/October, 1982, 2–10.

Hiatt, L. G. (1990). Continuing education seminar: Environmental design for the elderly. Sponsored by St. Luke's Hospital, St. Louis, MO, June.

Koncelik, J. A. (1976). *Designing the open nursing home* (Community Development Series, Vol. 27.) Stroudsburg, PA: Dowden, Hutchinson & Ross.

18

Nursing Home Family Care

Carl W. Bretscher

It has long been acknowledged that for residents of long-term-care facilities, the transition from community to institutional living is an adjustment of major proportions and involves intense and prolonged psychological trauma (Brooke, 1989). Less universally recognized is the traumatic impact of that transition upon many of these individuals' families.

The purpose of this chapter is (1) to identify specific issues that can be stressful for family members of nursing home residents and (2) to suggest ways in which the facility might offer families some genuine support and practical assistance. It rests upon the dual premise that, first, families of institutionalized older relatives have numerous, distressing, and often unmet needs and, second, that nursing homes are in a unique position to respond to those needs in positive and constructive ways.

The chapter's intent is to issue a call for nursing home family care as an openly acknowledged and energetically pursued institutional goal. Such an emphasis, consciously endorsed and vigorously implemented, holds the promise of rich dividends for family members themselves, the loved ones they care about, the caregiving staff, and the institution as a whole.

Viable facility response will need, however, to occur at two levels: the institutional or administrative level and the individual staff person level. The first has to do with official policy and philosophy, the second with the manner in which individual nursing home personnel relate to family members in one-to-one interactions. Both are crucial. Without the open commitment and consistent reinforcement by administration, staff will be hesitant and wary about implementing the kinds of interventions this chapter proposes. No matter how enlightened and well conceived the institution's philosophy or policy formulations about family care, little will come of them unless they are operationalized at the personal level by staff members in their direct dealings with residents' families.

Thus, a genuine nursing home response to family needs will have to originate with a firm and formal institutional decision to incorporate family care as a facility goal, indeed, to recruit residents' families as clients (Montgomery, 1983). It will then have to be clearly and convincingly communicated to staff members that "being there" for families and attending to family concerns are part of their job, and that staff time and energy expended with and for the benefit of family members are viewed as an extension, rather than interruption, of their caregiving role. (Grossberg et al., 1990).

What are some of the specific issues that are frequently troublesome for family members of nursing home residents that may be amenable to nursing home efforts to help? Table 18.1 lists some areas that have been found to be particularly stressful by family members who have shared their experiences and feelings with the author. Each stress-point will be elaborated upon in the remainder of this chapter, along with some potential therapeutic interventions.

PLACEMENT FALLOUT

The first point at which families experience anxiety and strain has to do with what this writer calls "placement fallout." It is the stress that commonly surrounds the decision to place a loved one in a long-term-care facility (Kasmarik & Lester, 1984). Many family members have told the author that it was the "hardest decision" they have ever been confronted with—hard to make and hard to live with. The nursing home decision is one that few, if any, ever want. Generally, it is made only after extended, often heroic, efforts to avoid it and tends to be experienced by families as capitulation and defeat. Frequently it is made in a crisis situation, at the worst possible time, when key family members are physically and emotionally drained. In addition, it is not uncommon for the decision to be made in a climate of family disharmony amid numerous financial, legal, and other practical complications.

TABLE 18.1 Common Stress Points for Families of Nursing Home Residents

Placement fallout
Distorted expectations
Resident advocacy
Role ambiguity
Visiting discomfort
Chronic grief
Behavioral sequelae
Decision-making quandaries
Death imminence

Perhaps worst of all, the determination to institutionalize a loved one is almost always accompanied by an enormous amount of emotional pain: intense feelings of inadequacy, failure, shame, fear, uncertainty, helplessness, anger, sadness, and guilt. Rather than quickly dissipating once the placement has been effected, much of the pain continues, often for months and even years, with unnerving "second thoughts," deepening sadness, unrelenting guilt and overwhelming feelings of hopelessness, loneliness, and personal loss. Family members, whether in the process of placing a relative in a long-term-care facility or already having done so, are often deeply hurting people.

Nursing home family care should begin by recognizing the psychological trauma frequently experienced by family members. The first response to such distressed individuals should be to offer genuine emotional support. This support should occur in the initial contacts with families and in early family orientation sessions. Ideally, the facility representative displays a willingness to spend time just empathically listening to the family's concerns regarding institutionalizing their loved one, what the decision-making struggle entailed, and what kinds of feelings family members are having to deal with. It is important that family members at this point not be pushed prematurely into the mechanics of the admission process. The family should be given adequate and repeated opportunity to share whatever they have a need to share and to be heard in a genuinely caring, nonjudgmental, and unrushed atmosphere.

Facility-sponsored family support groups would foster families' sharing with and receiving support from each other, besides lessening their sense of being so alone in their distress (Richards, 1986; Sancier, 1984). Care needs to be exercised by the facilitator that the group remain genuinely supportive in character, and not become a forum for the communication of facility policies and procedures.

Finally, the kind of support being offered through these more formal efforts needs to be supplemented and reinforced in an ongoing way by individual staff persons in their spontaneous day-to-day personal encounters with family members. This requires programming on the part of the facility to, first, sensitize staff personnel at all levels to the realities of the family experience and emotional trauma and, second, to train them in the skills of empathic listening and supportive responding (Grossberg et al., 1990).

DISTORTED EXPECTATIONS

A second source of distress for many families relates to their expectations of what the nursing home experience is going to be like. For some, these expectations may be grossly uninformed or misguided. More often, it is simply a case of vague uncertainty of what is to come. Either way, family members are commonly unprepared for and vulnerable to surprises, often of a disturbing nature, that inevitably await them. In general, people absorb shocks better if they have advance notice of their coming. Thus, another service long-term-care facilities can render is helping families anticipate things they may not be expecting. For instance, families need to be told early, to expect their loved ones to have a hard time adjusting to nursing home life and that they may not settle in quickly or easily; to show signs of unhappiness and anger; and to engage in complaining, accusatory, guilt-laying, and resistive behaviors.

Families need help in anticipating a possible decline in functional level or an increase in confusion and agitation on the part of their newly institutionalized relative. This may be due to the abrupt change of environment and the sudden introduction of new stimuli, unfamiliar surroundings, and altered routines. One guilt-ridden daughter who observed this kind of deterioration in her elderly mother exclaimed to the author, "My God, she's worse! What have I done?" Some advance preparation might have significantly mitigated her anguish.

It is also important for some families to be advised in advance of the difference between nursing home care and that of an acute care hospital. If, for example, the relative comes to the long-term-care facility soon after a hospital stay, family members may be shocked and angered to discover that, in the nursing home, the residents are expected and pushed to do as much as possible for themselves. Families usually will accept this treatment approach more easily if it, along with the rationale (the maximization of independence), has been explained in advance.

Long-term-care personnel can also alert families to expect difficulties in their own adjustment to the nursing home situation, to know that feelings of uneasiness, apprehension, frustration, sadness, anger, and guilt will likely surface, but that these are normal. Awkwardness and uncomfortableness with visiting their loved one can also be expected. Assistance to families in this regard will be discussed later.

As a general rule, the more family members anticipate these kinds of occurrences, the less stressful they will be and the more easily they will be accepted. Nursing homes provide a valuable service when staff gently but clearly prepare families for such unforeseen eventualities, thereby helping to reshape their expectations along more informed and realistic lines.

RESIDENT ADVOCACY

Another area of difficulty for many families, as well as a frequent cause of conflict with nursing home personnel, is their uncertainty as to how to respond to perceived deficiencies in their loved one's care. Family members may feel they have a justifiable complaint but be hesitant to express it, fearful of possible repercussions or not wishing to "cause problems." Others, similarly unhappy with some inadequacy in the treatment of their relative, may be very quick to respond but may do so in such inappropriate or provocative ways as to alienate the staff person they are confronting and, in effect, to defeat their own purpose.

This is another stress-point at which the long-term-care facility can appreciably serve its families, provided it does so early, preferably before the first such incident occurs. It is crucial that the facility recognize and accept the role of the family as the institutionalized relative's advocate. It is equally vital that this recognition be communicated candidly and convincingly to families from the moment the admission decision has been made. In the orientation process, families need to be given an unequivocal message that the nursing home expects them to have concerns about their loved one's care, to be displeased at times, and to have complaints. In fact, it wants them to act on their relative's behalf, voicing their concerns and working with the facility to have the deficiency or mistreatment addressed and corrected. Families need persuasive assurance that the facility not merely tolerates, but welcomes and encourages their active resident advocacy role.

Just as critical, however, is specific guidance to family members as to how they can most constructively exercise this role. They need direction as to whom to approach with their concerns and when, as well as how to pursue the issue in a manner that will be most effective and beneficial to the resident. Some facilities at the time of admission provide this information in written form or give family members a free copy of a booklet on "constructive confrontation" in the nursing home setting (Manning, 1989a).

Such a gesture not only equips families with useful practical information, but also forcefully communicates to them the genuineness of the facility's concern and commitment in this sensitive area.

ROLE AMBIGUITY

Upon placement, family members are often uncertain as to how much they still can or ought to be involved with the resident's care. Most sense they do have a role, but experience considerable ambiguity as to what that role is and how best to exercise it (Schwartz & Vogel, 1990). To meet this family need, communication, not only in initial meetings but in ongoing staff-family contacts, should continue. Family involvement is viewed by the facility and all its staff as a desired goal. More important than the articulation of this desire in words is its demonstration by concrete actions. One way to do so is to enlist family members' active partnership in the caring enterprise by asking for their input about care needs, the kinds of problems they encountered at home, and how they managed those problems. Drawing upon the family's knowledge of the resident's history, preferences, life style, vulnerabilities, and unique characteristics will not only provide staff with the "biographical expertise" (Bowers, 1988) that is essential to authentic personalized care, but will demonstrate the value the facility places on the family's knowledge. Continuous inclusion of family members in care planning conferences will serve the same purpose in an ongoing way.

Most important is the nursing home's identification for families of specific things they can do for and with their relative that will complement the facility's caregiving. A distinction has sometimes been offered between technical and nontechnical care; the former is provided by staff and the latter by family members. There are good arguments in support of both aspects of care by both (Bowers, 1988). Most helpful to families are concrete suggestions of meaningful things they can do, such as bringing in a pet or an object of sentimental value, perusing an old family photo album, playing favorite music, and so on. Through these efforts to foster continuing family involvement with their institutionalized loved one, not only will the resident's quality of life be enhanced, but also the family members' sense of usefulness and self-worth.

VISITING DISCOMFORT

One question that family members have frequently asked is, "How can I make my visits to my mother good, for her and for me? I know I should visit regularly, and I want to, but so often I come away feeling we're both worse off than if I hadn't gone at all. What can I do to make visiting better?"

Usually visiting can be enjoyable and rewarding, but often it can lack mutual satisfaction and, in some instances, be actually upsetting and painful. It is in the context of this frequently experienced awkwardness and frustration with visiting that another opportunity can be offered to the family. Nursing home staff can "free up" families in terms of their feelings about frequent and long visits. It is true, of course, that for many residents, time revolves around visits from their family members. The past may well be defined by their last visit, the present by their wish for a speedy return, and the future by their anticipated next visit (Brooke, 1989). Nevertheless, families need to be told that the quality of their visits generally has little to do with how often they come or how long they stay. Visits can be too long as well as too short. The less pressured the family member, the more rewarding will be the visit.

Nursing homes can also enhance the visiting experience by: providing pleasant visiting spaces with a bright and welcoming atmosphere (Brody, Dempsey, & Pruchno, 1990), having more flexible visiting hours, and informing family members as to their loved one's best time of the day (late afternoon is oftentimes the worst). Family members can also be counseled about the potential advantages of staggered one-to-one visits, thus avoiding the risk of the resident becoming overwhelmed or ignored when too many relatives or friends visit at once.

Guidance to families with regard to the content of their visits is especially essential. Family members often express concern about what they will say or talk about during a visit. Listening is an art, a skill to be learned and cultivated. Provision of family classes or training sessions in listening and communication skills, including that of nonverbal communication, would be another viable service of the long-term-care facility (Shulman & Mandel, 1988).

The value of reminiscing with the older resident also needs to be given prominence. Family members sometimes worry about or become impatient with their elderly relative's "living in the past" and forget that the past constitutes the major segment of the aged person's life. To discount or to discourage reminiscence is a serious injustice to the older individual and robs him of what can be of significant therapeutic benefit. Family members need to learn the value of deliberately incorporating elements of reminiscence and "life review" (Lewis & Butler, 1974) into their nursing home visits.

Suggestions to families regarding specific joint activities in which they might engage with their loved ones would also help to make visits more fulfilling. In addition to the possibilities enumerated in the previous section, helpful printed materials about nursing home visiting can be made available to families (Manning, 1989b).

Despite occasional difficult or uncomfortable visits, many of the noted suggestions can be helpful in quality visiting. The nursing home and its staff can do much to make visiting better for both the family and the resident.

CHRONIC GRIEF

Many nursing home residents are afflicted with an advanced dementing illness, such as Alzheimer's disease or a related disorder. The tragic consequence is that their personality or personhood is already gone, in effect dead, as if physical death had already occurred. This "death of the personality," as it has been called, imposes an unimaginable psychological burden upon close family members who must continue to see and deal with the living physical shell that once housed a loved one who is no longer (Guerriero, Austrom, & Hendrie, 1990). Mutual recognition, support, and meaningful interaction are no longer possible. What might be a visit for another family with other circumstances, in this instance becomes an obligation that has to be endured again and again. As described poignantly by a family support group member, "To visit my dad is like going to a funeral home, again and again, but they never close the casket!" This tragic experience of family members, long before death, is one of piercing, prolonged, and unrelenting grief.

Nursing home personnel need to be ready and able to respond to this unique, psychological family pain in the context of dementia. They cannot change the devastating reality, but they can be keenly aware of it. They need to view these family members as people in mourning and to relate to them as one would to a personal friend who was grieving the death of a significant other. Just being there for these distressed individuals, taking time to listen and validate their feelings, and by conveying a sensitivity to the special dimension of their anguish can provide significant emotional support. Not only recognizing, but encouraging the family's grieving can be of therapeutic value. Staff can commend family members for continuing to visit, gently emphasizing the importance of visits in the face of the heart-rending "quasi-death" of their loved one (Guerriero et al., 1990). They should also remind families of the receptivity of even the most severely intellectually impaired to genuine warmth and caring, as well as to appropriate nonverbal communication. Some families in this situation may benefit from being encouraged to become involved, if they are able, with other residents who are more cognitively intact but who lack caring family members who come and visit.

Facility-sponsored training programs are essential to sensitize staff members to the ongoing feelings and grief experienced by the families. The provision of special support groups for family members may be helpful. It may be beneficial to spouses to offer separate support sessions; one for spouses and another for other family members, because of some of the unique issues within the context of marriage.

BEHAVIORAL SEQUELAE

Families become distressed when they observe or become aware of problem behaviors in their institutionalized relatives. Even if they do not see it themselves, reports of episodes and inappropriate behaviors such as cursing, yelling and so on, may be upsetting. Such behaviors are not only disruptive to the nursing home environment, but also greatly disturb the resident population. These behaviors present a challenge for caregiving staff. The concern is the effect upon the families of residents who are behaving in such unacceptable ways.

Though the repercussions for families of such behavioral disturbances are many and varied, there are three that have been found to be particularly stressful. The first has to do with the often profound feelings of embarrassment, uneasiness, shame, guilt, dismay, and even shock if the behaviors have not been observed by the family before. Sometimes even anger may surface at the relative who may be perceived as being disruptive intentionally.

Second, family members of behaviorally disordered loved ones understandably tend to have serious concerns about the manner in which the long-term-care facility manages or treats such problem behaviors, especially when there is evidence or suspicion of excessive reliance upon physical and chemical restraints.

Third, families harbor what this author calls the "ultimate fear." Articulated more commonly than might be expected, this fear is that their behaviorally troublesome relative's continued residence at the facility will become at risk and eventually, if not abruptly, be terminated. What then?

With regard to the first of these concerns, it is vital that nursing home personnel deal with such families in a gentle, understanding, and emotionally supportive way. Families need help in understanding the reasons for the problem behaviors, to the extent these can be identified, plus the reassurance that staff members are experienced and comfortable with behavioral disturbances and are able to respond to them in a calm, informed, and professional manner.

In reply to families' warranted concern about treatment approaches to problem behaviors, the responsive facility will seek family input and include family members in planning intervention and management strategies. Families also need to be assured that restraint for the purpose of behavioral control is inconsistent with the facility's philosophy of care, and that the staff is trained and skilled in the use of more enlightened and humane behavioral management techniques and will energetically and consistently implement them. More detailed discussion of such measures appears elsewhere in this volume.

When it comes to families' fear of the termination of their loved one's residence due to unremitting behavioral problems, it is recognized that there will be those instances when such action may indeed be necessary. What is imperative in such cases is that the facility takes deliberate and patient steps in working with the staff and the family to exhaust every other alternative in striving to resolve the issue. If and when all efforts have failed and the removal of the resident is clearly mandated, it is crucial that the family be given ample time and that the nursing home staff actively assist in arranging for a suitable long-term-care facility or for acute treatment in a hospital geriatric psychiatry unit.

DECISION-MAKING QUANDARIES

Yet another stress-point for nursing home families is their frequent involvement in difficult decision making on behalf of their relative. This is more burdensome when the institutionalized relative's own intellectual capacity is significantly compromised.

Such decisions cover a broad range of concerns. There are little decisions such as whether to bring candy the resident likes but that may be harmful to him/her, whether to keep providing the cigarettes constantly begged for, or whether to take the resident out for the family Christmas gathering. There are bigger decisions relating to whether routine medical care will be given by a private physician or the facility's physician, or what measures will be taken to prevent falls or other unsafe behaviors. Heavier still are decisions regarding aggressively treating an acute illness, transferring him/her to a hospital, or possibly subjecting him/her to a surgical procedure or a course of electroconvulsive therapy. Most weighty are decisions relating to prolongation of life, the use or nonuse of resuscitation and other life-sustaining therapies, especially issues concerning withholding or withdrawal of hydration and nutrition (Kayser-Jones, 1990).

With family members often already guilt-ridden for their part in institutionalizing their relative, such decisions, generally loaded with ethical implications, can be overwhelming and can subject them to considerable, agonizing second thoughts, self-recrimination, and guilt. Since decisions regarding the weightier issues of treatment, life support measures, and the "right-to-die" dilemma are addressed extensively in another chapter of this volume, only a few general observations will be made here. The question is: What can the long-term-care facility offer families who are finding decision making perplexing and stressful? It is reassuring and perhaps also liberating to families to be told clearly that there is rarely an absolute right or wrong decision.

Nursing home staff should encourage family members to view the resident as the primary decision maker, to involve him/her to the fullest extent possible, and to respect his/her wishes. In the event that judgmental capacity is severely compromised or nonexistent, decisions should be guided by what is known about previous preferences and life philosophy. Staff should facilitate the family being as informed as possible about factors that might influence decision making such as alternatives, and potential benefits and risks, and should foster discussion between residents, families, health care professionals, and facility ethics committees. Staff may also need to encourage family members to consult with their clergy.

In contrast, there are instances when the rights and wishes of residents and/or their families collide with the values or religious principles of the facility and its health care professionals, particularly regarding artificial nutrition and hydration. Potential conflicts in this area can be minimized if the facility fully informs residents and families about related institutional policies in advance of the individual's admission (Miller & Cugliari, 1990).

Demonstrated staff support for family members after such decisions have been made can be especially benefical toward enabling them to live peacefully with their choices. It is a role for staff to assist families who are struggling with these difficult life decisions.

DEATH IMMINENCE

Though the goal of long-term-care facilities is to optimize the quality of life that remains for their residents, there is still much truth in the old perception that nursing homes are places where "people go to die." Death and dying are a real part of nursing-home life. Sometimes the death of the loved one comes suddenly and unexpectedly. Not uncommonly, however, the signs of its imminence become quite clear, and both staff and family are aware that the end is near. Family members are generally unprepared as to how to manage this "death watch," how to relate to the dying loved one, and how to cope with their own feelings.

This is the final opportunity for authentic family care on the part of the facility and its staff. Families generally benefit from openness and candor from the staff when death appears imminent. Because attending to the needs of a dying person may be more than many family members can handle, it is important they be given the fullest latitude in terms of how much or how little they will participate in the dying process. It is important for staff to be available to listen to family members during this time, to help them identify their associated feelings and to have them subsequently validated.

For family members who demonstrate a desire to be actively involved in the terminal care of their institutionalized relative, it would be helpful for the nursing staff to gently educate them with regard to potential changes in their dying loved one, such as changes in breathing patterns, drying of the mouth and lips, fluctuations in body temperature, and the like. Families need also to be prepared for possible psychological reactions the dying person may exhibit—anger, depression, withdrawal, and, hopefully, acceptance—and how to best respond to them. Family members also need to be alerted to the fact that the sense of hearing is frequently the last to be lost (Deininger, 1986). Consequently, speaking tenderly and reassuringly to the dying individual, reading some favorite poetry or Scripture text, or offering brief prayers may still be comprehended and have salutary value.

Even after the death of the resident, the staff can render an appreciated service by offering support groups for family survivors to assist in the grieving process, and to recall and affirm that individual's life. Such groups may also offer support for those unique family members who may feel guilty over not being able to mourn appropriately because they are, in effect, "grieved out," having already mourned over an extended period the loss, long ago, of the personhood of their loved one through a dementing illness.

CONCLUSION

In summary, this chapter has highlighted some of the stress points, and emotional and practical needs, of family members of relatives in long-term-care settings and has suggested ways in which the facility may respond with help and support. As it strives to implement them, within the realities and constraints of its own situation, it will be rendering a valuable and appreciated service to its families. But more, it will also be significantly enhancing the relationship between family members and facility staff persons, thus contributing to the effectiveness of the total caregiving team—to the benefit of the residents, the institution as a whole, and everyone concerned.

REFERENCES

Bowers, B. J. (1988). Family perceptions of care in a nursing home. *The Gerontologist 28*(3), 361–368.

Brody, E. M., Dempsey, N. P., & Pruchno, R. A. (1990). Mental health of sons and daughters of the institutionalized aged. *The Gerontologist 30*(2), 212–219.

Brooke, V. (1989). Nursing home life: How elders adjust. *Geriatric Nursing 10*(2), 66–68.

Deininger, I. (1986). Meaningful last days - better care for the dying. In D. H. Coons, L. Metzelaar, A. Robinson, & B. Spencer (Eds.), *A better life: Helping family members, volunteers and staff improve the quality of life of nursing home residents suffering from Alzheimer's disease and related disorders* (pp. 107–118). Columbus, Ohio: Source for Nursing Home Literature.

Grossberg, G. T., Hassan, R., Szwabo, P. A., Morley, J. E., Nakra, B. R. S., Bretscher, C. W., Zimny, G. H., & Solomon, K. (1990). Psychiatric problems in the nursing home: St. Louis University geriatric grand rounds. *Journal of the American Geriatrics Society 38*(8), 907–917.

Guerriero Austrom, M., & Hendrie, H. C. (1990). Death of the personality: The grief response of the Alzheimer's disease family caregiver. *American Journal of Alzheimer's Care and Related Disorders and Research*, March/April, *5*(2), 16–27.

Kasmarik, P. E., & Lester, V. C. (1984). A hard decision: When institutionalization is the best answer. In B. Hall (Ed.), *Mental health and the elderly* (pp. 165–184). Orlando, FL: Grune & Stratton.

Kayser-Jones, J. (1990). The use of nasogastric feeding tubes in nursing homes: Patient, family and health care provider perspectives. *The Gerontologist 30*(4), 469–479.

Lewis, M. I., & Butler, R. N. (1974). Life-review therapy: Putting memories to work in individual and group psychotherapy. *Geriatrics 29*(11), 165–174.

Manning, D. (1989a). *Socks—how to solve problems*. Hereford, TX: In-Sight Books.

Manning, D. (1989b). *Visiting in a nursing home*. Hereford, TX: In-Sight Books.

Miller, T., & Cugliari, A. M. (1990). Withdrawing and withholding treatment: Policies in long term care facilities. *The Gerontologist 30*(4), 462–468.

Montgomery, R. J. V. (1983). Staff-family relations and institutional care policies. *Journal of Gerontological Social Work 6*(1), 25–37.

Richards, M. (1986). Family support groups: Relationship bridges in nursing homes. *Generations 10*(4), 68–69.

Sancier, B. (1984). A model for linking families to their institutional relatives. *Social Work 29*(1), 63–65.

Schwartz, A. N., & Vogel, M. E. (1990). Nursing home staff and residents' families role expectations. *The Gerontologist 30*(1), 49–53.

Shulman, M. D., & Mandel, E. (1988). Communication training of relatives and friends of institutionalized elderly persons. *The Gerontologist 28*(6), 797–799.

19

Professional Caregiver Stress in Long-Term Care

Peggy A. Szwabo
Amy L. Stein

In this chapter the authors will address the components of stress in long-term-care facilities (LTCFs). Stress will be discussed in relation to the work setting and as it affects individuals personally, professionally, and in their role as employees. Conversely, if an individual's private life is stressful, it further impacts upon caregiving abilities and employee productivity.

Historically, long-term care has been viewed in negative and, perhaps at times, derogatory terms. It has been equated with a place to die, warehousing, and with poor and incompetent care provided by underqualified staff. Although positive strides have been made, the nursing home is potentially a stressful place to work, perhaps even more so than traditional medical settings. There is a wide range of research documenting that individuals who work in medical settings experience high levels of job-related stress (Heine, 1986; Jayaratne & Chess, 1984; Maslach, 1982; Packard & Motowidlo, 1987). Refer to Table 19.1 for stressful behaviors affecting employee performance. Thus, the negative perception of nursing homes coupled with identified stress in medical settings makes the nursing home a high-risk place to work. Nursing home work is both physically and emotionally demanding. Additionally, many employees work for near minimum wage. Many may have only a high school education with limited opportunity for

TABLE 19.1 Stressed Caregiver Behaviors Affecting the Employee and the Organization

High resistance to going to work and being at work every day

Anger and resentment

Guilt

Isolation and withdrawal

Work is frequently disorganized and not thorough

Increased physical complaints; i.e., colds, headaches, sleep disorders, etc.

Excessive use of alcohol or drugs

Marital and family conflict

Adapted from Burnout Among Nursing Home Personnel by C. Heine, 1986, *Journal of Gerontological Nursing, 12*, 14–18.

state-of-the-art training in long-term-care approaches and with few options for career advancement or for peer collegial recognition (Helper, 1987; Lyons, Hammer, Johnson, & Silberman, 1987; Pines & Maslach, 1978).

As important are the psychological ramifications of working in long-term care: staff must face their own fears of aging and death, deal with their own conflicts with their parents, and confront ethical issues about worth and time devoted to this aging, infirm resident population.

The relationship among personal stress, job performance, and job satisfaction has been studied. Stress has been linked to physical and mental responses, job dissatisfaction, absenteeism, and illnesses such as cardiac and gastrointestinal diseases (Anderson, Airo, Haslam, 1991; Caudill & Patrick, 1989).

To understand how stress is evidenced in long term-care, the concept of stress must be addressed. Stress is a part of the human condition and links medical and emotional disorders and social problems to the degree of stress people experience in their environments. Selye (1974) pioneered work on the stress response, which is the body's physical response to stress. A stimulus that evokes stress is a stressor. A physiological response occurs, regardless of the source. Chronic stress arousal can result in psychosomatic or psychophysiological disease. Stimuli such as caffeine, nicotine, or other drugs can also illicit stress responses. Physiological symptoms may include diarrhea, fatigue, headache, sleeplessness, aches and pains, and gastrointestinal symptoms. People under stress often have frequent illnesses or/and chronic conditions which are exacerbated. Chronic stress can play havoc with emotional responses leading to anxiety and depressive states. Psychosocial stimuli may precipitate a stress response by cognitive interpretations, that is, what the individual thinks about the event. Individuals vary in their interpretation of events. Some events most likely will be interpreted as a stressor by everyone, for example, being fired. Others will be interpreted individually, such as fear of public speaking or flying (Burns, 1980).

When stressed, the individual experiences a loss of mastery or control over events both internal (e.g., physical reactions or symptoms) and external (e.g., working short-staffed). Further, the loss of mastery triggers feelings of inadequacy and helplessness. This in turn leads to self-doubt, self-depreciation, and loss of self-esteem (Maslow, 1970). In work situations a person feeling helpless cannot ask for assistance or direction, causing poor performance, disorganized work, and increasing irritability.

Caregivers in the long-term-care institution experience daily stresses related to the caring for significantly impaired individuals. This stress may be transmitted to the residents in a nursing home, who may be the brunt of the staff person's reaction. Table 19.2 lists some staff behaviors which can affect the resident.

In addition, stressed caregivers may begin to stereotype the elderly (Solomon & Vickers, 1979). The belief in stereotypes leads to diminished expectations about the potential of the nursing home resident, lack of individualized care, and the internalization of this belief to the resident. These are important factors in the development of learned helplessness and stress-related symptoms.

Exchange theory helps to explain the development of learned helplessness in the LTC setting. If the caregiver does not maximize the emotional value from her/his contact in caring for the resident, she/he is unlikely to respond appropriately to the needs of that resident. Similarly, in an attempt to minimize the emotional costs of working in a situation that is perceived to be relatively devoid of psychological value, the caregiver is more likely to respond to his/her own needs and not those of the resident. The

---

TABLE 19.2 Stressed Caregiver Behaviors Affecting the Resident

---

Increased indifference to the resident

Loss of positive feelings for the resident

Stereotyping

Inability to deal with changes in routine

Infantilization of residents

Indiscriminate restraint usage

Physical and verbal abuse

Disregard of resident's rights

Adapted from "Burnout Among Nursing Home Personnel" by C. Heine, 1986, *Journal of Gerontological Nursing*, *12*, 14–18.

psychological value of the work can be enhanced through mechanisms that increase job satisfaction. Lack of psychological value for the caregiver increases interpersonal distance, which, in this setting, creates and reinforces learned helplessness.

In sum, exchange theory explains that behavior is learned and maintained by the individual's environment. Dysfunction can be said to exist when one fails to learn or reinforce adequate social skills or fails to extinguish symptoms causing behaviors. For change to occur, exchange theory suggests giving the staff person more effective ways to cope, for example, changing interpersonal consequences of behavior by identifying what is maintaining the behavior in the environment, and teaching new skills and behaviors.

As noted earlier, the observable consequences of stress are stress reactions, that is, adverse health and behavioral problems resulting from failure to cope effectively with environmental stress (see Figure 19.1). The early warning signs of stress are so subtle that these symptoms could be attributed to minor aggravations, for example, several bad days at work or food poisoning.

Issues specific to the nursing home work environment compound job-related stress. The nursing staff in long-term-care facilities are often faced with limitations in staffing patterns and budget allocations. In addition, architectural designs and psychosocial programs are often lacking or fragmented.

Environmental stress compounded with professional caregiving stress leads to emotional reactions. Nurses usually feel guilty and inadequate when they are not able to meet all of the residents' needs. These feelings of guilt increase with frequency when the nursing employee is faced with the overwhelming needs of the residents and not enough time or manpower to meet those needs. In its 1990 report, the National Committee To Preserve Social Security and Medicare (NCPSSM) cautioned that 88% of nursing homes are in need of additional nurses aides (NAs). This committee recommended the immediate employment of 286,000 additional nurses aides at a total cost of $2.6 billion (Mohler & Lessard (1991). In a similar vein, Fischer-Robertson and Cummings (1990) stressed that 50% to 150% more registered nurses (RNs) are necessary to meet future needs. The NCPSSM (1990) further estimated the costs of hiring 5,000 additional RNs and licensed practical nurses (LPNs) at $200 million. The dilemma not only is a monetary one, but also costly in time and staff-resident care. Experts recommend one caregiver for every 8 beds on the day shift, one caregiver for every 10 beds on the evening shift, and one caregiver for every 15 beds at night. This standard is presently being met by approximately 12% of the facilities nationwide (Fischer-Robertson & Cummings, 1990; Huey, 1990).

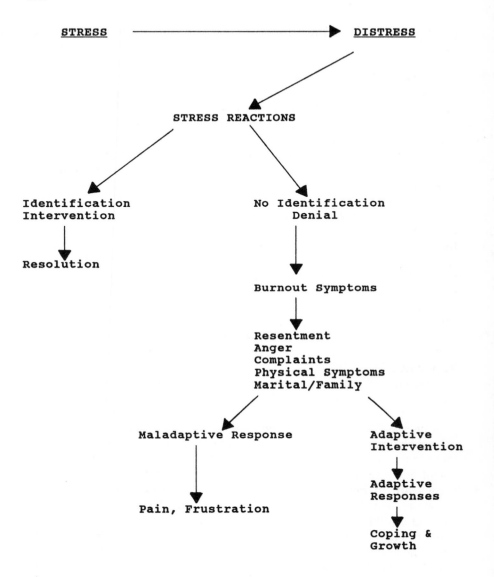

FIGURE 19.1 Stress-distress reactions.

Furthermore, isolation, withdrawal, and disorganized work habits are other behaviors frequently noted when the employee has high levels of stress associated with caring for the confused, dependent elderly (Wilson & Patterson, 1988; Hinshaw & Atwood, 1983). As anger and resentment increase with unrelieved job stress, nursing employees may also complain about the organization or management. The end product often is "burnout" and job stress among nursing caregivers. Maslach (1982) characterized burnout as physical, emotional, and spiritual exhaustion which ultimately involves the loss of concern with whom one is working (see Table 19.3).

Job stress and burnout are manifested in a number of ways, for example, increased absenteeism, tardiness, and increased turnover of personnel. Individuals exhibiting burnout behaviors ultimately affect other employees and the organization. These behaviors can also undermine the facility's mission and force the LTCF out of compliance with licensing regulations. High staff turnover rates have been associated with negative effects on staff and overall facility functioning. The problem of staff turnover has been a persistent economic and interpersonal difficulty for the nursing home industry (Knapp & Harissis, 1981; Schwartz, 1974).

The Health Care Financing Administration (HCFA) delineates a turnover rate for RNs at 63% and for NAs at 99% (Mohler & Lessard, 1990). Other studies report NA turnover rates of 200% or more annually (Fischer-Robertson & Cummings, 1990). Huey (1990), in an editorial on staffing statistics, noted the nursing home industry has an annual nursing staff replacement rate of 63% nationwide. This knowledge is vital to coordination of daily activities of care. Perhaps the most serious consequence of stress, anxiety, burnout, and high turnover in nursing home employees is how they ultimately affect the resident. Discontinuity of care and continual staff change is stressful to all, but more so to the cognitively impaired resident, who responds to structure, routine, and familiarity as a way to cope with progressive forgetfulness, disorientation, and confusion. When a familiar staff person leaves, the cognitively impaired resident may interpret as a loss and react to this loss (Heine, 1986; Waxman, 1984).

TABLE 19.3 Burnout Characteristics

Emotional, physical, and spiritual exhaustion
Detached, callous, depersonalized attitudes
Reduced personal accomplishments

Adapted from Maslach, C., 1982.

ASSESSMENT

Recognition of individual stress is the first step in lifestyle change. Many self-rating scales are available to assess personal stress levels: Maslach's Burnout Inventory (Maslach, 1982); Caregiving Hassles and Uplifts Scale (Kanner, Coyne, Schaefer, & Lazarus, 1981); and the Social, Readjustment Scale (Holmes & Rahe, 1970). Many "pop" psychology magazines, such as *Prevention, Psychology Today*, and *In Health*, as well as self-help literature are available to assess and manage stress. As with any assessment tool, it is useful only if used. Dealing with stress has a domino effect; what affects the individual also affects the family, job performance, and satisfaction levels.

Self-knowledge and self-assessment are integral parts of the process of managing stressful situations. Self-knowledge encompasses knowledge of what stress is and how it affects the individual, for example, defining what is stressful and the usual response to the stressor, physically, psychologically, and behaviorally. This self-assessment evaluates appropriate nutrition, exercise, leisure pursuits, time management, self-management style, ability to set limits, and use of stress-reduction techniques. When usual patterns of responding are consciously identified, change in responses can be initiated.

Too often, the individual may be unaware of his/her distress until situations are routinely tense and upsetting or until others react to that individual's behaviors. Out of concern, family or coworkers may confront this individual. Ideally, the distressed person will perceive the concerns voiced as another sign that change is needed.

INTERVENTION

Learning ways to reduce and handle chronic stress requires a change in life style. Distress and chronic stress have been previously demonstrated to cause a multitude of difficulties. This section will address self-change techniques and how individuals can apply these techniques. From an administrative and supervisory viewpoint, these strategies can be incorporated into employee orientation and into the facility's philosophy of practice to foster individual and group growth.

Stress reduction techniques can vary from very simple to highly specialized methods in the field of stress management or biobehavioral treatment. These techniques can be utilized individually or in group settings for staff and residents. The basic equipment required is motivation and willingness to change how one handles or does not handle stress. While stress reduction techniques are easy to learn, they also present a great challenge. Lifelong benefits can only be reaped through committed, continued application over time.

THE RELAXATION RESPONSE

Benson (1975) defined the relaxation response as the physiological change which occurs by altering one's state of consciousness without drugs. Relaxed states produce reduced breathing and heart rates. The relaxation response shows the psychological power to control the body's negative responses to stress. The technique illustrated in Table 19.4 has the best results when used daily for at least 15 to 20 minutes. This same response can be reached through prayer, yoga, meditation, or hypnosis.

Relaxation techniques require practice and mastery. Helpful adjuncts to assist in relaxing can be music, relaxation or meditation tapes, deep-breathing exercises, or thought-stopping techniques to alleviate intruding and upsetting thoughts. Once mastered, relaxation techniques can be applied during any stressful event. If mastery of relaxation techniques proves difficult, consultation with a skilled practitioner is warranted.

IMAGERY TECHNIQUES

Imagery techniques such as visualizations, guided imagery, active remembering, and listening to music are helpful in learning to relax and decrease stress.

TABLE 19.4 Relaxation Response Techniques

Have the individual sit quietly in a comfortable position, and suggest loosening any tight clothing.

Request individual to close their eyes.

Begin relaxation of muscles, starting with feet and progressing to the head.

Demonstrate breathing techniques by breathing slowly through the nose. Pace breathing as follows: breath in . . . out, and count "one." Breathe in . . . out, and count "two." Breathing should be easy and natural throughout, and deep into the abdomen.

Continue breathing techniques; these should be practiced 15 to 20 minutes.

When finished, have the individual remain quiet with their eyes closed, then, gradually opening them; remaining seated for the next several minutes.

Adapted from *The Relaxation Response* by H. Benson, 1975, New York: William Morrow.

Visualization is a technique in which the tension is given a symbol, such as knotted ropes. The participant unknots them through imagination. Colors can also be visualized. For example, the participant imagines red as tension and blue as calm, and then tries to change the red to blue.

Guided imagery can be a visual journey in which the participant visualizes a special place that is calm and has pleasant memories. The process includes detailed visual descriptions, enabling the participant to paint a soothing, relaxing picture in the mind's eye.

Active remembering is defined as the identification of stressful or troubling events and the release of those thoughts. The goal is to use thought-stopping techniques to effectively cease replaying troublesome situations.

Music has the ability to soothe, distract, change our moods and energy levels. Actively selecting soothing music allows distraction from stress. This can be easily used during breaks or in the car. Eventually, the music can be experienced without use of the tape in periods of stress. These techniques can provide the ability to control stressful responses; however, commitment, motivation, and practice are necessary to integrate them into a daily life style.

NUTRITION, EXERCISE, AND SELF-ENHANCEMENT

Since the body and mind are interrelated, creating a healthy life style will affect physical and emotional well-being. Components of a healthy life style should include following a nutritionally balanced diet and limiting "stress" foods such as excessive caffeine and sugar intake, chronic dieting, and skipped or hurried meals.

Exercise has also been found to be a stress reliever and a way to rid the body of minor irritations. Furthermore, exercise releases endorphins, the body's pain relievers, which assist in stress reduction (Fields & Basbaum, 1989).

To ensure a healthy life style, a wholistic approach of good nutrition, regular exercise, and development of self-enhancement skills is suggested. Aspects of self-enhancement include assessment of abilities to set limits and responses to setting limits, for example, saying "no" and subsequently not feeling guilty. Cognitive techniques, such as thought stopping, are effective in changing cognitive distortions. In brief, cognitive distortions are beliefs that result in negative or inappropriate feelings and behavioral responses. An example of a cognitive distortion is: "I should do this . . . if I don't I'm a failure." Identification of negative thoughts that affect moods and feelings is the basis of cognitive therapy. These changes are helpful in changing distorted thinking patterns into more realistic and healthier responses (for further reading on cognitive therapy see Burns, 1980).

STAFF SUPPORT THROUGH FACILITY INTERVENTIONS

Since organizational philosophy and support have been previously addressed, this section will review specific programs and strategies that can provide staff support.

Heine (1986) and others have recommended staff development and educational programs to continually update and enhance knowledge of caregivers who address resident care problems (Wilson & Patterson, 1988; Boyer, Bresloff, & Curley, 1986; Hinshaw & Atwood, 1983). Reviewing and upgrading of knowledge, skills, and techniques result in a higher level of nursing care offered with lower levels of stress. Additionally, development of resident-centered strategies with a multidisciplinary treatment team is effective in resolving difficult caregiving situations. Inclusion of the family, resident, and staff can provide a forum to establish realistic, comprehensive care and opportunities to view the resident as an individual with a unique background and not as a behavior problem (Brown, 1961).

Similarly, the Enhancement Project of Farmington, Maine, is an innovative program designed to improve the quality of resident care by providing extended training in psychosocial needs for certified nursing assistants (CNAs) (Boyer et al., 1986). CNAs were given special assignments focusing entirely on psychosocial care and communication activities with the residents. Pertinent articles, supervision, and specific activities were identified. The response to this experience demonstrated an increase in morale and more humanistic approaches in providing care to the residents. The CNAs reported increased self-confidence, increased sensitivity, and awareness of residents as individuals. Baldwin (1987) describes another such program using modules including didactic lectures, practical application, and consultation with geriatric psychiatric nurse clinicians. Her specific components included: stress management, dealing with aggressive behaviors, understanding mental illness, and therapeutic interventions with families and friends. She found that structured modules plus discussion by modeling appropriate behaviors were effective in staff reports of increased self-confidence, knowledge, and comfort levels in intervening in difficult situations.

CONCLUSION

Stress management is an integral component of the intervention in caregiver burnout. To begin resolution of stressful situations, it is essential to understand the impact of stress; first upon the individual, and second as the individual performs their job responsibilities and subsequently upon their reports of job satisfaction. Third, research demonstrates that quality of care provided is affected by job performance and satisfaction. Last, quality of care and staff performance directly affect the overall functioning of the facility. Handling stress and self-care is the responsibility of the individual. It is also the role of a professional caregiver to address the role of stress in work performance with colleagues. As a member of a treatment team, the caregiver may have the responsibility of confronting colleagues who are exhibiting symptoms of stress. Administrators and supervisors have responsibilities to identify and implement strategies and develop institutional supports to address and reduce burnout and job stress.

When the above is implemented, comphrehensive successful interventions can be incorporated to decrease personal and work-related stress.

REFERENCES

Anderson, M., Airo, T., & Haslam, B. (1991). How satisfied are nursing home staff. *Geriatric Nursing*, March/April, 85–87.

Baldwin, B. (1987). Innovation in mental health training programs for nursing home staff [Abstract]. *Proceedings of the 3rd Congress of the International Psychogeriatric Association, 3*, p. 61.

Benson, H. (1975). *The relaxation response.* New York: William Morrow.

Boyer, M., Bresloff, L., & Curley, D. (1986). The enhancement project: A program to improve the quality of residents' lives. *Geriatric Nursing*, July/Aug., 192–195.

Brown, E. (1961). *Newer dimensions of patient care.* New York: Russell Sage Foundation.

Burns, D. (1980). *Feeling good: The new mood therapy.* New York: William Morrow.

Caudill, M., & Patrick, M. (1989). Nursing assistant turnover in nursing homes and need satisfaction. *Journal of Gerontological Nursing, 15*(16), 24–30.

Fields, H. L., & Basbaum, A. I. (1989). *Endogenous Pain Control Mechanisms.* In P. D. Wall & R. Melzack (Eds.), *Textbook of Pain.* Edinborogh: Churchill & Livingstone, Chapter 11, 206–217.

Fischer-Robertson, J. & Cummings, C. C. (1990). What attracts and keeps nurses in long term care? *Geriatric Nursing*, Nov./Dec., 284.

Gray-Toft, P., & Anderson, J. (1985). Organizational stress in the hospital: Development of a model for diagnosis and prediction. *Health Services Research, 19*(6), 753–774.

Helper, S. (1987). Assessing training needs of nursing home personnel. *Journal of Gerontological Social Work, 11*(112), 71–79.

Heine, C. (1986). Burnout among nursing home personnel. *Journal of Gerontological Nursing, 12*(3), 14–18.

Hinshaw, S., & Atwood, J. R. (1983). Nursing staff turnover stress and satisfaction: Models, measurements and management. *Annual Review of Nursing Research*, 133–153.

Holmes, T. H., & Rahe, R. H. (1970). The social readjustment scale. *Journal of Psychosomatic Research, 41*, 121–132.

Huey, F. L. (1990). Editorial: Shocking staffing statistics. *Geriatric Nursing*, Nov./Dec., 265.

Jayaratne, S., & Chess, W. (1984). Job satisfaction, burnout and turnover: A national study. *Social Work*, NASW Inc., Sept./Oct., 449–453.

Kanner, A. D., Coyne, J. C., Schaefer, C., & Lazarus, R. S. (1981). Comparison of two modes of stress measurement: Daily hassles and uplifts versus major life events. *Journal of Behavioral Medicine, 4* (1), 3–9.

Knapp, M., & Harissis, K. (1981). Staff vacancies and turnover in British old people's homes. *Gerontologist, 21*, 76–84.

Lyons, J. S., Hammer, J. S., Johnson, N., & Silberman, M. (1987). Unit specific variation in occupational stress across a general hospital. *General Hospital Psychiatry, 9*, 435–438.

Maslach, C. (1982). *Burnout—The cost of caring.* New York: Prentice-Hall.

Maslow, A. H. (1970). *Motivation and personality.* New York: Harper & Row.

Mohler, M. M., & Lessard, W. J. Jr. (1990). *Nursing staff in nursing homes. What will it take to remedy the insuffiency and what will it cost?* Paper presented at 43rd annual meeting of the Gerontological Society of America, Boston, MA.

Mohler, M. M., & Lessard, W. J. (1991). Nursing staff in nursing homes: Additional staff needed and cost to meet requirements and intent of OBRA 89 (pp. 1–24). Washington, D.C.: A publication of the National Committee to Preserve Social Securing and Medicare, Revised 5, 1991.

Packard, J., & Motowidlo, J. S. (1987). Subjective stress, job satisfaction and job performance of hospital nurses. *Research in Nursing Health, 10*, 253–261.

Pines, A., & Maslach, C. (1978). Characteristics of staff burnout in mental health settings. *Hospital and Community Psychiatry, 29*(4), 233–237.

Selye, H. (1974). *Stress without distress.* Philadelphia: J. B. Lippincott.

Schwartz, A. N. (1974). Staff development and morale building in nursing homes. *The Gerontologist, 14*, 50–53.

Solomon, K., Vickers, R. (1979). Attitudes of health care workers toward old people. *Journal of the American Geriatric Society, 27*, 186–191.

Waxman, H., Carner, E., & Berkenstock, G. (1984). Job turnover and job satisfaction among nursing home aides. *The Gerontologist, 24* (5), 503–509.

Wilson, R. W., & Patterson, M. A. (1988). Perceptions of stress among nursing personnel on dementia units. *The American Journal of Alzheimer's Care and Related Disorders and Research*, July/Aug., *3*(4) 34–39.

PART III
Ethical and Legal Issues

20

Surrogate Management

Barbara J. Gilchrist
George H. Zimny

INTRODUCTION

In June 1990, the U.S. Supreme Court issued its decision in the Nancy Cruzan case, which focused national attention on the question of who is allowed to decide to terminate treatment for persons unable to speak for themselves. On the heels of this decision, the U.S. Congress passed the Patient Self Determination Act, effective December 1, 1991, which requires all health care providers receiving Medicare or Medicaid funds to provide information to patients about powers of attorney, living wills, and other rights regarding medical care. Each of these events reflects a growing concern, especially among the elderly population, for maintaining control, including refusal or termination, over the type of health care that will be provided when individuals are no longer able to make or express their own decisions. Also of concern are control and direction of other personal and financial matters.

These concerns are particularly important for elderly persons who may require the services of a nursing home. Estimates of the risk of institutionalization for persons 65 years old and older range from 36% to 65%. By the year 2000, the estimated number of people who will be residents of nursing homes is 2.0 million. By 2040, that estimate is set at 4.6 million. Of particular importance here are the statistics that indicate that

84% of nursing home residents do not have a spouse living, only 63% have children, and 62.6% suffer from disorientation or memory impairment (Aging America, 1987–1988).

This chapter explains the advance legal planning and other legal tools available to individuals to help address the need to maintain control over their health care and to protect them from abuse and unfair advantage. Nursing homes, too, need to be informed about these tools, because their residents may have or may need to have such tools and because of the requirement to provide information to residents imposed on nursing homes by the Patient Self Determination Act.

ADVANCE LEGAL PLANNING

There are a variety of legal tools available for maintaining control after incapacity, and we have categorized them all as forms of surrogate management. For our purposes, here, we have defined surrogate management as a formal relationship established for the purpose of allowing another person or entity to make decisions for an adult who has or expects to have significantly limited physical or mental capacity. The relationship may be established by the individual while he or she has capacity—advance planning—or by a court or governmental body when the individual does not have legal capacity. Also, for our purposes, legal incapacity exists when a person is unable by reason of any physical or mental condition to receive or evaluate information or to communicate decisions to such an extent that the person lacks the ability to manage financial resources and/or meet requirements for essential personal needs.

Adequate planning in advance of incapacity allows the individual to make choices about which forms of surrogate management are the most appropriate and to choose the agent to whom authority is being given. This advance legal planning can be an effective way to resolve the issue of control and protection. However obvious the value of advance planning may be, the process requires an individual to acknowledge and accept his/her own vulnerability to diminished physical and mental abilities and to his/her own mortality. Not everyone is able or willing to go through this process prior to the onset of debilitating disease or injury (Lower, 1988). In the absence of advance planning, a court or other governmental entity may impose surrogate management, usually in the form of a guardianship, with the court deciding who will be in charge and what health care decisions can and cannot be made on behalf of the now incapacitated individual.

PURPOSES

There are several purposes for surrogate management that benefit an individual who has lost or expects to lose some or all of his or her mental or physical capacities. These purposes are: to delegate decision-making authority; to prevent abuse, neglect or unfair advantage; and to protect and manage the assets and personal affairs of the individual. In the context of long-term care, the institution also benefits in that nursing home personnel can confidently look to an identified and legally authorized person who can provide direction to the nursing home and make decisions on behalf of the resident.

None of the surrogate management tools is perfect, and each includes risks and disadvantages to the individual who is making the choice or who has a guardianship imposed on him or her. These issues are addressed more specifically below when each tool is described.

VOLUNTARY LEGAL TOOLS

Voluntary forms of surrogate management are available in every state and are controlled by the law of the particular state. Not every form exists in every state, and the specifics as to when each becomes effective, the parameters of the authority that can be transferred, and the requirements for proper execution vary from one state to another. At this time, there is no clear legal answer to whether a surrogate management document properly prepared in one state will be honored in another.

The fundamental requirement for voluntary forms of surrogate management in every circumstance is that the individual must have the legal capacity to understand the consequences of the actions he or she is choosing to take at the time that the document is executed. The most common forms that are found in most states are described below.

Will

A will is a document in which a person states how his/hjer assets are to be distributed after death. In the absence of a will, the assets in a decedent's estate will be distributed in accordance with the state law of inheritance. The terms of the will have no effect until the principal has died, the will has been submitted to the court, and an executor or personal representative has been appointed. The assets in the estate are subject to the claims of creditors, and the debts of the estate must be paid prior to any distribution to the beneficiaries or heirs of the estate. Assets may pass to the intended beneficiary outside of any court process if the individual has taken advantage of certain transfer-on-death arrangements. The two most common examples of a transfer-on-death arrangement are the naming of a beneficiary on a life insurance policy and joint ownership. Other transfer-on-death arrangements and joint ownership are described in more detail below. All transfer-on-death arrangements take precedence over the terms of a will and the state law of inheritance.

Wills may contain trust provisions, described more fully below, such that assets are given to a trustee rather than outright to a potentially incapacitated surviving spouse. Wills may also contain a nomination of a guardian for the surviving spouse in the event of that person's incapacity (Lower, 1988). Although this nomination is not binding on the probate court, it is to be taken into account when the court is deciding who to appoint. This may be an important consideration given the prevalence of impaired individuals residing in nursing homes who do not have a spouse or children to assist them.

Living Will (Health Care Declaration)

A living will is a document in which a person states his or her wishes regarding the termination or withdrawal of treatment in the event that the person is no longer able to express his or her wishes, the condition is terminal, death is imminent, and ongoing treatment would prolong the dying process. Although many people think of living wills as a directive to stop treatment, the statements in the living will should be tailored to reflect each individual's personal wishes, which might be a desire for all forms of treatment to be continued or that certain treatment be stopped only after a specified period of time or under specified conditions.

Living wills are viable only under the very limited circumstances described above (St. Mary's L.J., 1989). The statements in the living will must be honored by health care providers and do take precedence over any authority given under a health care power of attorney.

Durable Power of Attorney

A durable power of attorney is a document in which the principal gives someone else the authority to act on the principal's behalf in financial and/or medical matters. This grant of authority may be very broad and general or may be very narrow and specific in the terms of the powers given. The authority given to the other person continues after the principal becomes incapacitated.

Many state laws provide standard forms that may be used to establish a durable power of attorney. Some states, such as Missouri, have not yet passed a state statute recognizing the right of an individual to appoint an agent for health care decisions. This does not mean that a Missouri resident cannot appoint an agent for health care decisions. Nor does it mean that the authority granted by the principal under a health care power of attorney will not or should not be honored by health care providers. It does, however, mean that there will continue to be questions for everyone involved in the care of a now incapacitated person as to the limits of the authority of the named agent.

Durable powers of attorney are one of the most important documents for planning purposes, because they allow an individual to make the choice of who is to make a variety of health care decisions, not just decisions made at the end of life, when the principal is no longer able to make these decisions for themselves (St. Mary's L.J., 1989). These documents are also inherently very dangerous, because the authority given may be easily abused if the principal becomes incapacitated. There is no monitoring system that oversees the activities of the agent on a regular basis. Unless someone else, such as a friend, family member, or care provider, brings a problem to the attention of the courts, the agent may misuse the authority given with impunity.

Joint Ownership

Joint ownership is a legal relationship in which two or more persons are co-owners of an automobile, real estate, a bank account, or any other investment that has a title. Each person has full rights of ownership and control, even if only one person contributes the funds. Upon the death of one of the owners, the survivor owns the entire asset without having to go through the probate process.

Joint ownership is very easy to establish and is an effective way to avoid probate and give someone else the ability to manage assets. It also has the potential for very serious negative and unintended consequences. For example, an older person may add someone else's name to his/her bank account simply by filling out a form with the bank. The new joint owner may withdraw the money from the account without the older person's permission. Similarly, an older person may add someone's name to their house title simply by obtaining a quitclaim deed form and filing the document with the recorder of deeds. In the event that the new joint owner was married at the time his or her name was added and later goes through a divorce proceeding, the house will be part of the joint owner's marital assets. A joint owner may suffer financial problems and be sued. Any creditor with a judgment against the joint owner may place a lien on the older person's house.

The addition of someone's name to the title of any asset may also be viewed for purposes of eligibility for Medicaid nursing home benefits as a gift or, more technically, a transfer of assets for less than fair value. If such a transfer has been made within 30 months of an application for these benefits, the individual may be found ineligible for a period of time not to exceed 30 months.

Trust

A trust is established by transferring assets to a trustee (who may be a person or institution) in trust for the grantor's or some other beneficiary's benefit. A trust may be established while the grantor is living or at death through the terms of a will. The terms of the trust are usually specifically stated in a lengthy trust document, and the trustee has management authority but no ownership rights. The management authority continues after the grantor or other beneficiary becomes incapacitated, and there may be provisions in the trust for distribution of the assets outside of any probate process at the death of the grantor.

Trusts are very effective tools for ensuring proper management of assets in the event of incapacity. However, the costs of having a trust document prepared and the fees charged to the estate by the trustee for managing the assets may be prohibitive, unless the value of the trust assets is large enough to generate enough interest to pay these fees as well as to provide support for the intended beneficiary.

Transfer-on-Death

There are a variety of transfer-on-death arrangements available for use which do not require any court involvement to make the transfer effective. Joint ownership and trusts, described above, are two examples. A person may also register the title to an automobile so that, at the owner's death, the title can be transferred to a specified beneficiary. A bank account, certificate of deposit, or any other investment may also be set up so that the account or investment is paid out to a specified beneficiary upon proof of death of the owner. Beneficiary deeds for real property may also be executed, so that title to the property will be transferred at death to a named beneficiary.

Each of these transfer-on-death arrangements is easily established by executing the necessary document with the institution that has charge of the asset or title in question. At the death of the owner, the beneficiary simply must provide that same institution with a death certificate and proof of their own identity, and the assets will be released or the title changed. There is no probate proceeding involved, and creditors may not make claims against the asset. With the exception of joint ownership, none of these transfer-on-death arrangements gives present ownership or access to intended beneficiary. The owner maintains complete control over the asset until death and can rescind or alter a transfer-on-death arrangement at any time unless incapacitated.

INVOLUNTARY LEGAL TOOLS

When an individual becomes incapacitated and has not taken advantage of one or more of the voluntary surrogate management tools or when a tool is inadequate under the circumstances, there are three possible surrogate management arrangements that can be imposed. The first, representative payee, is uniform on a national basis and allows for the management of certain financial benefits. The second and third, guardianships and conservatorships, are controlled by state law. Like the voluntary tools, the process of establishing guardianship and conservatorship, the terminology used, and the expectations of the guardian or conservator vary from one state to another.

Representative Payee

The Social Security Administration, Railroad Retirement Board, and the Veterans Administration will approve the issuance of benefits to someone other than the beneficiary upon proof that the beneficiary is not able to manage his/her own funds. This representative payee is required to use the funds for the benefit of the beneficiary and must respond to a questionnaire on an annual basis.

This is a very effective method for protecting an incapacitated beneficiary of Social Security or other benefits and may preclude the need for a conservatorship if these benefits are the only source of income for the incapacitated person. It is also an easily abused grant of management authority. Very little proof is required to establish this arrangement, and the annual questionnaire is not an effective method for monitoring the use of the funds by the representative payee.

Guardianship

As used here, a guardian is someone appointed by the court to make and carry out decisions about the personal care of an incapacitated person, usually called a ward. A guardianship is established after a petition has been filed with the court and a hearing, in some form, has been held to determine whether the individual is, in fact, incapacitated and who should be named as the guardian. If the court does determine that a person is incapacitated, that person loses all civil rights, such as the right to determine where to live, to request or refuse medical treatment, to vote, and to make a contract. The guardian is not financially responsible for the ward but has the authority and responsibility to ensure that the ward is residing in the least restrictive environment appropriate for his/her needs and that the ward receives whatever personal care or treatment required. Most courts require an annual or biennial report from the guardian on the status of the ward.

Conservatorship

A conservator is someone appointed by the court to manage and control the financial affairs of an incapacitated person. The procedure for establishing a conservatorship is the same as a guardianship, and, oftentimes, the two are done together. A conservator has the authority and responsibility to manage the ward's funds for the benefit of the ward. Most courts require a periodic accounting of the use of the funds by the conservator and the status of the assets.

Unlike the case for most other forms of surrogate management, there is a monitoring system for guardianships and conservatorships. Courts have a responsibility for monitoring the performance of guardians and conservators that they, the courts, appoint to care for the personal and financial well-being of wards. Monitoring commonly involves the court requiring reports from the guardians and conservators, which are then reviewed by the court. However, the care and quality of monitoring by courts varies from one state to another and from one court in a particular state to another court in the same state (Zimny, Gilchrist, Grossberg, & Chung, 1991). Some state laws leave monitoring up to the discretion of the judge while others, notably California, require an annual visit to the ward by a court investigator. Even with monitoring, abuses by guardians and conservators do occur, as reported in the popular press (Gest, 1985; Topolnicki, 1989) and by Federal bodies (Subcommittee on Health and Long Term Care of the House Select Committee on Aging, 1987). Administrators and staff of nursing homes, as part of the care they provide to residents, should be alert to the possibility of abuse of their residents by guardians and conservators as well other surrogate managers appointed by residents themselves.

CONCLUSION

Advance planning by choosing and executing one or more surrogate management tools can be an effective way to maintain control over health care after an individual has become incapacitated. These tools are available in every state, and benefit both the incapacitated resident and the health care providers in a long-term-care setting. Great care should be taken, however, in choosing the tools most appropriate for the individual and in choosing an agent who will have authority to act for the individual in the future. Nursing homes, in turn, should be aware of the tools already chosen by their residents and be alert to the development in their residents of the need for surrogate management tools.

REFERENCES

Aging America: Trends and projections. U.S. Senate Special Committee on Aging, American Association of Retired Persons, Federal Council on the Aging, U.S. Administration on Aging (1987–88 Edition). Washington, D.C., U.S. Department of Health & Human Services.

American Bar Association Commission on the Mentally Disabled and Commission on Legal Problems of the Elderly (1989). Guardianship: An agenda for reform. Washington, DC.: ABA.

Callahan, D., Strauss, P. (1990). *Estate planning for the aging or incapacitated client.* PLI. New York: Practicing Law Institute.

Estate planning for the non-taxable estate. (1989). 211 St. Mary's Law Journal, 367.

Gest, T. (1985, February). Ripping off estates—An epidemic of abuse. *U.S. News & World Report,* p. 25.

Lower, J. (1988). *Estate planning for older clients of modest means,* 67 Mich. Bar Journal 1122.

Subcommittee on Health and Long-Term Care of the House Select Committee on Aging. (1987). *Abuses in guardianship of the elderly and infirm: A national disgrace, A report by the chairman, 100th Cong., 1st Sess. 37* (committee print). Washington, DC: Author. U.S. Govt. Printing Office.

Topolnicki, D. (1989, March). The gulag of guardianship. *Money,* 140–152.

Zimny, G. H., Gilchrist, B. J., Grossberg, G. T., & Chung, S. (1991). Annual reports by guardians and conservators to probate courts. *Journal of Elder Abuse and Neglect,* 61–74.

21

The Right to Die

The Ethicist's Perspective

Jean de Blois

A Pastor's Viewpoint

Herbert E. Hohenstein

THE RIGHT TO DIE AND ETHICAL DECISION MAKING
—Jean de Blois

Introduction

Ethical decision making in health care is understandably a difficult task. Frequently, patients, families, and others are confronted with decisions about health care interventions that may not offer clear benefit or that require judgments based on partial knowledge. Moreover, many persons are confused about the factors to be considered when making decisions of an ethical nature. This is particularly true when considering the use or nonuse of life-sustaining therapies. Because these decisions have such significant consequences for all involved, it is imperative that as much precision be brought to the decision-making process as possible. A significant obstacle in this endeavor is raised by the repeated and unreflected use of "right to die" language. The intention of this chapter is to bring clarity to the decision-making process by (1) analyzing and clarifying the meaning of "right to die" claims and (2) explicating the principles and criteria for use in the appropriate ethical assessment of life-sustaining therapies.

RIGHT TO DIE: CLARIFYING THE CLAIM

"Right to die" language is common parlance today. For example, when the case of Nancy Cruzan went to the U.S. Supreme Court, newspaper headlines read: "High Court to Hear First 'Right to Die' Case." Media reports of Dr. Jack Kevorkian's assistance in Janet Adkins' suicide were laced with "right to die" rhetoric. And accounts of the legislative proposals to legalize physician-assisted suicide and active euthanasia often describe these propositions as "right to die" measures. The problem, of course, is that "right to die" is used in each instance as if the meaning of the phrase is clear. This, however, is not the case. Thus, clarification is in order.

Let us begin by observing a simple fact: death is not something that we need to claim as a right. It is part of the human condition and will be experienced by every person. There is no need to claim a right to that which is inexorably a part of what it means to be human. Thus, those who argue for a "right to die" generally have something else in mind. What Janet Adkins, Dr. Jack Kevorkian, and advocates of assisted suicide and euthanasia assert should not be described as the "right to die." For what they seek to claim is a right to choose death, to intend and effect death, either by direct action or by omission of some action. Accordingly, proponents of this view argue that respect for individual autonomy and regard for the dignity of the person require that death be induced on request. They would have us believe that, in the face of human suffering, the killing action is the only humane, beneficent, and dignity-affirming action.

Arguments of this kind are based on a number of erroneous and misleading assumptions. First, advocates of death by choice seem to hold that personal autonomy has few, if any, limits. Accordingly, the individual can choose to do anything as long as that choice does not injure others. Second, proponents of this "right" imply, and sometimes explicitly claim, that the experience of suffering renders life devoid of meaning and value. They hold that the measure of human dignity is the amount of control that one can exert over the circumstances of life. How can the suffering or dying patient maintain some semblance of control in what many argue is a situation that inevitably "robs the person of dignity?" Mistakenly, the conclusion often is: "I will do it to myself, before it is done to me." Death by design is the ultimate exercise of control and is, therefore, a dignity-affirming choice. Finally, those who claim the right to kill and/or be killed deny that human actions have proximate as well as ultimate effects. They hold that the actions of Jack Kevorkian should be evaluated ethically only on the basis of their intended outcome, benignly described as relief of suffering. Of little or no concern to advocates of death by choice is the fact that the actions chosen do have proximate effects on both the individual performing them (e.g., Dr. Kevorkian becomes "Doctor Death") and on the broader community of persons within which the actions take place (e.g., the community becomes less sensitive to the needs of those who suffer and less disposed to try to meet their needs in appropriate ways).

These are quite different claims than those made by the parents of Nancy Cruzan. They did not seek to kill Nancy. Rather, they asked that an ineffective and burdensome life-sustaining therapy be withdrawn and that their daughter be allowed to die. However, use of "right-to-die" language by the media and others in reporting and discussing the Cruzan case caused a great deal of confusion in the minds of many. Because of this confusion, "right to die" language should be abandoned. We should speak, rather, of the right to make one's own decisions about health care, the duty to preserve life, and the right to refuse life-sustaining treatment under certain circumstances.

THE RIGHT TO MAKE ONE'S OWN DECISIONS

It is reasonable to claim the right to make one's own decisions about treatment options, particularly those concerning life-sustaining interventions. The appropriateness of this claim derives from the fact that the individual person bears primary responsibility for health and that decisions about health and health care should be consistent with other life choices, personal beliefs, commitments, goals, and values. Within the Judeo-Christian tradition, recognition of this responsibility is expressed by the language of stewardship. Accordingly, decisions about the use/nonuse of life-prolonging medical interventions are weighed in light of a number of assumptions. First, life is a gift, and the person is steward rather than owner of the gift. Stewardship responsibilities set the parameters wherein personal autonomy is exercised. Some actions are clearly beyond the limits of responsible stewardship, for example, actions that intend and cause death. Second, human life has a purpose or mission that is pursued primarily through relationship with others. In general, the capacity for relationship requires the integrated functioning of the human organism. Each person particularizes life's mission by adopting goals, commitments, and values which are consistent with individual gifts, interests, limitations, and talents. Decisions about treatment options should be made in light of careful evaluation of the proposed therapies' potential to allow for integrated functioning, allowing the individual some ability to pursue life's purpose. Third, because life is a basic good and the occasion for experiencing all other goods, the individual has a duty to preserve life. But the duty is a limited one. The limits are set by the ability to strive for the purpose of life. When illness or injury so compromise the capacity for integrated functioning that the person is unable to pursue effectively life's mission, death need no longer be resisted. Finally, persons are social by nature, members of human community. In making decisions about the use/nonuse of life-sustaining interventions, recognition of this communal reality gives rise to two further considerations. First, the moral right to make decisions resides with the individual person and with the family or community when the individual is incapacitated. Second, decisions made regarding the treatment of an individual are made in a communal context. Thus, the needs, resources, and burdens of the broader community must be taken into account in the decision-making process.

ETHICAL CRITERIA FOR DECISION MAKING

When individuals are faced with decisions about the use or nonuse of life-sustaining interventions, decisions should be made which reflect and support the life commitments, beliefs, and goals of the person. The following criteria are offered as guides for decision making in a manner consistent with the assumptions outlined above.

In the presence of a fatal pathology, when the treatment or intervention in question is ineffective and/or its use or the effects of its use cause serious burdens for the person and/or the community of persons, it can be withheld or withdrawn even if death will ensue. A fatal pathology is any disease, illness, or injury which will cause death if allowed to run its course. A fatal pathology can be acute, for example, heart attack, cancer of the lung, pneumonia, or it can be chronic, for example, kidney failure, diabetes, Alzheimer's disease. When a fatal pathology is present, the question to be asked is: is there a duty to intervene and preserve life? That question is answered by assessing the following. Will the intervention be effective? Effectiveness should not be measured merely in terms of the ability to maintain physiologic life. Rather, a treatment's effectiveness should be assessed in terms of its ability to preserve, promote, or restore integrated function, allowing the person some capacity to strive for life's purpose. For example, if an elderly but reasonably healthy person has pneumonia and use of an antibiotic promises to return her to health, there is an obligation to use it. However, if the person with pneumonia is irreversibly comatose and use of the antibiotic can only maintain the person in a comatose condition, there is no such obligation to use it. In this case, the antibiotic can be forgone even though death will result from the untreated pneumonia. The effectiveness of any treatment or intervention must be measured in light of the overall, integral well-being of the person. If a therapy offers little or no possibility for allowing the person to pursue life's purpose, even if in a limited way, then there is no duty to utilize the therapy.

There may be times, however, when an effective therapy can be foregone. This conclusion may be reached upon evaluating the degree of burden associated with use of a given therapy. If an effective intervention imposes burden to the extent that the person is unable to pursue life's purpose in a meaningful way, the therapy may be refused, even if death will ensue. For example, a person contemplating a proposed course of surgery and chemotherapy for treatment of cancer may decide to forgo the treatment because of the unacceptable side effects, limitations, or financial costs associated with the treatment plan, even though undergoing treatment may add two or three years to life.

In summary, appropriately understood, decision making about the use or nonuse of life-sustaining therapies is an exercise of stewardship over life. In general, the individual has an ethical obligation to preserve life insofar as there is a reasonable possibility to pursue life's purpose in a way meaningful to the person. When a fatal pathology is present and the proposed life-sustaining intervention cannot offer the person that possibility, either because it is ineffective or because it causes serious burden, the therapy can be withheld and/or withdrawn even though death will ensue.

DECISION MAKING FOR THE DECISIONALLY INCAPACITATED

With increasing frequency, decisions about the use/nonuse of life-sustaining therapies must be made on behalf of persons who are no longer able to participate in the decision-making process themselves. While the locus of decision making may change, the goal of and criteria for decision making remain the same. When an individual can no longer make his own health care decisions, for whatever reason, the moral right to make such decisions resides with the community of persons, in particular with family, loved ones, and caregivers. Decisions made on behalf of the individual should be consistent with past life commitments, goals, and values, and should aim at allowing the person to continue to pursue life's purpose in meaningful and fulfilling way. In other words, decisions should be made which further the legitimate best interests of the person in question.

Toward this end, many people are advocating use of some form of advance directive for future health care decisions, usually a living will or durable power of attorney for health care. While both mechanisms allow persons to make explicit their preferences about future health-related decisions, neither should be understood as a replacement for sound ethical decision making by family and care givers.

CONCLUSION

Patients and families need assistance and guidance in the difficult task of assessing the appropriate use or nonuse of life sustaining therapies. While caregivers can facilitate the decision-making process in a number of ways, they should pay particular attention to the following. First, slogans such as "right to die" should be avoided, because their use obfuscates the issues which must be addressed in making appropriate treatment decisions. Second, caregivers should help patients and families focus on how proposed therapies may or may not serve the overall well-being of the patient. Too often, possible outcomes are evaluated only in terms of limited physiologic effects (e.g., an antibiotic will cure pneumonia). Finally, caregivers should emphasize the need to assess life-prolonging treatment options in light of the ethical criteria for decision making outlined above.

THE RIGHT TO DIE: A PASTOR'S VIEWPOINT
—Herbert E. Hohenstein

A Pastor's Viewpoint

1. Where am I coming from?
2. What does the Bible say?
3. What does a segment of my national church body say?

The above questions deal, of course, with the much publicized and, frequently, sometimes even hastily, discussed and debated issue of the right to choose to die. What about the right to die? As an individual, I struggle for answers to that question first for myself, as I recognize my own desire to die with dignity, and second, as I attempt to counsel and advise my parishioners who share with me that same desire.

As I am a Lutheran pastor, the Bible is my first and primary resource for guidance on ethical issues. Therefore, I will summarize some of the relevant Biblical data that bear on these questions.

SOURCES FROM THE BIBLE

What does the Bible say about the right to die? The Bible, especially the Hebrew Scriptures, makes it abundantly clear that individuals have no right to live, if by "right" we mean that which is earned, merited, deserved, and inalienable to our human nature. According to the Bible, life is a gracious gift from God, preserved by God, and returned to God at death.

Two conclusions may be drawn from this teaching. First, life is not ours to do with as we please. We exercise only temporary stewardship of our precious gift from God. Second, since all of life belongs to God, the distinction between the sacred and the secular, which is sometimes made, is both inaccurate and artificial. Every decision reached, whether about life or death, is fraught with religious, ethical significance, meaning, and overtones.

The Bible also most emphatically proclaims the right to die, but not in the sense that we usually understand that phrase. What the Bible attests is that by sinning against God, humans have earned the right to die, and that therefore death is inalienable to our sinful nature. Simply stated, we have the right to die because we have broken God's laws, the inevitable consequence of which is death (Genesis 3). Or, as Saint Paul puts it in Romans 6, "The wages that sin pays is death." Thus, according to the Bible, sin is the supremely terminal disease because it causes all others, has no cure, and inescapably results in death.

But does the Bible speak of the right to die as we commonly use those words? It does not, at least not explicitly. What, then, do the Scriptures say? First, that God alone decides, controls, and commands our departure from this life. Psalm 90, Verse 3, proclaims: "You, oh God, turn us back to the dust and say: 'Return you children of the ground.'" Do these words imply that God alone should decide where, when, and how we should die? Second, God commands us not to kill. "You will not commit murder," He says (Exodus 20:13). Exceptions to that command, at least in the Hebrew Scriptures, are capital punishment and waging of holy wars.

What about the Christian Scriptures? Personally, this writer finds no passages in the New Testament that explicitly allow one human to take the life of another, regardless of the circumstances.

What is found is this: first, the words of Jesus. "Love the Lord your God with all your heart, soul, strength, and mind, and your neighbor as yourself" (Matthew 22:37-39). To do that, implies Jesus, is to fulfill all of God's laws.

A second word from Jesus, who spoke to his followers on the night before his death, is, "I leave you with only one command, that you love one another as I loved you" (John 15:12). The word translated "love" here refers to the love of God, a love that is totally self-giving and unconditional and a love that, for Christians, finds its highest and supreme expression in the self-offering of Jesus on the cross for the salvation of the world.

From the words of Jesus, we now turn to the words of Saint Paul. In his letter to the Romans, the Apostle writes that "love fulfills all laws" (Romans 13:10), a conviction that most surely echoes the words of Jesus to which I have just referred.

Let me now offer a summary of the Biblical data as I understand it: First, the Bible does not speak of a "right to live." Life is a gracious gift from God, preserved by God, and returned to God at death. Second, the Bible does speak of a "right to die," but not in the sense that we understand this phrase. We have the right to die because of our mortal nature and because we have rebelled against God. Third, according to the Bible, there is one supreme law or principle that must control and govern all decisions of both life and death, and that is the law of God-like, unconditional, self-giving love.

Now to address the third question: What does a segment of the Luthern national church body say about the right to die? The following quotation is from the document entitled "Death and Dying," prepared by an ethical task force of the American Lutheran Church in July of 1977. (In January of 1988, the American Lutheran Church merged with the Lutheran Church in America and the Association of Evangelical Lutheran Churches in America. I am a member of that body. The following quote is not to be understood as an official position or a church dogma, but as a statement for guidance, discussion, and reflection.)

SUSTAINING LIFE

When death is judged to be certain and imminent, we affirm that grave injustice to the respect and memory of persons is rendered if extraordinary technology is applied. Our highest concern is for the total person rather than technological curiosity and mechanical performance. We are confronted with values of human and personal life in the face of every death.

Wherever life support systems can be used to improve the quality of personal and biological life, we heartily affirm their use.

We affirm that in many instances, heroic and extraordinary means used to prolong suffering of both the dying person and the loved ones are unkind. Wherever personality and personhood are permanently lost, artificial supportive measures often are seen as unfair to the dignity of the person and an extreme cost that is burdensome to the family. Families in these cases need not feel a burden of guilt for refusal to try unusual, heroic, and extraordinary life support.

We affirm that direct aid to the irremediably deteriorating and hopelessly ill person hastening a swifter death is wrong. While direct intervention in many cases may appear "humane," deliberate injection of drugs or other means of terminating life are acts of intentional homicide. This deliberate act is far removed from decisions which allow people to die—like shutting off a life-supporting machine or even withholding medication. Permission for the normal process of death is an act of omission in the spirit of kindness and love within limits of Christian charity and legal concerns. Direct intervention to cause death, known as direct euthanasia, cannot be permitted.

In summary, my interpretation about the right to die: first, I endorse the comments I have just quoted because I believe they are consistent with the Biblical data I have shared with you. Second, I am convinced that decisions regarding the right to die must be made on an individual basis. I find it difficult to imagine any set of rules or laws that could or should govern every case, circumstance, or situation. Third, as I struggle to decide thorny, controversial ethical questions, including the right to die, both for myself and those whom I seek to counsel, I keep asking this question: "What, under the circumstances, is the most loving word to speak, the most loving deed to do, for the temporal, eternal, physical, mental, moral, and spiritual welfare of all involved?"

Having asked that question, having prayed over it, having consulted others whose views, competence, and expertise I respect, I then reach a decision. On the basis of that decision, I speak, I act, and I counsel in the firm conviction that God approves, and if not, then I have His forgiveness. It is the only way I can live and then die at peace with myself, others, and my God.

REFERENCES

Gibbs, N. (1990, March 19). Love and let die! *Time Magazine,* pp. 62–71.

Miller, D. L. (1990, August 8). Pulling the plug of life. *The Lutheran,* pp. 6–18. (Available from Evangelical Lutheran Church in America, 8765 Higgins Road, Chicago, IL, 60631-4183.)

Nelson, J. B. (1976). *Rediscovering the person in medical care.* Minneapolis, MN: Augsburg-Fortress Publishing House.

Ramsey, P. (1977). *The patient as person.* New Haven, CT: Yale University Press.

Report on Euthanasia With Guiding Principles. A Report of the Commission on Theology and Church Relations, Lutheran Church-Missouri Senate as prepared by its Social Concerns Committee, October, 1979. St. Louis, MO: Concordia Publishing House.

The American Lutheran Church (1977). *Death and dying.* [An analysis offered by the Task Force on Ethical Issues in Human Medicine, Office of Research and Analysis.] Minneapolis, MN: Augsburg-Fortress Publishing House.

Thielicke, H. (1976). *The doctor as judge of who shall live and who shall die.* Minneapolis, MN: Augsburg-Fortress Publishing House.

Vaux, K. (1978). *Will to live and will to die.* Minneapolis, MN: Augsburg-Fortress Press.

Wennberg, R. N. (1989). *Terminal choices.* Grand Rapids, MI: William B. Erdmans Publishing Co.

22

OBRA: An Opportunity or a Disaster for Long-Term Care?

Raymond F. Rustige

INTRODUCTION: COBRA OR PANACEA?

The two extreme reactions to the Omnibus Budget Reconciliation Act of 1987 (OBRA) were headlined recently in long-term-care magazines. The first said: "OBRA IS A COBRA—How are you going to pay for it?" The second said: "AHCA URGES PROVIDERS: 'Make best use of OBRA.'"

The disaster-mentality article continued to say that there are two fangs in OBRA: compliance and cost. Both of these will be deadly. The opportunity-perspective article holds great promise for residents and providers. In that article, McCleod (1990) indicates that "it can lead us to a true outcome-oriented regulatory system."

The effects of OBRA will continue to unfold during the 1990s. At the present moment, the surveyor's experiences are being formulated. Evaluative studies and other research endeavors will bring a clearer picture.

Formerly, the Conditions of Participation focused on structure and process rather than outcomes. Now the goals and objectives expected from care planning are gaining center stage. As McLeod observes: "The good care practices and the underlying philosophy were not dreamed up in a

276

Washington conference room. They have been in place in many nursing facilities throughout the country for years."

In summary, OBRA brings an outcome-oriented regulatory system that focuses on residents and gives an organization power to define its own performance.

LEGISLATIVE HISTORY: INTENT AND REALITY

In 1982 the Health Care Financing Administration (HCFA) entered into a $1.6 million contract with the Institute of Medicine (IOM) to conduct a full-range study of nursing home regulatory issues. The IOM report, *Improving the Quality of Care in Nursing Homes* (1986), report recommended sweeping changes in regulation and reimbursement. Highlighted recommendations include:

• The regulatory distinctions between skilled nursing facilities (SNFs) and intermediate-care facilities (ICFs) should be eliminated.
• A new condition of participation should be required for resident assessment.
• Regulations should be more resident centered and outcome oriented.
• New residents' rights standards should be added.
• Standards in social services should be strengthened.
• New standards should be added on nurses aide training.
• Positive incentives for good performance should be incorporated into the survey and certification process.

Following the release of the IOM Study, a national coalition of industry and consumer advocacy groups was formed—the National Coalition for Nursing Home Reform (NCNHR). When the 99th Congress failed to pass appropriate legislation, the NCNHR created a consensus blueprint for action. Congress enacted OBRA 1987, which was signed by the President on December 22, 1987 (Public Law 100-203). This bill included elements of the IOM Study and the NCNHR's consensus blueprint.

OBRA REGULATIONS

Here are highlights of the new regulations now in effect:

• Quality Assessment and Assurance—Requires facilities to provide services and activities to maintain the highest practicable physical, mental, and psychosocial resident well-being.
• Team Plan of Care—Prepared by a team of professionals, each resident's care plan describes his or her needs and how they will be met. Regulations suggest that family members should be included together with the

resident where practicable. Though this is not required, "non" professionals (nursing assistants, dietary workers, housekeepers, etc.) offer significant insights due to their immediate knowledge of the residents— and should be included in care planning. Administrative support by presence, when possible, is excellent leadership.

- Resident Assessment—Regular, ongoing updates refine the care plan. At the same time, a Minimum Data Set (MDS) and the Resident Assessment Protocol Summary (RAPS), while demanding extensive documentation, may provide important data for research.

  The resident assessment process includes the MDS which contains core elements and common definitions for comprehensive resident assessment. Part two is RAPS which provides additional assessment items and background information about residents, their strengths, preferences, and needs.
- Preadmission Screening and Annual Resident Review (PSARR)—Admission of mentally ill or mentally retarded persons would be restricted to those in need of nursing services. This provision does not apply to those with a primary diagnosis of Alzheimer's or dementia.
- Elimination of ICF/SNF Distinction—Establishes a single set of nursing home standards for the one category of service.
- Twenty-Four-Hour Nursing Coverage—Requires the presence of an RN eight hours a day for seven days a week with licensed nurse coverage around the clock.
- Nursing Assistant Training—Ongoing training, education, and competency evaluations are required. States must develop a registry of aides who are certified, with information about any neglect/abuse or misappropriation of resident property.
- Social Service—A full-time professional social worker Bachelor of social work (BSW) is required for facilities with 120 beds or more.
- Resident's Rights—Included in the listing are choice of physician, participation in care plan, freedom from restraints, privacy and confidentiality, and prior notice of room change. A written description of legal rights must include protection of personal funds and a complaint filing statement.
- Transfer and Discharge Rights—Involuntary transfer or discharge is allowed only for the resident's welfare or safety of others. Facility must give proper notice and prepare the resident for transfer.

ADMINISTRATORS' RESPONSE TO OBRA

Initial reactions at this time from an information telephone survey of administrators show a cautious optimism. One corporate vice president with facilities in six states summarized his experience as, "our solid facilities will do well with the new requirements, but I'm disappointed that HCFA refuses to perform in a consultative role." Another administrator of a large facility with predominantly Medicaid residents saw OBRA as "having well-intentioned objectives, yet still not providing adequate reimbursement mechanisms."

On the positive side, administrators indicated that there was a heightened awareness of quality assurance due to the emphasis on resident outcomes. Many cited the increased importance of team care plans and the resulting rise in staff morale. Most administrators responded that they were already fulfilling the mandates relative to resident rights, but saw some potential image enhancement for nursing homes by stressing these considerations. Of particular note was the positive response toward the reduction in the use of restraints.

On the negative or cautious side, administrators pointed primarily to the need for adequate reimbursement to fulfill OBRA's expectations. While there was some mention of costs for additional staffing, most singled out the staff time required for the MDS and RAPS documentation. While administrators praised the restraint reduction requirement, costs for more staff and appropriate training and safeguards were noted. Again, while appreciating the emphasis on residents' rights, the reality or residents remembering the presentation and detailing as required was a downside. Others noted that the surveyors need appropriate training in their role as enforcers to strike an appropriate balance, since HCFA has downplayed consultation.

WHO WILL PICK UP THE TAB?

As noted, the major expressed concern of administrators is inadequate reimbursement for OBRA's requirements. However, OBRA clearly says that the "States and the U. S. Department of Health and Human Services (DHHS) must take into account the costs of complying with the nursing home reforms." In addition, the Boren Amendments call for "reasonable and adequate compensation to provide the enhanced quality of care envisioned by OBRA."

Numerous lawsuits are in process, challenging the states relative to inadequate reimbursement. The long-term-care community closely watched *Virginia Hospital Association v. Baliles*, in which hospitals tested providers' ability to sue the government for adequate reimbursement. The U. S. Supreme Court in June 1990 upheld the providers' rights to challenge inadequate Medicaid reimbursement rates.

At the present writing, a settlement has been reached in a Boren suit that was filed in Michigan. Provisions to providers will be based on an inflation factor plus 1%, according to the Health Care Association of Michigan. The added reimbursement would approximate $25 million per year.

Providers in Kansas are the latest to challenge their state's reimbursement system. In this case, the basis for the suits is a one-year rate freeze plus inadequate coverage of costs associated with the implementation of OBRA. Kansas had boosted rates by only a few cents per day, which providers said missed the boat completely in terms of actual costs.

A current suit in California has a more complicated bent. The state of California is being sued by The National Senior Citizens Law Center for refusing to implement OBRA. The state contends that its current system of nursing home certification is equivalent to OBRA, while being more efficient. Most recently, the California Association of Health Facilities (CAHF) has entered the case to protect the interest of the state's facilities. CAHF wants to ensure adequate funding for any new provisions.

The financial crunch is similar in the state of Missouri. The projected Medicaid maximum rate is $55.92 per day, an increase of $1.72 per day. A recent cost analysis indicated a $3.80-per-day increase for OBRA implementation (Present, 1990), or a shortfall of $2.08 per day. Major per-day costs included $1.15 for increased nurse staffing, $1.14 for resident assessments, and $0.82 for eliminating SNF/ICF distinctions.

These are just a few examples of the financial constraints being felt throughout the country. Both national associations, the American Health Care Association (AHCA) and the American Association of Homes for the Aging (AAHA), have adequate reimbursement for OBRA as a priority on their agendas.

OUTCOMES: RESEARCH OFFERS RESULTS

Due to the newness of OBRA, research efforts are in the formative stages. However, several studies serve as an example of what current and future research may demonstrate.

A system, so far used only at Veterans Administration (VA) nursing homes, may become a mainstay because of OBRA's mandate to make outcome surveillance a prerequisite to reimbursement (Rajecki, 1991). This quantitative method, called "outcome analysis," was developed by Daniel Rudman, M.D., professor of medicine at the Medical College of Wisconsin and associate chief of staff at the VA Medical Center, Milwaukee.

Rudman and his colleagues assigned a profile of scores to four types of adverse outcomes: death; calorie and protein undernutrition; bedsores; and loss of activities of daily living (ADLs). The scoring method was tested at three VA nursing homes in the Great Lakes area. The VAs' computerized patient assessment instrument (PAI) provided the baseline for the study.

The researchers examined the prevalence, incidence, and rate of change in the four outcomes. The ultimate findings revealed the bad news that there was a continuing decline for residents with greater functional impairment. However, there was the good news that the problems could be alleviated through aggressive interventions. This kind of outcome analysis should be able to assist in identifying both excellent and problem facilities.

Another study centers on the potential impact of PSARR. The intent of this process is to identify persons with mental illness who do not require nursing services and who therefore would be inappropriate for nursing home placement. However, there is the risk of displacing the mentally ill from nursing homes with no other viable housing options (Freiman, 1990).

Freiman and associates utilized data from the 1985 National Nursing Home Survey (NNHS) and analyzed the OBRA regulation for current nursing home residents. Residents with any type of mental illness were identified. Then, a determination of the need for nursing services was made. The assumption was made that all persons with mental illness who do not need nursing services would be candidates for placement elsewhere. Each person in the NHHS data base was evaluated according to the OBRA selection criteria. Then, the number of persons were counted who had mental illness, did not have a primary diagnosis of dementia, and did not need nursing services. The range of estimates of the number of residents possibly displaced from nursing homes would be from 37,890 to 65,600.

This study concludes that "OBRA mandates an elaborate screening process to determine who among the mentally ill should be retained in nursing homes, which have little incentive to keep them, and who should be removed, without regard to the availability of alternatives."

CONCLUSION: ONE SMALL STEP NOW

While there may be two extreme reactions to OBRA now, future evaluations may show that the outcome orientation approach is "One small step now—A potential giant step for long-term care!"

REFERENCES

Freiman, M., Arons, B. S., Goldman, H. H., & Burns, B. J. (1990). Nursing home reform and the mentally ill. *Health Affairs*, Winter, 47–60.
Institute of Medicine (1986). *Improving the quality of care in nursing homes.* Washington, D.C. National Academy Press.
McLeod, K. (1990). Policy perspective. *Provider*, September, 9–10.
Present, R. (1990). *The Cost of OBRA Implementation.* [Presentation to Catholic System Directors for Aging Services.] St. Louis, MO: Ernst & Young.
Rajecki, R. (1991, January). Outcome analysis underlies rating system. *Contemporary Long-Term Care*, 34–36.

Index

Index

Springer Publishing Company

THE ELDERLY WITH CHRONIC MENTAL ILLNESS

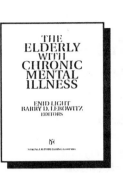

Enid Light, PhD
Barry D. Lebowitz, PhD, Editors

"In this volume we attempt to encourage research in this area in two ways. First, the authors of the chapters address many of the complex theoretical and methodological issues...Second, each of the contributors suggests and explores emerging lines of promising research and makes recommendations regarding the refinement and elaboration of research areas that have already been undertaken."

—From the Introduction

1991 384pp 0-8261-7280-6 hardcover

CARING FOR THE PSYCHOGERIATRIC CLIENT

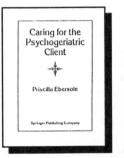

Priscilla Ebersole, PhD, RN

Written with warmth and sensitivity, this book is a practical manual for understanding and managing a broad range of common behavioral and psychiatric problems among the elderly.

"...an ideal hands-on text...a holistic approach that goes far beyond the usually narrow, disease-specific approach to care."

—American Journal of Nursing

1987 304pp 0-8261-6420-X hardcover

Ⓢ *Springer Publishing Company*

AGING AND MENTAL DISORDERS
International Perspectives

Manfred Bergener, MD, **Kazuo Hasegawa,** MD,
Sanford T. Finkel, MD, and **T. Nishimura,** MD, Editors

Broad, current international coverage ranging from general social issues of aging—to the ways various mental disorders affect the elderly, treatment, services and government policies, and education/training. Provides a state-of-the-art look at this field, as well as an indication of likely future research directions.

Partial Contents: **Part I: Transcultural Perspectives on Aging.** Aging in Japan, *D. Maeda* • Mental Function and Health Status of Centenarians, *A. Homma, et al.* • Quality of Life: Affect and Mood in Later Life, *E.W. Busse* • The Epidemiology of Dementia and Depression in Later Life, *A.S. Henderson, et al.* **Part II: Perspectives on Mental Disorders: Diagnosis.** Depression versus Dementia in the Elderly, *B.V. Reifler* • Depression and Suicide in Late Life, *M. Shimizu* • Psychological Assessment and Rating Scales: Depression and Other Age-Related Affective Disorders, *S.-L. Kivela* • Age-Associated Memory Impairment—Diagnosis, Research, and Treatment, *G.J. Larrabee, et al.* • Approaches in the Experimental Neuropsychology of Dementia, *L.W. Poon, et al.* **Part III: Perspectives on Mental Disorders: Treatment and Management.** Alzheimer's Disease: Risk Factors and Therapeutic Challenges, *L. Amaducci, et al.* • Use of Psychotropics in the Elderly in the United States: An Overview, *G.T. Grossberg, et al.* • Pharmacotherapy in Later Life: Eastern Principles, *F. Kuzuya & K. Kono* **Part IV: Organization of Services and Government Policy.** Model for Diagnosis and Treatment of Psychological and Somatic Disturbances in the Elderly: A German Perspective, *M. Bergener* • Assessment Units and Other Care Facilities for Patients with Dementia, *G. Bucht & P.-0. Sandman* • Organization of Psychogeriatrics in Western Countries: A Critical Study, *J. Wertheimer* • Geriatric Psychiatry Services in N. America, *R. Eastwood & J.S. Kennedy* • Coping with Dementia in Sweden, *A. Norberg* • Geriatric Psychiatry Day Hospital: A Treatment Program for Depressed Older Adults, *A.B. Steingart* • Long-Term Care, Psychogeriatrics, and Government: Regulation in the United States, *S.I. Finkel* **Part V: Education and Training.** Education and Old Age Psychiatry: The UK Experience, *R. Jones* • Nursing Issues in Psychogeriatrics, *A. Norberg* • Development of Subspecialization for Geriatric Psychiatry in the United States, *G. Cohen*

1992 416pp 0-8261-7030-7 hardcover

Springer Publishing Company

RECAPTURING COMPETENCE
A System's Change for Geropsychiatric Care

Gail S. Fidler, OTR
in collaboration with **Barbara Bristow**, MSW

Describes the concepts and procedures used to transform a state long-term nursing care facility for the chronically mentally ill elderly into a comprehensive geropsychiatric treatment and rehabilitation hospital.

"The material presented herein is the result of a three-year initiative to transform a state mental health institution from a nursing home care facility to a comprehensive geropsychiatric treatment and rehabilitation hospital focusing on early return to community living. This endeavor involved the generation of fundamental changes in the institution's organization and administrative functions, its clinical policies and practices, its definition of patient needs, intervention strategies, and priorities. These alterations finally brought about significant change in both patient and staff expectations regarding autonomy, achievement, and productivity." —**From the Introduction**

Contents: Guiding Principles and Philosophy of Patient Care • The Therapeutic Community and Participatory Management • The Non-Human Environment: Its Meaning and Uses • Interdisciplinary Functional Skills Assessment Methodology • Program Planning • Team Building in the Psychiatric Hospital • Perspectives on Change

1992   160pp   0-8261-7760-3   hardcover

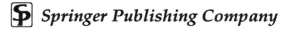 *Springer Publishing Company*

WHO IS RESPONSIBLE FOR MY OLD AGE?

Robert N. Butler, MD
and Kenzo Kiikuni, Editors

An insightful, international perspective on the "new gerontology." Emphasis is given to the notion that self-reliance among the aging cannot be achieved without active participation on the part of the entire community. Contributors to this work include James Birren, Rosalynn Carter, Betty Friedan, and Maggie Kuhn.

1992 288pp 0-8261-8140-6 hardcover

ANXIETY DISORDERS ACROSS THE LIFESPAN
A Developmental Perspective

Cynthia G. Last, PhD

The purpose of this volume is to bridge the gap between what we know about childhood and adult anxiety disorders. Reflects the growing interest with psychiatry and psychology to view mental disorders from a developmental or longitudinal perspective.

Springer Series on Behavior Therapy and Behavioral Medicine, Volume 26

1992 232pp 0-8261-6460-9 hardcover